ADVANCES IN CLINICAL AUDIOLOGY

Edited by **Stavros Hatzopoulos**

Advances in Clinical Audiology
http://dx.doi.org/10.5772/63685
Edited by Stavros Hatzopoulos

Contributors

Milaine Sanfins, Stavros Hatzopoulos, Gro Gade Haanes, Raphael R. Ciuman, Andrzej Dobrucki, Maurycy Kin, Bartlomiej Kruk, Payton Lin, Henryk Skarzynski, Piotr Skarzynski, Agnieszka Szczepek, Piotr Kielczynski, Yoshiharu Soeta, Christiane Marques Do Couto, Izabella Dos Santos Brites, Pedro Menezes, Kelly Andrade, Gabriella Peixoto, Aline Carnaúba, Klinger Costa

Published by InTech

Janeza Trdine 9, 51000 Rijeka, Croatia

Publishing Process Manager Ana Simcic
Technical Editor SPi Global
Cover InTech Design team

First published April, 2017
Printed in Croatia
Legal deposit, Croatia: National and University Library in Zagreb

Additional hard copies can be obtained from orders@intechopen.com

Advances in Clinical Audiology, Edited by Stavros Hatzopoulos
p. cm.
Print ISBN 978-953-51-3043-7
Online ISBN 978-953-51-3044-4

For EU product safety concerns:
IN TECH d.o.o., Prolaz Marije Krucifikse Kozulić 3, 51000 Rijeka, Croatia,
info@intechopen.com or visit our website at intechopen.com.

Meet the editor

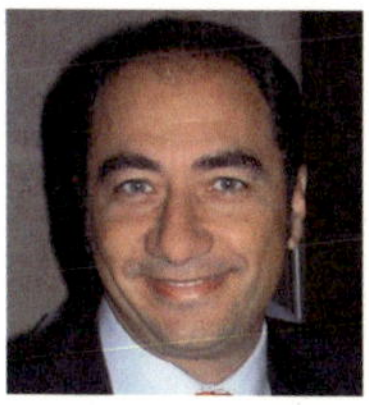

Dr. Stavros Hatzopoulos is a faculty member of the Audiology and ENT clinic, University of Ferrara, Italy, since 1994. His background is in biomedical engineering, audiological engineering, and hearing science (BS, from the University of Southern California; MSc from Texas A&M University; PhD from Worcester Polytechnic Institute in Massachusetts). He received his habilitation as an associate professor in 2014. He is the author of more than 175 book chapters, peer-review papers, and congress presentations. He has participated in numerous European Concerted Action Projects in the areas of otoacoustic emissions, genetics, and nanotechnologies. He currently serves as the editor of the Portal on Otoacoustic Emissions and as the audiology section editor in the Journal of Hearing Science.

Contents

Preface

The objective of the present book is to diffuse information related to a number of technological and procedural advances in the area of clinical audiology. This book was made possible through the generous contribution of 20 authors.

The format for this book is purely educational, targeting graduate courses in audiology, speech pathology and hearing science, and neurosciences and basic graduate courses in ENT. The authors have been asked to present a generous background of their topic, in the "Introduction" section of their chapter, and an extensive list of technical terms used throughout the chapter.

The book is divided into six sections as follows:

1. **The Cochlea and Cochlear Modeling:** In this section, there are two chapters, one describing the functionality of the cochlear dynamics and the other describing a possible modality (model) by which the cochlea performs the amplification of the incoming stimuli and generates the well-known tonotopical frequency map.
2. **Advances in Clinical Procedures:** The three chapters of this section describe new procedures for the assessment of hearing loss related to otoacoustic emissions, speech-evoked brainstem responses, and wideband tympanometry.
3. **Cochlear Implants:** The two chapters in this section discuss the temporal filter banks in cochlear implants and a new surgical procedure for the treatment of partial deafness (i.e., a cochlea which presents acceptable hearing levels at its apical region).
4. **New Aspects of the Auditory Function (Psychoacoustics):** The two chapters in this section discuss the possible evidence of an autocorrelation mechanism (related to loudness and annoyance) in the auditory system and various aspects of the auditory fatigue.
5. **Aging:** The two chapters in this section discuss issues of amplification in an aged auditory system and the various methodologies of intervention for hearing loss in the old age.
6. **Ototoxicity:** The single chapter in this category is a broad excursus into the various drug side effects related to cochlear-induced stress.

It was my intention to use multimedia material wherever possible, but for the majority of contributors, this was not feasible, during the publication time. We were only able to locate a few interesting videos on wideband tympanometry, and the web references are included in the Appendix section of the relative chapter.

Acknowledgments

I would personally like to thank all the contributing authors, the InTech personnel, and specifically Ms. Ana Simcic for her continuous and generous assistance during the preparation of the volume.

Stavros Hatzopoulos, PhD
Clinic of Audiology and ENT,
University of Ferrara, Italy

Section 1

Introduction

Chapter 1

Introductory Chapter - Genealogy of Audiology

Stavros Hatzopoulos

Additional information is available at the end of the chapter

http://dx.doi.org/10.5772/67437

1. Introduction

The twenty-first century clinical Audiology has not been very creative in terms of novel breakthroughs, since the majority of clinical novelties, we routinely used today, were discovered in the 1970s and the 1980s. The trend, which can be observed in the last few decades, is an amelioration of our technological approaches/strategies to restore an impaired hearing function with hearing aids, middle ear prostheses, and cochlear implants. New and novel procedural developments have not surfaced yet to clinical practice.

A Scopus literature search within the last 5 years shows, for example, that there are developments in procedures related to (i) cortical-evoked potentials, such as the speech-evoked auditory brainstem responses (see the relative chapter in this volume) and (ii) various protocol developments in the area of steady-state responses (ASSR), with applications to the newly charted area of electrically evoked SSRs [1, 2]. Important aspects of novel hearing restoration strategies including gene therapy [3], stem cells [4, 5], and related intracochlear distribution nanotechnologies [6, 7] are still at best in a preclinical phase.

From my personal experience as an educator, I have found that very few of our colleagues and graduate students have a clear idea about the origins of Audiology. This book deals with the latest advances in this field, which can only make sense if we recall briefly our point of origin.

2. Genealogy of the term "Audiology"

As we start 2017, clinical Audiology celebrates a historical span of 71 years, according to Kenneth Berger. In 1976, Berger published an article [8] in the *Journal of the American Audiology Society (AAS)*, where he presented his findings regarding the time occurrence of the term "Audiology." The first printed reference of the term originates back in 1946. In the 1946,

Journal of Speech Disorders on page 218 appears a brief announcement that the "Speech Clinic at the U.S. Naval Hospital, Philadelphia, is the permanent Naval center for rehabilitation and for research in Speech and Audiology."

Interestingly, according to Berger [8] the term "Audiology" cannot be attributed to a specific individual, a notion which contracts what I have learned in my academic training in the US, where it was considered common knowledge that Raymond Carhart was the father of Audiology. Berger [8] reports the following: *"the original creator of the term (Audiology) remains unknown, but possible originators are considered: (i) Mayer BA Schier; (ii) Willard B Hargrave ; (iii) Stanley Nowak; (iv) Norman Canfield; (v) Raymond Carhart* [9]. *In a biographical profile by Robert Galambos, Hallowell Davis* [10] *is credited with coining the term in the 1940s, when he said that the then-prevalent term "auricular training" sounded like a method of teaching people how to wiggle their ears."* It is interesting to note that from these six pioneering contributors, four (Carhart and Davis excluded) were related to technical fields (electroacoustics).

3. Deviations of the term "Audiology"

From the mid-1970s, several terms have appeared in print, regarding clinical activities which were deviated from the classical categorization of "Audiology." Typical examples are the following terms: "Hearing Science" [11]; "Clinical Auditory Science" [12]; "Auditory NeuroScience" [12], and so on. It is still difficult to define and discriminate these terms, since the Audiological training is very different around the globe. For example, in most European countries, Audiology is a medical specialization, while the Speech and Hearing Science is associated with communication department curricula. So in an attempt to define all terms, one can assume that activities related to Hearing Science/Auditory Science have a "research inspiration" objective (more research or education oriented) derived from basic Neurosciences, while the terms Audiology or Clinical Audiology refer to a basic clinical activity of assessing the hearing of a human subject.

To summarize, my objective in conjunction with the contributions and collaboration of the participated authors for this "Advances" volume was to collect material from a Hearing Science perspective, which could be applied to the everyday clinical Audiological reality.

4. What "advances" can be?

Considering the long history of Audiology and Hearing Science, it is only natural that numerous and fundamental volumes exist (as the all-time reference by Katz [13]) in English and in many other languages. So it was an interesting challenge to chart the latest "advances" in the field and to find the best way to diffuse the new information to students and professionals.

The term "**advances**" implies a further development on a specific topic. For the area of Audiology, this would mean developments in the following thematic areas: (i) clinical hearing assessment procedures, (ii) rehabilitation strategies, (iii) hardware development (more precise equipment, better sensors, lower noise, etc.), (iv) telemedicine/teleconsultation concepts, and (v) new methods of long-distance learning and undergraduate/graduate course delivery. Any of these areas could have been the exclusive topic of the present volume.

For practical reasons (and with the hopes that other future books can follow covering the remaining thematic areas), the focus of the present volume is limited to the first two major thematic areas, namely to developments in assessment procedures and rehabilitation strategies (cochlear implants).

Author details

Stavros Hatzopoulos

Address all correspondence to: sdh1@unife.it

Clinic of Audiology and ENT, University of Ferrara, Ferrara, Italy

References

[1] Deprez H, Gransier R, Hofmann M, vanWieringen A, Wouters J, Moonen M. Characterization of cochlear implant artifacts in electrically evoked auditory steady state responses. Biomedical Signal Processing and Control 2017;31:127–138.

[2] Santos TS, Silva JJ, Lins OG, Melges DB, Tierra-Criollo CJ. Detection efficiency of auditory steady state responses evoked by modulated noise. Hearing Research 2016;339:125–131.

[3] Akil O, Seal RP, Burke K, Wang C, Alemi A, During M, Edwards R, Lustig L. Restoration of hearing in the VGLUT3 knockout mouse using virally mediated gene therapy. Neuron 2012;75:283–293.

[4] Ohlemiller KK, Jones SM, Johnson KR. Application of mouse models to research in hearing and balance. JARO 2016;17:493–523.

[5] Stark D, Rosenberg AR, Johnson D, Knight K, Caperon L, Uleryk E, Frazier AL, Sung L. Patient-reported measures of hearing loss and tinnitus in pediatric cancer and hematopoietic stem cell transplantation: A systematic review. Journal of Speech Language and Hearing Research 2016;59:1247–1252.

[6] Plontke SK, Gotze G, Rahne T, Liebau A. Intracochlear drug delivery in combination with cochlear implants. Current aspects. HNO 2016;64:797–807.

[7] Wise AK, Tan J, Wang YJ, Caruso F, Shepherd RK. Improved auditory nerve survival with nanoengineered supraparticles for neurotrophin delivery into the deafened cochlea. PLoS One 2016;11(10).1–17.

[8] Berger KW. Genealogy of the words "audiology" and "audiologist". Journal of the American Audiology Society. 1976;2(2):38–44.

[9] Raymond C. Papers, 1938–1975. Northwestern University Archives, Evanston, Illinois. 1912–1975. The material can be downloaded from this link: http://findingaids.library.northwestern.edu/catalog/inu-ead-nua-archon-1226.

[10] Hallowell D. A Biographical Memoir by Robert Galambos (in the National Academy of Sciences). 1896–1992. Can be downloaded from this link: http://www.nasonline.org/publications/biographical-memoirs/memoir-pdfs/davis-hallowell.pdf

[11] John D.D, Jean HL. (editors). Bases of Hearing Science (third edition). Williams and Wilkins, Baltimore 2002.

[12] Kraus N, McGee T. Auditory event related potentials. Handbook of Clinical Audiology. Baltimore: Williams & Wilkins; 1994. pp. 406–423.

[13] Katz J. (editor). Handbook of Clinical Audiology (fifth edition). Williams & Wilkins, Baltimore 2001.

Section 2

Advances in Clinical Procedures

Chapter 2

Speech-Evoked Brainstem Response

Milaine Dominici Sanfins, Piotr H. Skarzynski and
Maria Francisca Colella-Santos

Additional information is available at the end of the chapter

http://dx.doi.org/10.5772/66206

Abstract

The auditory brainstem response (ABR) is a clinical tool to assess the neural functionality of the auditory brainstem. The use of verbal stimuli in ABR protocols has provided important information of how the speech stimuli are processed by the brainstem structure. The perception of speech sounds seems to begin in the brainstem, which has an important role in the reading process and the phonological acquisition speech ABR assessment allows the identification of fine-grained auditory processing deficits, which do not appear in click evoked ABR responses. The syllable /da/ is commonly used by speech ABR assessment due to it being considered a universal syllable and allows it to be applied in different countries with good clinical assertiveness. The speech ABR is a objective, fast procedure that can be applied to very young subjects. It be utilized in different languages and can provide differential diagnoses of diseases with similar symptoms, as an effective biomarker of auditory processing disorders present in various diseases, such as dyslexia, specific language impairment, hearing loss, auditory processing disorders, otitis media, and scholastic difficulties. Speech ABR protocols can assist in the detection, treatment, and monitoring of various types of hearing impairments.

Keywords: speech, speech perception, electrophysiology, frequency-following response, speech-ABR

1. Introduction

The auditory processing information can be analyzed by an assessment of the auditory evoked potentials (AEP). Among the different types of AEPs, there is the auditory brainstem response

(ABR) The ABR is a clinical tool to assess the neural functionality of the auditory brainstem [1]. Until recently, assessment using clinical ABR protocols was carried out only with nonverbal stimuli, such as clicks, tone-bursts, and chirps. The ABR responses (i) permit the analysis of the integrity of the auditory pathways and (ii) can establish electrophysiological thresholds in order to identify basic neural abnormalities and to evaluate patients who did not provide reliable responses in the standard behavioral audiological assessment [2].

Although the use of the click-evoked ABR has been widely used clinically, it is still necessary to unravel how verbal sounds are coded in the brainstem. Recent technological advances have enabled the inclusion of verbal stimuli in the ABR commercial equipment. The use of verbal stimuli in ABR protocols provided important information of how the speech stimuli are processed by the brainstem structure, which actively participates in the analysis of the complex verbal stimuli [3].

The verbal stimulus most widely used in speech ABR is a syllable composed of a consonant and a vowel (CV) [4]. The consonant perception is performed by the distinction between vocal production times and sound of consonant that guarantees the intelligibility in the process of human communication and the proper development of language.

The perception of speech sounds seems to begin in the brainstem, which has an important role in reading process and phonological acquisition [5–7]. An effective and objective way to investigate this process will be the assessment of speech ABR that allows the identification of fine-grained auditory processing deficits associated with real-world communication, skills which do not appear in click responses, and it also can be used for early identification of auditory processing impairments in very young children [8]. Above all, speech ABR can be used as an objective measure of the hearing function. One of the great advantages of this method is that it is not influenced by environmental issues, which can disrupt the behavioral assessments [2]. Even the best behavioral tests can confound the subject by factors such as attention, motivation, alertness/fatigue, and by co-occurring disorders, such as language impairments, learning impairments, or attention deficits [9].

Understanding the neural processing of speech sounds at the brainstem level provides knowledge regarding the central auditory processes involved in normal hearing subjects and also in clinical populations [10]. Moreover, altered responses of speech ABR may be associated with impaired speech perception in noise. These changes can cause a negative impact on communication and serious consequences for academic success [8]. According to Sinha and Basavaraj [11], the major application of speech ABR can be in diagnosing and categorizing children with learning disability in different subgroups, assessing the effects of aging on central auditory processing of speech, assessing the effects of central auditory deficits in hearing aid, and cochlear implant users.

2. Assessment

Speech ABR has an important feature, that is, the specific aspects of acoustic signal are preserved and reflects the neural coding in figure [representation of 40 ms of syllable /da/ (gray) stimulus and responses (black)] [4]. Furthermore, this assessment permits to understand the neural basis of the auditory system, even if it is normal or deficient stimulus and responses (black)] [4] (**Figure 1**).

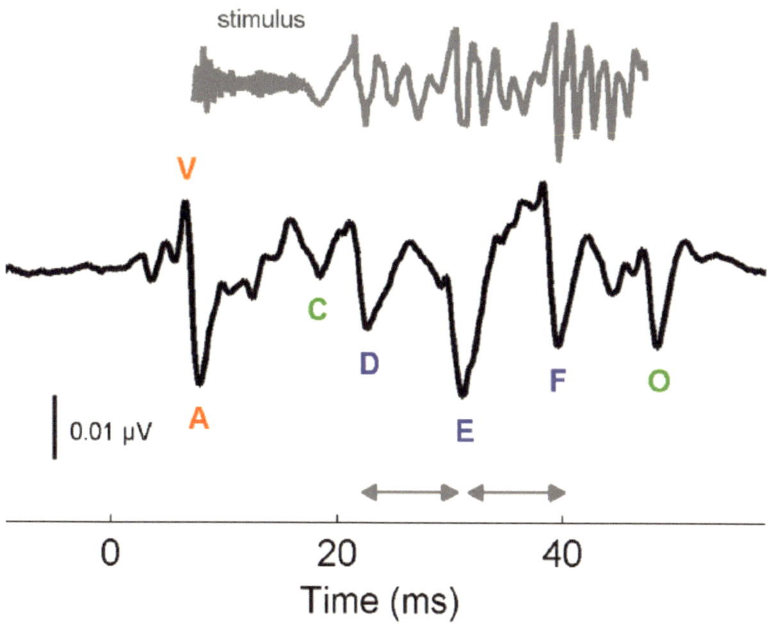

Figure 1. Representation of 40 ms of syllable /da/ (*gray*) stimulus and responses (*black*) [4].

The verbal stimulus used in the speech ABR assessment, normally, is the syllables /ba/, /da/, or /ga/. The verbal assessment provides information about how the speech syllable is encoded by auditory system. The trace of the speech ABR response can be dismembered in two parts: the onset and the frequency following response (FFR). The first part represents the consonant and the second part the vowel [10].

The best-known model used is elicited with the synthesized syllable /da/ provided by a computer software. The use of synthesized speech allows acoustic parameters to be controlled and constant and ensures the quality of the stimulus that will be presented to the listener and/or the patient [12]. This stimulus modality was developed by the group of Dr. Nina Kraus at Northwestern University. The stimulus consisted of the consonant /d/ (transient portion—onset) and the short vowel /a/ (sustained portion—following frequency response). When elicited by the stimulus /da/, the subcortical response emerges as a waveform of seven peaks—V, A, C, D, E, F, and O—wherein the single wave with a positive peak is the complex of wave V. Waves V and A reflect the onset response, wave C the transition area, waves D, E, and F the periodic area (the frequency following response), and wave O the offset response (**Figure 2**) [4, 13, 14]. A typical response is shown in **Figure 2** (electrophysiological response representation of synthesized syllable /da/. Investigator's personal data based on the assessment of a normal hearing, performed with the BioMARK™ software) [13].

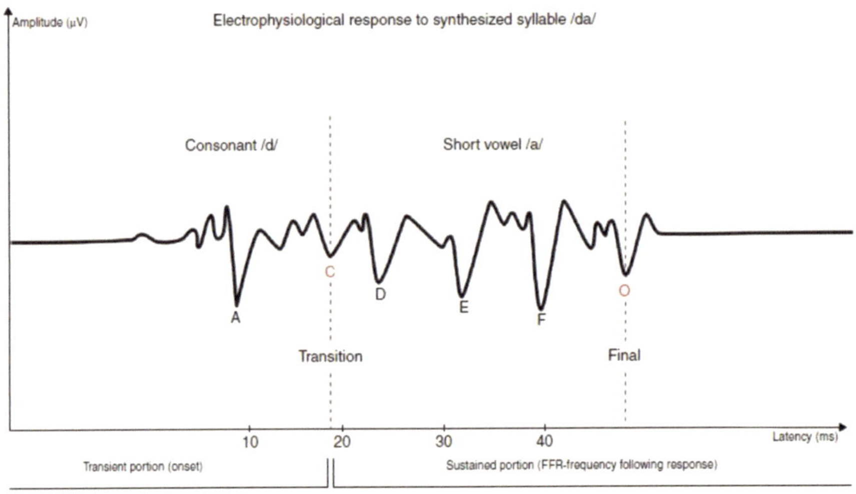

Figure 2. Electrophysiological response representation of synthesized syllable /da/. Investigator's personal data based on the assessment of a normal hearing, performed with the BioMARK™ software [13].

It is important to describe that the onset component seems to be elicited around 10 ms and is considered the transient portion of sound stimulus reflecting the decoding of fast temporal changes inherent in the consonant [15]. The component FFR is called sustained portion and seems to be elicited around 18–50 ms. This component reflects the encoding of periodic and harmonic structure of vowel sound related to harmonic vowels [11] and is also related to encoding of the elements of fundamental frequency and its modulations (first and second formants) [4, 15].

Another feature of speech ABR responses is that there is no variation between intra and inter subject, maintaining stable the morphological characteristics [16, 17].

The speech sounds are present more frequently in the daily lives of every human being. A long-term of auditory experience can improve the performance of the whole auditory system. Therefore, a subject who has a good processing of speech sounds has better electrophysiological responses for this type of stimulus, showing that auditory experience might modify the basic sensorial coding of the whole auditory pathway [18–21]. On the other hand, a subject who has auditory deprivation may have significant electrophysiological changes in the auditory system, as can be seen in children with history of otitis media.

3. Parameters

There are several searches about the coding processing of verbal sound occurs and to insert speech ABR as part of clinical routine.

The syllable /da/ is commonly used speech for ABR assessment due to it being considered a universal syllable and allows it to be applied in different countries with good clinical assertiveness [4]. However, previous studies show that there is difference response in subjects from different culture [22] since each language has its own characteristics and peculiarities that can contribute or not to a suitable processing of speech sounds.

The majority of the studies was performed with native English speakers, which is explained by the fact that Dr. Kraus, the leading researcher and creator of the speech stimulus, did her work at Northwestern University, USA [1, 4]. However, additional studies have been initiated in numerous languages such as Arabic, Brazilian Portuguese, French, Greek, Hebrew, Indian, Japanese, and Persian [1, 11, 13, 22–32].

In each laboratory and/or institution, researchers choose their own parameters that will be applied on clinical investigation. Below are some items that should be thought about at the time of creation of the assessment parameters.

3.1. Equipment and software

Sanfins and Colella-Santos analyzed which equipments and software were often used for assessment of speech ABR. Biologic Navigator Pro (Natus) is the most used equipment followed by Neuroscan equipment (Biolink). As regards the software, the *BioMark* (Biological Marker of Auditory Processing) and *Neuroscam Stim 2* are the main packages available [1].

3.2. Electrode montage

The position of the electrodes follows the traditional ABR assessment (click ABR). Neurophysiological responses can be recorded with an active electrode positioned on the vertex (Cz), the reference electrodes on the ipsilateral mastoid, and the ground on the contralateral mastoid, using one channel with surface electrodes fixed, according to the 10–20 system [33]. Automatic switching function of the reference signals and the amplifier ground based on the stimulated ear should be activated on the equipment. The electrode on the left ear can be connected to input 2/channel 1, and the electrode on the right ear can be connected to ground connection cable. During the recording session, impedance should be maintained at below 5 kΩ and inter-electrode impedance below 3 kΩ [22].

3.3. Stimulated ear

Research shows that there is an asymmetry for the auditory processing of verbal sounds that occur in the brainstem and extend to auditory cortex when evaluating the differences between the responses obtained from the presentation of acoustic stimuli on the right and left ears [34, 35].

Regarding the stimulated ear, the great majority of studies performed the assessment of ABR with speech stimuli elicited only on the right ear, which can be explained by the advantage of right ear in encoding speech by contralateral projection to the left hemisphere [24, 26, 29, 31, 32, 36–44].

However, some researchers have written that stimulus presentation can be performed on the ear with better threshold confirmed by pure tone audiometry [45]. In a systematic review about the applicability of speech ABR [1], it was possible to see that in 14.3% of articles, stimulation was performed monaurally; however, between the left ear and right ear stimulation, there is scientific evidence that even if there is a proven right ear advantage in the processing of speech, the left ear can participate in this process, but with less intense electrophysiological responses [28, 36, 46]. Therefore, an analysis of responses from both ears could help in the diagnosis process as well as therapeutic monitoring.

Importantly, there is a tutorial about ABR of complex sounds that notify that the monaural stimulation is preferred for children, while the binaural stimulation is more realistic than monoaural [4].

Ahadi et al. [25] presented the sound stimulus on three conditions: monaural right, monaural, and binaural left. They showed that the magnitude and strength of speech ABR responses depend on the stimulus presentation mode, and the binaural presentation of speech syllable enables better visualization of the response, however,

3.4. Stimulus

The speech ABR assessment allows to apply different types of sound stimulus. The syllable / da/ is most well known and applied more often in studies [11, 13, 15, 22, 25, 28, 29, 32, 36, 39, 45, 47]. However, there are researchers who used disyllables as /baba/ [27] or even other syllables composed by consonant-vowel as /ba/ [23, 30, 31].

The presentation rate parameter is related to the duration of the sound stimulus; in the case of speech ABR, it is related to the size of the sound stimulus speech. The frequent value found in the studies is 10.9/s, however, no reports of the use of 11.1/s. In a study of literature review, it is noted that in about 19% of the previous studies on the assessment of speech ABR, this parameter is not described by the researchers [1].

Considering the length parameter, it is observed that the most frequently found values were 40 and 170 ms [1]. There is a relation between the presentation rate and duration, so the higher, the shorter will be the presentation rate [45, 48]. Song et al. [16] used both acoustic stimuli and concluded that short (40 ms) and long stimulus (170 ms) reflect the coding of speech in the brainstem in a reliable way, thus enabling that neural changes can be monitored through an objective electrophysiological measure.

The type of polarity of the sound stimulus is one of the most consistent parameters across studies on the assessment of speech ABR. Approximately, 90.5% of the previous studies have used alternating polarity [13, 22, 23, 28, 29, 39, 45, 47, 49, 50]. The choice for this type of polarity should be the reduction of artifacts and cochlear microphonic [51].

Regarding the intensity used in the assessment of speech, ABR suggests the use of 60–85 dB SPL [4, 15]. It is noted that, as it is an assessment process, the sound should be applied in an audible and comfortable intensity to the patient. The majority of studies has used the intensity of 80 dB SPL [1].

The speech stimulus requires approximately 4000 and 6000 sweeps in order to get a robust and replicable response, differently, the click stimulus or tone burst that needs around 2000 sweeps to get a good quality of response [4]. The number of sweeps is one of the most diverse parameters across studies [1]; however, the majority of researches used two blocks of 3000 free sweeps artifacts [13, 22, 25, 28, 36, 39–41, 47, 49]. Both trials were averaged to create a calculated wave of 6000 sweeps. The traces of both recordings were added, and the responses of the resultant waves were identified and analyzed in **Figure 3** (electrophysiological response representation of two blocks of 3000 sweeps and calculated wave of 6000 sweeps. Investigator's personal data based on a subject's assessment performed with BioMARK™ software).

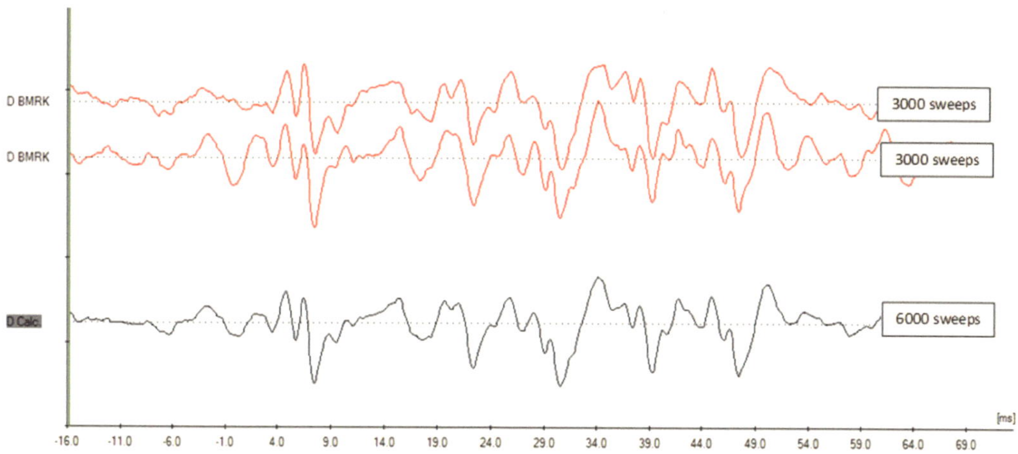

Figure 3. Electrophysiological response representation of two blocks of 3000 sweeps and calculated wave of 6000 sweeps. Investigator's personal data based on a subject's assessment performed with BioMARK™ software.

3.5. Transducer

The literature recommends that earphones are not to be used once this device can increase the chances of artifacts. Thus, the recommendation is to use the insert earphones. In cases of insert earphones are not possible to be used, there is the possibility to do the test with loudspeakers. It is important to consider that the responses are not so reliable as ones with insert earphones. The evaluator should be very careful in positioning the patient and the loudspeakers, and these loudspeakers should be equidistant between the right and left ears [4]. In addition, previous study has presented speech stimulus through individual hearing aid with excellent results with free and high-quality artifact [23].

3.6. Assessment of condition

As the traditional ABR assessment, the patients are instructed to keep their bodies relaxed with no movements in order to minimize the myogenic artifacts. [24]

Researchers reinforce that the attention can influence the FFR portion of speech sounds [52]. Therefore, the majority of researches has allowed the patient to watch a movie with reduced sound intensity or with subtitle [16, 23, 40, 41, 50], which seems that it keeps them quiet and relaxed during the assessment. Other researchers allow the patient to choose between watching a movie or sleep during the assessment process [24, 45].

Different parameters are being used. The parameters most cited in the literature about the assessment of speech ABR and with good clinical results are presented below in **Chart 1** (Speech ABR parameters). Note that there is a well-written tutorial by Skoe and Kraus [4] with detailed, clear, and objective information about the functioning and clinical application of speech ABR. This tutorial can be a material support to those interested in unraveling this new and effective electrophysiological assessment method.

Parameters	Setting
Equipment	Biologic navigator pro
Software	BioMARK
Electrode montage	Cz, M1, and M2
Stimulated ear	Right ear
Stimulus	Speech
Stimulus type	Syllable /da/
Stimulus duration	40 ms
Stimulus polarity	Alternating
Stimulus intensity	80 dB SPL
Stimulus rate	10.9/sec
Number of sweeps	6000
Replicability	Twice for 3000 sweeps
Transducer	Insert
Assessment condition	Watch a movie

Chart 1. Speech ABR parameters.

4. Criteria of normality

Before presenting the criteria of normality, it is important to understand the influence of the maturational process and gender in response to speech ABR.

4.1. Maturation

The response of ABR with nonverbal stimulus is mature around 18 months, while the speech ABR appears to be mature by the age of 5 [10]. This way a procedure can be used in young and school-age children, helping in the differential diagnosis of diseases with similar symptoms

[14]. Further studies are being conducted to regulate the normal values for different age range and confirm the age of maturation of central auditory system for verbal sounds.

According to Yamamuro et al. [39], age affects the coding of sounds by a single stimulus or the complex and neural timing and auditory skills are improved over the years. The responses of speech ABR in a child of 5 years are not so different from a child's responses in the age group of 8–12 years , whereas a child's responses in the age group of 3–4 years are very different in morphological aspect as related to the latency time.

Source	Latency (ms)				Amplitude (μv)				VA measures			
	Test		Retest		Test		Retest		Test		Retest	
	Mean	SD	Mean	SD	Mean	SD	Mean	SD				
V	6.65	0.27	6.68	0.27	0.13	0.05	0.13	0.04				
A	7.62	0.35	7.62	0.37	0.20	0.06	0.21	0.06				
C	18.60	0.68	18.47	0.68	0.03	0.06	0.03	0.05				
D	22.67	0.59	22.67	0.58	0.13	0.07	0.14	0.07				
E	31.12	0.53	31.2	0.57	0.22	0.06	0.21	0.07				
F	39.70	0.57	39.71	0.50	0.14	0.09	0.13	0.08				
O	48.26	0.43	48.34	0.39	0.15	0.06	0.16	0.06				
Slope VA (μv/ms)									0.35	0.11	0.37	0.12
Area VA (μv × ms)									0.16	0.05	0.15	0.05

Song et al. [16] performed their study with 45 adults with normal hearing (29 females) (19–36 years old; 24.5 ± 3.0).

Note: Parametric study in normal adults.

Table 1. Parametric study (mean and standard deviation) by syllable /da/, 40 ms, (silence) performed in adults with normal hearing (Song et al. [16]) on the right ear in two different conditions (test and retest).

4.2. Gender influence

Previous studies of literature have shown that there are differences of responses in the auditory perception between genders with better performance in female in the entire trajectory of the peripheral auditory and central nervous system [53, 54]; however, when the focus of analysis is the speech ABR, it was observed that women have better responses (higher values for amplitudes and lower values for latencies), and it was only the initial portion of the speech stimuli of the coding process when compared to men [55]. Differences in speech ABR responses between genders were explained by the premise that the synapses of the afferent and efferent systems of the auditory system are strongly influenced by the hormone estrogen activity [56].

4.3. Normative data

There are some studies that are used as parametric models for the analysis of speech ABR. Normative data for young adults (19–36 years old) with normal hearing and analysis of all the waves are presented in **Table 1** (parametric study [mean and standard deviation] by syllable / da/, 40 ms, [silence] performed in adults with normal hearing—Song et al. [16]—on the right ear in two different conditions—test and retest [16]). Two studies for children and adolescents will be presented: (i) composed of children between 8 and 12 years of age with normal hearing and with the analysis of waves V, A, C, and F and VA complex in **Table 2** (parametric study [mean and standard deviation] by syllable /da/, 40 ms, [silence] performed in children with normal hearing—Russo et al. [15]—on the right ear [15]) and (ii) composed of children and adolescents between 8 and 16 years of age with normal hearing and examination of all the waves in **Table 3** (parametric study [mean and standard deviation] by syllable /da/, 40 ms [silence] performed in children and adolescent with normal hearing—Sanfins et al. [22]—on the right and left ears [22]).

Source	Latência (ms)		Amplitude (μv)		VA measures	
	Right ear		Right ear		Right ear	
	Mean	SD	Mean	SD	Mean	SD
V	6.61	0.25	0.31	0.15		
A	7.51	0.34	0.65	0.19		
C	17.69	0.48	0.36	0.09		
F	39.73	0.61	0.43	0.19		
Slope VA (μv/ms)					0.13	0.05
Area VA (μv × ms)					1.70	1.23

Russo et al. [15] studied 36 and 38 children and adolescent (17 females) with normal hearing (8–12 years old).

Note: Parametric study in normal children.

Table 2. Parametric study (mean and standard deviation) by syllable /da/, 40 ms (silence) performed in children with normal hearing (Russo et al. [15]) on the right ear.

The majority of studies about speech ABR assessment was performed with monoaural stimulus on the right ear [13, 24, 29, 39, 49, 50]. The choice for the assessment only on the right ear is related to the advantage of the left hemisphere for processing of language sounds. Associated with this fact, earlier research has shown that there are no statistically significant differences between the responses on the right and left ears in subjects with normal hearing and typical development. However, there are many conditions to be studied through the speech ABR, and it is important to consider whether there are differences in responses between the ears.

Thereby, the responses on the right and left ears were presented in the population of children and adolescents with normal hearing and normal development so that it can be used as a comparison with the responses obtained in subjects with different pathologies.

It is noted that the parametric studies provide a direction to the researchers. It is fundamental to know the parameters of collection and analysis of each reference author before the use of this data. Each research center or clinic should carry out its own normative study for the different age groups.

Source	Latency (ms)				Amplitude (μv)				VA measures			
	Right ear		Left ear		Right ear		Left ear		Right ear		Left ear	
	Mean	SD	Mean	SD	Mean	SD	Mean	SD				
V	6.50	0.21	6.51	0.21	0.12	0.06	0.11	0.06				
A	7.46	0.33	7.48	0.36	0.22	0.09	0.21	0.07				
C	18.33	0.42	18.41	0.46	0.10	0.08	0.11	0.10				
D	22.21	0.66	22.36	0.44	0.14	0.09	0.13	0.08				
E	30.89	0.50	30.78	0.61	0.30	0.39	0.23	0.09				
F	39.37	0.55	39.20	0.47	0.24	0.29	0.19	0.09				
O	48.00	0.75	47.95	0.54	0.21	0.30	0.16	0.12				
Slope VA (μv/ms)									0.37	0.14	0.35	0.13
Area VA (μv × ms)									0.33	0.13	0.31	0.13

Sanfins et al. [22] studied 40 children and adolescent (25 females) with normal hearing (8–16 years old; 10.95 ± 2.0).

Note: Parametric study in normal children and adolescent.

Table 3. Parametric study (mean and standard deviation) by syllable /da/, 40 ms (silence) performed in children and adolescent with normal hearing (Sanfins et al. [22]) on the right and left ears.

5. Clinical applicability

5.1. Auditory training

Auditory training is able to induce neurophysiological changes that can be observed by an evaluation of speech ABR. According to Killion et al. [57], an auditory training program promotes gains in both speech perception in quiet environments such as in noisy environments and improves short-term memory skills and attentional processes.

According to Hayes et al. [58] children with learning problems can benefit from an auditory rehabilitation program through auditory training. Research has shown that these children have a delay in responses of speech ABR, more specifically, the values of onset portion—wave A, and the assessment of speech ABR may be able to ascertain whether the auditory training program was effective, monitoring the benefits of rehabilitation in children and in young adults [15, 16].

Further studies are needed in the elderly population to determine if this type of assessment can be effective in monitoring this population. Anderson et al. [49] reported that the elderly usually have a hearing loss, thus an auditory training program should be recommended along the selection and adaptation of hearing aid suitable for need each elderly.

Auditory training and amplification are ideal to improve the auditory function and, especially, to improve the process of speech perception. In this context, the assessment of speech ABR could have an important role to demonstrate quickly, clearly, and objectively what are the real gains of interventions. Researchers have emphasized that the assessment of speech ABR is considered a biological marker of auditory training, being able to identify subjects who will have the benefit of an auditory training program [58, 59].

5.2. The aging process

The elderly has a reduced neural synchrony in the encoding of speech sounds, especially when the speech sounds are produced in the presence of background noise. The assessment of speech ABR is able to monitor the difficulty in understanding speech in noise reported by the elderly. The fitting process allows speech sounds to be heard more clearly. Thus there has been a change of morphology and the latency values of the speech responses ABR [24, 36, 45].

5.3. Differential diagnosis

Research shows that the literacy process depends on an efficient functioning of the auditory processing in the brainstem. The assessment of speech ABR could accurately predict early and possible changes in the processes of reading, writing, and literacy in preschool children [41, 60, 61].

Children with learning, speech, and hearing impairments not only suffer from background noise and competitive sounds but also have some difficulty in the perception of speech sounds in quiet environments [62]. This difficulty can be arising from changes in temporal processing that can impact the perception of speech. In this context, the speech ABR is a biological marker of auditory processing disorder, being able to identify children with predisposition to these changes [4].

Children with dyslexia often have impairments in the perception of speech sounds that can affect their reading skills [63]. According Hornickel and Kraus [64] good readers have a stable neural representation of sound and that children who have inconsistent neural responses are likely at a disadvantage when learning to read. Thus, the speech ABR can help identify and separate these children, enabling a more appropriate intervention.

Besides that, another application of speech ABR can be in diagnosing and categorizing children with learning disability in different subgroups, assessing the effects of aging on central auditory processing of speech, and assessing the effects of central auditory deficits in hearing aid and cochlear implant users [11].

Understanding the neural processing of speech sounds at the brainstem level may provide knowledge regarding the central auditory processes involved in normal hearing subjects and also in clinical populations [10]. Moreover, altered responses of speech ABR may be associated with impaired speech perception in noise. These changes might have a negative impact on communication and have serious consequences for academic success [8].

5.4. Musician

Currently, there is an increasing interest in the influence of musical experience related to language processing. The intense musical training in the long term seems to cause an anatomical and physiological change and improves the working memory in cognitive processes, the control of emotions, and perception of sound stimuli [65].

The brain stem has an important role in the encoding of speech sound stimuli and temporal processing [66]. Temporal processing contributes to the perception of duration of the consonants and the identification of notes and musical scales [66, 67]. The literacy process, including the process of reading, writing, and language, is also influenced by the temporal processing [68]. The detection of small and rapid changes of the sound stimulus is associated with the rhythm, the frequency of the sound stimulus, phonemic discrimination, duration, and discrimination of pitch [69]. Understanding how music influences the encoding of speech sounds can be used for more information about the learning process [64]. One way to analyze this is through the responses of speech ABR.

5.5. History of otitis media

Otitis media is one of the most common childhood diseases, affecting about two-third of children in the first 5 years of life [70, 71]. This period is important for the development of oral and written language. Otitis media can cause functional sequelae of the middle ear structures and can induce a temporary mild-to-moderate hearing loss. The latter can remain for a few days or for several weeks [72, 73]. Concomitantly, the accumulation of fluid in the middle ear interferes the speech perception, causing a distortion in the perception of acoustic signals and reduces the speed and accuracy of verbal decoding [74]. When hearing fluctuation occurs early in life, that is the critical period for linguistic development, a limited acquisition of speech and language occurs. As a result communication problems may appear, such as language developing impairment, auditory processing deficits, cognitive impairment, and psychosocial development and impairment in the acquisition of literacy skills [75, 76].

Inadequate auditory stimulation in childhood can lead to long-term alterations of the auditory structures in the central auditory nervous system [73]. Research shows that children suffering from secretory otitis media in their first 6 years of age and underwent a surgery for bilateral ventilation tubes placement demonstrates neurophysiological modifications of speech perception when compared with typically developing children and adolescents.

6. Conclusion

The assessment of speech ABR could accurately predict early and possible changes in the processes of reading, writing, and literacy in preschool children.

The speech ABR is objective, fast, and can be applied from early childhood. It is equally effective in different languages and can provide differential diagnoses of diseases with similar symptoms, as an effective biomarker of auditory processing disorders that may be present in various diseases, such as dyslexia, specific language impairment, hearing loss, auditory processing disorders, otitis media, and scholastic difficulties.

It is a science with great possibility of research with different approaches to assist in detection, treatment, and monitoring of various diseases.

Glossary

ABR>	Auditory brainstem response
AEP>	Auditory evoked potentials. General term to evoked potential when using an auditory stimulus
CV syllable>	Formed by a consonant and a vowel that produces a phoneme
10–20 International System	A standard system for electrode location
FFR>	Frequency Following Response. The second part of the speech—ABR responses that reflect the vowel.
Synthesized speech>	Artificial production of human speech
Onset portion>	The first part of the speech—ABR responses that reflect the consonant

Acknowledgements

This work was supported by the Project "Integrated system of tools for diagnostics and telerehabilitation of sensory organs disorders (hearing, vision, speech, balance, taste, smell)" acr. INNOSENSE, co-financed by the National Centre for Research and Development (Poland), within the STRATEGMED program.

Author details

Milaine Dominici Sanfins[1*], Piotr H. Skarzynski[2,3,4] and Maria Francisca Colella-Santos[5]

*Address all correspondence to: msanfins@uol.com.br

1 Faculty of Medical Science, State University of Campinas, Campinas, Brazil

2 World Hearing Center, Warsaw, Poland

3 Department of Heart Failure and Cardiac Rehabilitation, Medical University of Warsaw, Warsaw, Poland

4 Institute of Sensory Organs, Kajetany, Poland

5 Human Development and Rehabilitation Department, Faculty of Medical Science, State University of Campinas, Campinas, Brazil

References

[1] Sanfins M, Colella-Santos M. A review of the clinical applicability of speech-evoked auditory brainstem responses. Journal of Hearing Science. 2016;6 (1):9–16.

[2] Sanfins MD. Auditory neuropathy/auditory dys-synchrony: a study with the hearing impaired students of three special schools in the city of São Paulo [dissertação]. São Paulo: University of São Paulo, Faculty of Medicine; 2004. doi:10.11606/D.5.2004.tde-19092014-101620

[3] Blackburn CC, Sachs MB. The representation of steady-state vowl /eh/ in the discharge paterns of cat anteroventral cochlear nucleus neurons. Journal of Neurophysiology. 1990;63:1303–1329.

[4] Skoe E, Kraus N. Auditory brainstem response to complex sounds: a tutorial. Ear and Hearing. 2010;31:320–324.

[5] Dhar S, Abel R, Hornickel J, Nicol T, Skoe E, Zhao W, et al. Exploring the relationship between physiological measures of cochlear and brainstem function. Clinical Neurophysiology. 2009;120(5):959–966.

[6] Basu M, Krishnan A, Weber-Fox C. Brainstem correlates of temporal auditory processing in children with specific language impairment. Developmental Science. 2010;13(1):77–91.

[7] Hornickel J, Skoe E, Nicol T, Zecker S, Kraus N. Subcortical differentiation of stop consonants relates to reading and speech-in-noise perception. Proceedings of the National Academy of Sciences of the United States of America. 2009;106(31):13022–13027.

[8] Kraus N, Hornickel J. cABR: a biological probe of auditory processing. In: Geffner DS, Ross-Swain D, editors. Auditory processing disorders: assessment, management, and treatment. 2nd ed. San Diego: Plural Publishing; 2013. pp. 159–183.

[9] Baran JA. Test battery considerations. In: Plural, editor. Handbook of (central) auditory processing disorders. 1. San Diego: Plural; 2007. pp. 163–192.

[10] Johnson KL, Nicol T, Zecker SG, Kraus N. Developmental plasticity in the human auditory brainstem. Journal of Neuroscience. 2008;28(15):4000–4007.

[11] Sinha SK, Basavaraj V. Speech evoked auditory brainstem responses: A new tool to study brainstem encoding of speech sounds. Indian Journal of Otolaryngology and Head and Neck Surgery. 2010;62(4):395–399.

[12] Kent R, Read C. Análise acústica da fala2015. 504 p.

[13] Sanfins M, Borges L, Ubiali T, Colella-Santos M. Speech auditory brainstem response (speech ABR) in the differential diagnosis of scholastic difficulties. Brazilian Journal of Otorhinolaryngology. 2015 Nov 6. pii: S1808–8694(15)00187–1. doi: 10.1016/j.bjorl.2015.05.014

[14] Johnson KL, Nicol TG, Kraus N. Brain stem response to speech: a biological marker of auditory processing. Ear and Hearing. 2005;26(5):424–434.

[15] Russo N, Nicol T, Musacchia G, Kraus N. Brainstem responses to speech syllables. Clinical Neurophysiology. 2004;115:2021–2030.

[16] Song JH, Nicol T, Kraus N. Test-retest reliability of the speech-evoked auditory brainstem response. Clinical Neurophysiology. 2011;122(2):346–355.

[17] Banai K, Kraus N. The dynamic brainstem:implications for APD. In: McFarland and A. Cacace (eds). Current Controversies in Central Auditory Processing Disorder. Plural Publishing Inc: San Diego, CA. 2008. pp. 269–289.

[18] Strait DL, Kraus N, Parbery-Clark A, Ashley R. Musical experience shapes top-down auditory mechanisms: evidence from masking and auditory attention performance. Hearing Research. 2010;261(1–2):22–29.

[19] Strait DL, Slater J, O'Connell S, Kraus N. Music training relates to the development of neural mechanisms of selective auditory attention. Developmental Cognitive Neuroscience. 2015;12:94–104.

[20] Musacchia G, Strait D, Kraus N. Relationships between behavior, brainstem and cortical encoding of seen and heard speech in musicians and non-musicians. Hearing Research. 2008;241(1–2):34–42.

[21] Parbery-Clark A, Tierney A, Strait DL, Kraus N. Musicians have fine-tuned neural distinction of speech syllables. Neuroscience. 2012;219:111–119.

[22] Sanfins MD, Borges LR, Ubiali T, Donadon C, Hein TAD, Hatzopoulos S, et al. Speech-evoked brainstem response in normal adolescent and children speakers of Brazilian Portuguese. International Journal of Pediatric Otorhinolaryngolgoy. 2016;90:12–19.

[23] Bellier L, Veuillet E, Vesson JF, Bouchet P, Caclin A, Thai-Van H. Speech auditory brainstem response through hearing aid stimulation. Hearing Research. 2015;325:49–54.

[24] Fujihira H, Shiraishi K. Correlations between word intelligibility under reverberation and speech auditory brainstem responses in elderly listeners. Clinical Neurophysiology. 2015;126(1):96–102.

[25] Ahadi M, Pourbakht A, Jafari AH, Jalaie S. Effects of stimulus presentation mode and subcortical laterality in speech-evoked auditory brainstem responses. International Journal of Audiology. 2014;53(4):243–249.

[26] Rocha-Muniz CN, Befi-Lopes DM, Schochat E. Sensitivity, specificity and efficiency of speech-evoked ABR. Hearing Research. 2014;317:15–22.

[27] Wagner R, Torgesen J, Rashotte C. Development of reading-related phonological processing abilities: new evidence of bidirectional casuality from a latent variable longitudinal study. Development Psychology. 1994;30 (1):73–87.

[28] Rana B, Barman A. Correlation between speech-evoked auditory brainstem responses and transient evoked otoacoustic emissions. Journal of Laryngology and Otology. 2011;125(9):911–916.

[29] Karawani H, Banai K. Speech-evoked brainstem responses in Arabic and Hebrew speakers. International Journal of Audiology. 2010;49(11):844–849.

[30] Akhoun I, Moulin A, Jeanvoine A, Menard M, Buret F, Vollaire C, et al. Speech auditory brainstem response (speech ABR) characteristics depending on recording conditions, and hearing status an experimental parametric study. Journal of Neuroscience Methods. 2008;175(2):196–205.

[31] Akhoun I, Gallégo S, Moulin A, Ménard M, Veuillet E, Berger-Vachon C, et al. The temporal relationship between speech auditory brainstem responses and the acoustic pattern of the phoneme /ba/ in normal-hearing adults. Clinical Neurophysiology. 2008;119(4):922–933.

[32] Friendly RH, Rendall D, Trainor LJ. Learning to differentiate individuals by their voices: infants' individuation of native- and foreign-species voices. Developmental Psychobiology. 2014;56(2):228–237.

[33] Jasper H. The ten-twenty system of the international federation. Electroencephalography and Clinical Neurophysiology. 1958;10:371–375.

[34] Abrams D, Nicol T, Zecker S, Kraus N. Auditory brainstem timing predicts cerebral asymmetry for speech. The Journal of Neuroscience. 2006;26(43):11131–11137.

[35] Hornickel J, Skoe E, Kraus N. Subcortical laterality of speech encoding. Audiology & Neuro-Otology 2009;14:198–207.

[36] Elkabariti RH, Khalil LH, Husein R, Talaat HS. Speech evoked auditory brainstem response findings in children with epilepsy. International Journal of Pediatric Otorhinolaryngology. 2014;78(8):1277–1280.

[37] Kösem A, Gramfort A, van Wassenhove V. Encoding of event timing in the phase of neural oscillations. NeuroImage. 2014;92:274–284.

[38] Shamma S, Fritz J. Adaptive auditory computations. Current Opinion in Neurobiology. 2014;25:164–168.

[39] Yamamuro K, Ota T, Iida J, Nakanishi Y, Matsuura H, Uratani M, et al. Event-related potentials reflect the efficacy of pharmaceutical treatments in children and adolescents with attention deficit/hyperactivity disorder. Psychiatry Research. 2016;30 (242):288–294.

[40] Hornickel J, Lin D, Kraus N. Speech-evoked auditory brainstem responses reflect familial and cognitive influences. Developmental Science. 2013;16(1):101–110.

[41] Hornickel J, Knowles E, Kraus N. Test-retest consistency of speech-evoked auditory brainstem responses in typically-developing children. Hearing Research. 2012;284(1–2):52–58.

[42] Rocha-Muniz CN, Befi-Lopes DM, Schochat E. Investigation of auditory processing disorder and language impairment using the speech-evoked auditory brainstem response. Hearing Research. 2012;294(1–2):143–152.

[43] Anurova I, Renier LA, De Volder AG, Carlson S, Rauschecker JP. Relationship between cortical thickness and functional activation in the early blind. Cerebral Cortex. 2015;25(8):2035–2048.

[44] Song JH, Banai K, Russo NM, Kraus N. On the relationship between speech- and nonspeech-evoked auditory brainstem responses. Audiology and Neuro-Otology. 2006;11(4):233–241.

[45] Mamo SK, Grose JH, Buss E. Speech-evoked ABR: effects of age and simulated neural temporal jitter. Hearing Research. 2015.

[46] Engineer CT, Perez CA, Carraway RS, Chang KQ, Roland JL, Kilgard MP. Speech training alters tone frequency tuning in rat primary auditory cortex. Behav Brain Res. 2013;8, pp.1–10.

[47] Tahaei AA, Ashayeri H, Pourbakht A, Kamali M. Speech evoked auditory brainstem response in stuttering. (Cairo): Scientifica.. 2014;2014:328646.

[48] Hamaguchi K, Tschida KA, Yoon I, Donald BR, Mooney R. Auditory synapses to song premotor neurons are gated off during vocalization in zebra finches. eLife. 2014;3:e01833.

[49] Anderson S, Parbery-Clark A, White-Schwoch T, Kraus N. Auditory brainstem response to complex sounds predicts self-reported speech-in-noise performance. Journal of Speech Language and Hearing Research. 2013;56(1):31–43.

[50] Song JH, Banai K, Russo NM, Kraus N. On the relationship between speech- and nonspeech-evoked auditory brainstem responses. Audiology and Neurotology. 2006;11(4):233–241.

[51] Gorga M, Abbas P, Worthington D. Stimulus calibration in ABR measurements. In: Jacobson J, editor. The auditory brainstem response. San Diego: College-Hill Press; 1985.

[52] Galbraith G, Olfman D, Huffman T. Selective attention affects human brain stem frequency-following response. Neuroreport. 2003;14:735–738.

[53] Jerger J, Hall J. Effects of age and sex on auditory brainstem response. Archives of Otolaryngology. 1980;106:387–391.

[54] Sininger Y, Cone-Wesson B, Abdala C. Gender distinctions and lateral asymmetry in the low-level auditory brainstem response of the human neonate. Hearing Research. 1998;126(1–2):58–66.

[55] Krizman J, Skoe E, Kraus N. Sex differences in auditory subcortical function. Clinical Neurophysiology. 2012;123(3):590–597.

[56] Tremere L, Pinaud R. Brain-generated estradiol drives long-term optimization of auditory coding to enhance the discrimination of communication signals. The Journal of Neuroscience. 2011;31:3271–3289.

[57] Killion M, Niquette P, Gudmundsen G, Revit L, Banerjee S. Development of a quick speech-in-noise test for measuring signal-to-noise ratio loss in normal-hearing and hearing-impaired listeners. The Journal of the Acoustical Society of America 2004;116:22395–22405.

[58] Hayes E, Warrier C, Nicol T. Neural plasticity following auditory training in children with learning problems. Clinical Neurophysiology. 2003;114:673–684.

[59] Russo NM, Nicol TG, Zecker SG, Hayes EA, Kraus N. Auditory training improves neural timing in the human brainstem. Behavioural Brain Research. 2005;156(1):95–103.

[60] Anderson S, Parbery-Clark A, White-Schwoch T, Kraus N. Aging affects neural precision of speech encoding. Journal of Neuroscience. 2012;32(41):14156–14164.

[61] Wible B, Nicol T, Kraus N. Atypical brainstem representation of onset and formant structure of speech sounds in children with language-based learning problems. Biological Psychology. 2004;67(3):299–317.

[62] Ziegler J, Pech-Georgel C, George F, Lorenzi C. Speech-perception in-noise deficits in dyslexia. Developmental Science. 2009;12:732–745.

[63] Bogliotti C, Serniclaes W, Messaoud-Galusi S, Sprenger-Charolles L. Discrimination of speech sounds by children with dyslexia: comparisons with chronological age and reading level controls. Journal of Experimental Child Psychology. 2008;101:137–155

[64] Hornickel J, Kraus N. Unstable representation of sound: a biological marker of dyslexia. The Journal of Neuroscience. 2013;33 (8):3500–3504.

[65] Owen, M. J., Norcross-Nechay, K., & Howie, V. M. (1993). Brainstem auditory evoked potentials in young children before and after tympanostomy tube placement. Journal of Pediatric Otorhinolaryngology: 25, 105–117.

[66] Lukhanina EP, Karaban IN, Burenok Iu A, Mel'nik NA, Berezetskaia NM. Effect of cerebrolysin on the electroencephalographic indices of brain activity in Parkinson's disease. Zhurnal Nevrologii i Psikhiatrii Imeni S.S. Korsakova. 2004;104(7):54–60.

[67] Li M, Kuroiwa Y, Wang L, Kamitani T, Omoto S, Hayashi E, et al. Visual event-related potentials under different interstimulus intervals in Parkinson's disease: relation to motor disability, WAIS-R, and regional cerebral blood flow. Parkinsonism & Related Disorders. 2005;11(4):209–219.

[68] Jiang C, Kaseda Y, Kumagai R, Nakano Y, Nakamura S. Habituation of event-related potentials in patients with Parkinson's disease. Physiology and Behavior. 2000;68(5): 741–747.

[69] Wang L, Kuroiwa Y, Li M, Kamitani T, Wang J, Takahashi T, et al. The correlation between P300 alterations and regional cerebral blood flow in non-demented Parkinson's disease. Neuroscience Letters. 2000;282(3):133–136.

[70] Chhetri S. Acute otitis media: a simple diagnosis, a simple treatment. Nepal Medical College Journal. 2014;16:33–36.

[71] Kong K, Coates H. Natural history, definitions, risk factors and burden of otitis media. Medical Journal of Australia. 2009;191:S39–S43.

[72] Bess F, Humess L. Patologias do sistema auditivo. Porto Alegre: Artmed: Fundamentos de audiologia; 1998. pp. 155–195.

[73] Bahare K, Farhad F, Maryam E, Zahra HD. Auditory processing abilities in children with chronic otitis media with effusion. Acta Oto-Laryngologica. 2016:136. pp. 456–459.

[74] Katz J, Tillery K, Mecca F, (tradução). Uma introdução ao processamento auditivo. In: Lichitg I, Carvallo R, editors. Abordagens atuais. São Paulo: Pró-Fono; 1997. pp. 145–172.

[75] Borg E, Risberg A, McAllister B, Undermar B, Edquist G, Reinholdson A, et al. Language development in hearing-impaired children. Establishment of a reference material for a language test for hearingimpaired children. LATHIC. International Journal of Pedriatric Otorhinolaryngology. 2002;65(1):15–26.

[76] Shriberg L, Flipsen PJ, Thielke H, Kwiatkowski J, Kertoy M, Katcher M, et al. Risk for speech disorder associated with early recurrent otitis media with effusion: two retrospective studies. Journal of Speech, Language, and Hearing Research. 2000;43(1): 79–99.

Chapter 3

Wideband Tympanometry

Thais Antonelli Diniz Hein, Stavros Hatzopoulos,
Piotr Henryk Skarzynski and
Maria Francisca Colella-Santos

Additional information is available at the end of the chapter

http://dx.doi.org/10.5772/67155

Abstract

The wideband tympanometry (WBT) assesses the middle ear function with a transient wideband stimulus in order to capture the middle ear behavior at a wide range of frequencies. Data in the literature suggest that the WBT has more sensibility to detect middle ear disorders than the traditional tympanometry. In this context, pathologies, which might be more easily identified/monitored by WBT, include otosclerosis, flaccid eardrums, ossicular chain discontinuity with semicircular canal dehiscence, and negative middle ear pressure with middle ear effusion. The chapter presents information on classical tympanometry, the multifrequency tympanometry equivalent coded as WBT, clarification of terms used in WBT measurements, and a short overview of clinical applications in infants and adults.

Keywords: acoustic immitance, tympanometry, wideband tympanometry, acoustic reflectance, acoustic absorbance

1. Introduction to tympanometry

Sound stimuli can be modified by alterations of the middle ear functionality; therefore, an assessment of the middle ear function is fundamental for a proper evaluation of hearing impairment. Acoustic immittance is a general term referring to measurements related to tympanometry and acoustic stapedial reflexes, which can provide information about the middle ear (ME) status. Tympanometry measurements represent alterations in the sound absorbance characteristics of the ME system (composed by the tympanic membrane + the middle ear), as the pressure in the external acoustic canal is modified. Clinically, these pressure values range from +200 to -400 daPa. According to Shanks and Lilly [1], the most accurate measurements are those in the low pressure end.

The ME ossicular structures drive the incoming sound stimuli from the eardrum (maleus) to the inner ear (footplate of the stapes). In terms of acoustic energy transmission, there is a physical problem interfacing the middle and the inner ear. The middle ear propagation medium is gaseous while the inner ear medium is liquid. To optimize the propagating stimulus energy, it is necessary to adjust the ME impedance so that the stimulus at the stapes undergoes an *"optimal power transference into the inner ear"* also called *"minimum impedance reflection."* This operation is termed as *"the middle ear impedance matching transformer"* [2, 3] and describes the efficiency by which the acoustic sound energy at the stapes is transformed into an acoustic pressure wave inside the helix structures of the inner ear, without significant energy losses.

There is a specific terminology in the ME measurements: There is an excellent review of these terms by Block and Wiley [4] and by Hall and Chandler [5]. Most of the ME measurements refer to *acoustic immittance* values, which describe the *easiness* by which a sound stimulus can propagate across a medium (air or liquid). Most media impose a resistance to any type of propagation energy. According to this concept, the structures of the ME impose a *resistance* to the propagation of the sound energy, and this opposition/resistance is termed as *acoustic impedance* $Z(\omega)$. By definition, the reciprocal value of acoustic impedance is *acoustic admittance* $Y(\omega)$. In this context an acoustic immittance measurement can refer to either $Z(\omega)$ or $Y(\omega)$ and the measurement is conducted with the same manner. The $Z(\omega)$ and $Y(\omega)$ variables are complex and they are characterized by a real and an imaginary part. In clinical terms, this characteristic means that the values of these depend on the frequency (ω) of the propagating stimulus. There is another measurement called "static immittance" which refers to measurement under a normal atmospheric pressure (i.e., not varying) and according to Hall and Chandler [5] clinically this can be measured at 226 Hz.

Traditional tympanometry assesses the impedance of the middle ear at the frequency of 226 Hz. The measurement modality is described in **Figure 1**, and it is conducted with a sensitive probe, which seals completely the ear of the patient. Once the 226 Hz tone is emitted, the pressure variation in the external acoustic meatus displaces the eardrum. This causes the tone absorption of the ME to vary, and a sensitive microphone incorporated in the probe evaluates the total admittance of the system [2].

Tympanometry provides quantitative information about the presence of fluid in the ME, about the mobility of the tympanic-ossicular system, and about the volume of the external acoustic meatus. While it is an effective procedure to identify ME changes in children, adults, and seniors, it has its limitations. For example, there are reported cases in the literature of myringotomy surgeries where the 226 Hz tympanometric data were reported as normal [6]. Assessment outliers like these myringotomy cases, are probably caused by a lack of specific norms for the different types of populations under assessment. It is well known that the eardrum and the external acoustic meatus of neonates and children are anatomically different than those from adult subjects. In this context, the ME impedance norms of one population do not describe well the norms of the other.

Data in the literature suggest that in infants of approximately 6 months of age, the high-frequency ME transmission is more efficient. Tympanometry measurements with a high-frequency tone (1000 Hz) can be more sensitive to identify ME changes than those conducted with a 226 Hz probe tone [6–8]. High frequency tympanometry has been shown to be reliable and highly reproducible. But the data in the literature also suggest that the 1000 Hz protocol cannot always identify all children with ME alterations. As a result, discrepant data between studies are reported, as well as reports describing an interpretation difficulty of the 1000 Hz impedance tracing [9, 10]. The 1000 Hz tympanometry trace is different than the traditional trace of 226 Hz. For many subjects the 1000 Hz trace presents a double peak and its clinical interpretation can be quite complicated [11].

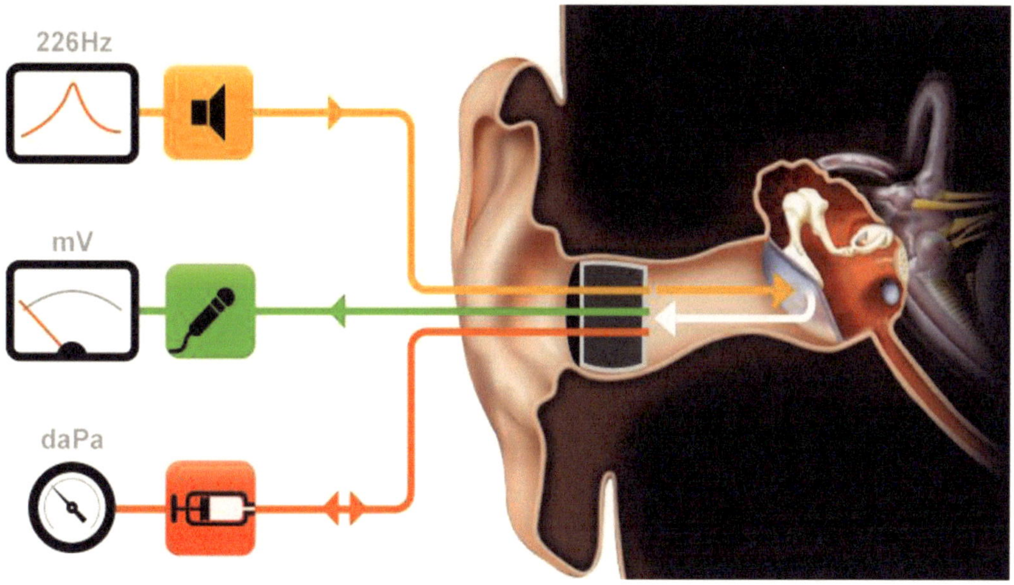

Figure 1. The tympanometry probe (shown with three major components) seals the ear of the patient. The components shown include the microphone, the pressure regulation system, and a speaker transducer.

A differential diagnosis for the evaluation of middle ear function is essential for infants presenting ME disorders, as in the case of temporary conductive hearing losses. This aspect is critical, because there is high incidence of unsuccessful results (FAIL) in neonatal hearing screening programs. These results are frequently caused by changes in the ME status and affect significantly the time and spectral characteristics of the transiently evoked otoacoustic emissions (TEOAEs), which are routinely used in the hearing screening protocols [12–15].

2. Wideband tympanometry

2.1. Description and instrumentation

As described in the previous section, the traditional tympanometry probe-tone at 226 Hz evokes different results depending on the anatomical characteristics of the ME cavity, which can influence the test results. The use of a wideband stimulus (i.e., acoustic click, chirp) has been shown to be more efficient and precise for a ME assessment. Because of the presence of multiple frequencies in the transient stimuli, wideband tympanometry (WBT) is less susceptible to myogenic noise, which originates from the patient movements [3, 16].

The WBT evaluates the ME function with a transient stimulus (click or chirp) testing frequencies from 226 to 8000 Hz, in small incrementing steps. Assessment of ME function over such a broad bandwidth provides detailed information on the ME status and can assist considerably any needed diagnosis.

Currently, there are two families of devices in the market, which offer WBT measurements: (i) the Otostat, and the HearID systems from Mimosa Acoustics, USA; and (ii) the Titan system from Interacoustics, Denmark. As in the traditional tympanometry, WBT is performed by placing a sealing probe into the external auditory canal. The probe contains a microphone, a pressure system, and a speaker transducer. The Mimosa devices are PC-independent, while the Titan requires a PC connection to perform the WBT measurements. **Figure 2** shows the WBT data from the Otostat system, displayed on a PC running the Otostation data management software. All the other figures in the text are generated using WBT data from the Titan device.

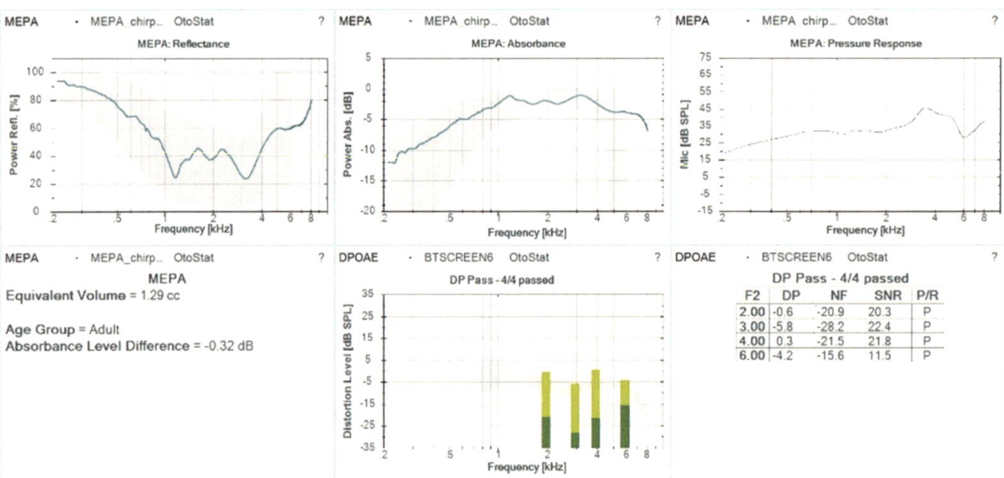

Figure 2. WBT data from the Otostat system (Mimosa Acoustics). The panels indicate WBT reflectance, absorbance, and pressure response × tested frequency (the Otostat uses a chirp stimulus). The lower panels show the distortion product OAEs in terms of spectrum and S/N ratios at the four tested frequencies. The WBT + OAE combination favors a good assessment of the ME function in neonates, and it can be used to avoid many REFER or FAIL results.

Interacoustics follows the philosophy of presenting the WBT data not in the traditional 2D manner but in a 3D format, depicting pressure (y-axis), frequency (x-axis), and absorbance (z-axis). An example of this 3D representation is shown in **Figure 3(A)** and **(B)** where neonatal WBT responses are depicted. The 3D graph can rotate, so the user can identify patterns in the 3D contour, which might be of interest. So far there are no data in the literature connecting the 3D pattern variations with some clinical observations. The main reason for this is the enormous amount of data (and the large number of variables represented) in the 3D graph.

http://dx.doi.org/10.5772/67155

Higher absorbance values suggest a more efficient ME (**Figure 3A**). Lower values suggest some sort of energy impediment in the ME structure, with a very good probability of a hearing impairment (**Figure 3B**). Interacoustics offers in the 3D graph, an absorbance scale which is color-coded with maxima in the blue and minima in the red color region. The scale is subject-dependent and it is not normalized (thus serves only as a visual aid).

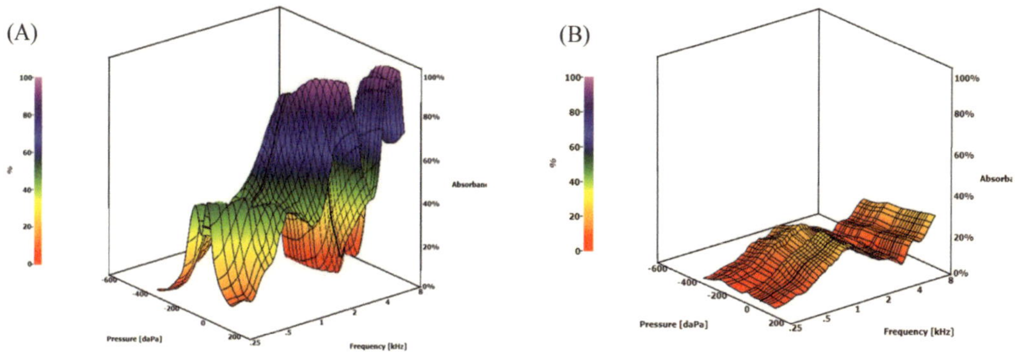

Figure 3. (A): Neonate normal WBT data. The subject passed a TEOAE screening test and it is considered as normal. The 3D curve is color-coded, showing good values in blue (high absorbance) and lower or possibly problematic absorbance values in red. The scale is relative to this subject and it is used for a visual aid. In the Appendix there are links from where the readers can download a video (avi file) showing how this 3D structure can be rotated or collapsed, in order to obtain specific frequency information. (B) Neonate WBT data from a infant who failed the TEOAE screening test. The 3D curve is color-coded, showing lower or possibly problematic absorbance values in orange red. The scale is relative to this subject and it is used for a visual aid. In the Appendix there are links from where the readers can download a video (avi file) showing how this 3D structure can be rotated or collapsed, in order to obtain specific frequency information.

2.2. Absorbance and related measurements

It is possible to collapse a number of frequencies and obtain absorbance data over an averaged frequency range (wideband averaged tympanogram), which might offer better clinical estimates for well babies and NICU residents. The WBT average range used in infants is from 800 to 2000 Hz, because it is optimized for ME transmission anomalies such as ME negative pressure and ME with effusion. In this frequency range these pathologies generate 3D graphs presenting major and significant differences between normal and abnormal ears.

According to Interacoustics, the WBT average range in adults is defined from 375 to 2000 Hz. Using average WBT data in this range it is possible to discriminate well WBT responses between children and adults. Interacoustics suggests to average the WBT data starting from 375 Hz and not from 226 Hz, since the latter frequency does not offer a high discriminative value.

It is also possible to obtained absorbance information at the resonance ME frequency, which corresponds to the frequency where mass and stiffness contribute equally to the absorbance (response with a zero phase). The resonance frequency can be useful in the diagnosis of ME abnormalities such as the disjunction of the ossicular chain or otosclerosis. For cases of ossicular chain discontinuity or of other pathologies presenting a dominant ME mass, the resonance frequency of the middle ear tends to be reduced. In the case of otosclerosis, the resonance frequency shifts to higher frequencies [17, 18]. Monitoring the resonant frequency seems to be promising as a method to follow the clinical progression of otosclerosis. It is also possible to obtain the "resonance frequency tympanogram," which is useful in the differentiation between cases of ossicular disruption and a flaccid eardrum [17–19].

From the 3D-WBT graph, it is possible to obtain information about the absorbance at a particular frequency measured in ambient pressure or at the pressure of the middle ear (see Appendix section for a video showing how this is accomplished). The acoustic absorbance (A) is defined as the ratio of (absorbed sound power)/to (incident sound power). Pathologies that can be further monitored or identified with this data modality are: otosclerosis, flaccid eardrums, ossicular chain discontinuity, and semicircular canal dehiscence and babies with negative middle ear pressure and middle ear effusion [20, 21]. The WBT devices from Mimosa Acoustics utilize the concept of acoustic reflectance. Reflectance is the amount of energy reflected by the system in relation to total energy propagating through the system, and it is measured in percentage. The reader might find useful terminology reviews by Hall and Chandler [5] and by Stinson [22].

Several publications indicate that the graph of absorbance allows a better differentiation between middle ear diseases than the traditional tympanometry. There are groups of patients where the pressurization of the ear can be difficult or unwise. Thus, an absorbance test held in nonpressurized conditions will be useful for monitoring middle ear state immediately after surgery, with perforated eardrum during neonatal hearing screening. In several studies performed in ambient pressure proved to be able to detect changes in middle ear function significantly for infants and neonatal measurements [23, 24]. In the case of patients with ventilation tubes in the eardrum, data from Groon et al. [25], suggest that: (i) for any leak larger than 0.25 mm there are absorbance alteration effects up to 10 kHz; (ii) above 1 kHz these effects are unpredictable; and (iii) absorbance values were mostly increased in the lower frequency bands (0.1–0.2 and 0.2–0.5 kHz).

Data from Keefe and Simmons [26] suggested that the absorbance measurements, if they are conducted at peak pressure level, are more sensitive to ME pathologies and complications. Analytically they have reported "comparing tests at a fixed specificity of 0.90, the sensitivities were 0.28 for peak-compensated static acoustic admittance at 226 Hz, 0.72 for ambient-pressure WBT, and 0.94 for the pressurized WBT. Pressurized WBT was accurate at predicting conductive hearing loss with an area under the receiver operating characteristic curve of 0.95."

3. Clinical applications

3.1. Otosclerosis

Otosclerosis is a disease that affects the ME and causes progressive hearing loss, occurring predominantly in women (predominant age range 20–30 years). In most cases, the disease manifests bilaterally through calcification and an abnormal growth of the Stapes. In patients with otosclerosis, the absorbance measures can identify an eardrum-ossicular system rigidity with more details. During the progression of the disease, the fixation of the stapes in the oval window worsens, making the ME transmission of energy very difficult [17, 27].

WBT provides more detailed and specific information on the eardrum-ossicular system and allows a differential diagnosis of otosclerosis. According to the data from Shahnaz et al. [18], the most prominent change in the absorbance pattern following an otosclerosis surgery is a sharp and deep drop in absorbance values in the range between 700 and 1000 Hz. There is also a secondary wider and smaller increase in absorbance, following the surgery, between 2000 and 4000 Hz. **Figure 4** shows a typical absorbance profile of an otosclerosis patient. The peak absorbance value has been shifted to higher frequencies, approximately at 2.8 kHz.

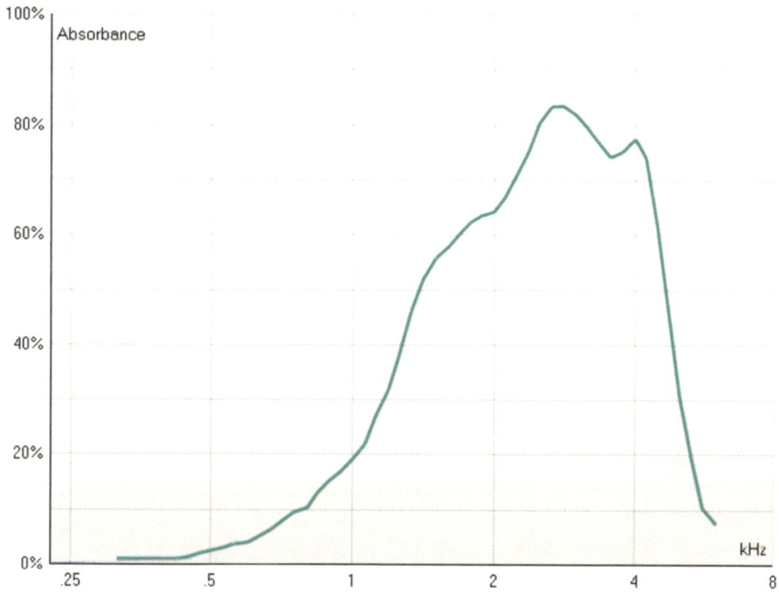

Figure 4. The characteristics of the absorbance graph (which is obtained by collapsing the pressure axis in the 3D-WBT graph) of the case of a patient presenting otosclerosis.

3.2. Immittance in neonates

Growth and thus changes in auditory canal occur rapidly in the first 6 months of life when they reach adult size. Among the possible outcomes in neonatal hearing screening program, there are false positives that may result from differences in the development of ear structures that harm the impedance mechanism [23, 28]. Due to the presence of amniotic fluid, meconium mesenchyme or the external auditory canal may cause temporary changes in hearing. These alterations increase the mass, stiffness, and resistance of the eardrum-ossicular system and consequently alter the middle ear of impedance and efficient sound of conduction [29, 30].

At birth, the neonatal external and middle ear are not fully developed. The external auditory canal is surrounded by a thin layer of elastic cartilage [31]. When performing the pressurization, as occurs in typical tympanometry, the diameter of the external auditory canal can increase or decrease depending on the applied pressure. As the infant grows, the ossification of the external canal increases its rigidity. It also increases the length of the canal, which decreases the canal's resonance frequency [23]. The eardrum will eventually decrease in thickness, will increase in size, and will modify its inclination. Changes occur in the ME as well. Data from Proctor [32] and Holborow [33] show that the neonatal Eustachian tube is shorter [30 mm], and almost horizontal [32]. The Eustachian tube opens effectively but closes more slowly, resulting in tubal inefficiency. The Eustachian tube develops slowly reaching full maturity at the age of 7 years with increased length and steepening. This may explain higher prevalence of otitis media associated with upper respiratory tract infections in early childhood [33, 34].

A number of studies have shown [23, 28, 35] that the majority of the significant modification to the values of wideband absorbance occurs is the first 6 months of life, due to the development of the external and middle ear. During this period, there is an "absorbance immaturity" at low frequencies and an absorbance significant increase in the high frequencies. After this period, the absorbance measurements start to approach the absorbance values reported from adult subjects. **Figure 5** shows a typical neonatal average absorbance (0.8–2.0 kHz) curve, from an infant who has passed the neonatal screening TEOAE test.

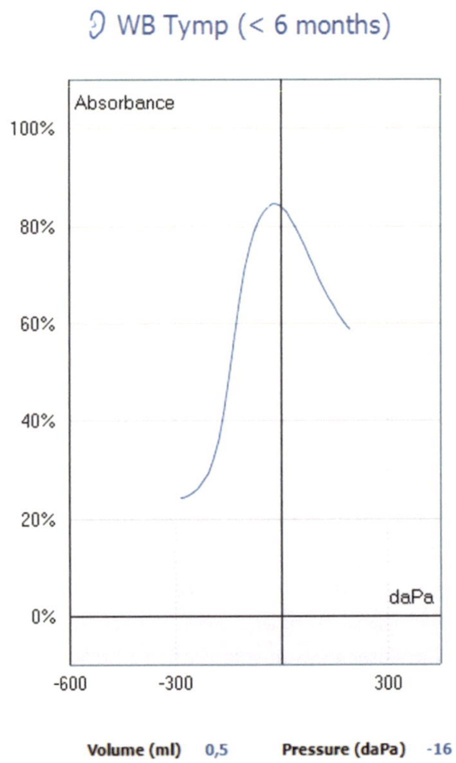

Figure 5. Example of wideband averaged tympanogram in a neonate with a normal function ME and a PASS from the TEOAE assessment.

http://dx.doi.org/10.5772/67155

Because of the difference in the size of the ear canal, between an adult and a neonate, the absorbance measurements between these populations differ considerably. In the neonates, absorbance shows low values at the low frequencies and then a decrease approximately at the frequency of 6.0 kHz [36–38]. The latter also depends on the stimulus bandwidth. Some commercial systems like the Titan from Interacoustics use a stimulus bandwidth of 8 kHz.

Many references in the literature, i.e., [36–38], use and report reflectance values in their WBI assessment. **Figure 6(A)** and **(B)** shows normative neonatal data from reflectance and absorbance curves (10–95 percentiles). The reader can see that the reflectance curve can be deduced from the inverse of the absorbance curve.

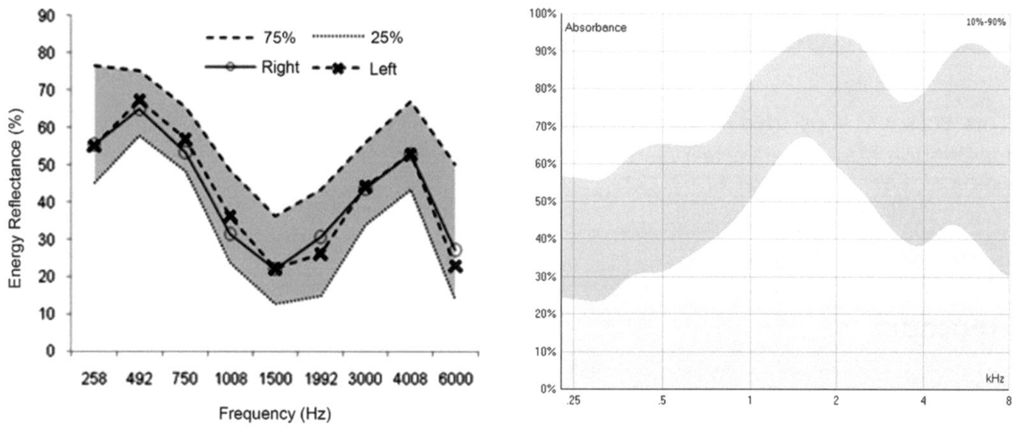

(A) (B)

Figure 6. (A) This graph shows the normal Reflectance zone (25–75 percentiles) for neonatal WBT responses, as reported by Silva et al. [37]. The reflectance curve shows low averaged values (<25%) at the mid frequencies 1.0–2.0 kHz. Two peaks are shown, one at approximately 0.5 kHz (65%) and the other at 5.0 kHz (55%). Due to the fact that different systems were used for the generation of (A) and (B), the data in (A) are not perfectly inverse of the data of (B). (B) This graph shows the normal absorbance zone (10–90 percentiles) for neonatal WBT responses, in the Titan device. The absorbance curve shows low values (<50%) at frequencies <1.0 kHz and above 6.0 kHz. Two absorbance peaks are shown one at approximately 2.8 kHz (85%) and 5.0 kHz (82%).

4. Consensus on the terminology and research objectives

During the 2012, Eriksholm Workshop [39] sponsored by the Oticon Foundation (November 5–7, 2012), an array of consensus statements was developed, regarding the emerging field of wideband immittance measurements. These are summarized below:

(1) The term wideband acoustic immittance (WAI) describes all measurements referring to impedance or power-based variables as the power reflectance.

(2) The term transmittance, which has been defined as (1 minus power reflectance), should be used any more. It should be substituted by the term absorbance, defined as (1 minus power reflectance).

(3) The term aural acoustic immittance was chosen to describe measures of impedance and admittance in the current American National Standards Institute standard for devices to measure aural acoustic immittance (American National Standards Institute S3.39-1987-R2012).

(4) Future publications or datasets should mention: population means, population variance, effect size, and sensitivity and specificity for detecting pathologies. The frequency resolution of measurements should be specified in all research reports.

(5) The WAI data should be interpreted in light of the patient history, the physical examination, and other auditory tests.

Acknowledgements

This work was supported by the project "Integrated system of tools for diagnostics and telerehabilitation of sensory organs disorders (hearing, vision, speech, balance, taste, smell)" acr. INNOSNESE, cofinanced by the National Centre for Research and Development (Poland), within the STRATEGMED program.

Appendix

Readers have the possibility to see how the Titan data (**Figure 3A** and **B**) can be manipulated in 3D, in order to observe other aspects of the 3D-WBT graph, collapsing one axis in order to see the absorbance at a particular stimulus frequency. The corresponding videos can be downloaded from the OAE Portal at the address:

http://www.otoemissions.org/index.php/en/?option=com_content&view=article&id=261

Glossary of terms

- *Acoustic absorbance* (A): The amount of acoustic energy absorbed by the ossicular chain, during the stimulus propagation. It is defined as the ratio of (absorbed sound power)/to (incident sound power) or as (1 – Reflectance^2).
- *Acoustic admittance* $Y(\omega)$: The inverse of Impedance (i.e., the facility of propagation in a medium). It is also a complex variable and stimulus frequency dependent.
- Acoustic immittance: Measurement of the sound energy flow in a medium. The immittance can be either in terms of acoustic impedance (resistance) or acoustic admittance (easiness).
- *Acoustic impedance* $Z(\omega)$: "Resistance" that a sound stimulus experiences while passing through various media. It is a complex variable and stimulus frequency dependent.
- *Acoustic reflectance*: The acoustic energy, reflected backwards, when an acoustic stimulus propagates forward in a medium (i.e., through the ossiculare chain). It is defined as (1-A).

http://dx.doi.org/10.5772/67155

- *Aural acoustic immittance*: Term chosen to describe measures of impedance and admittance in the current American National Standards Institute standard for devices to measure aural acoustic immittance.
- *ME*: Middle ear.
- *MEPA*: Middle Ear Power Analysis, a term which has been coined for the Mimosa Acoustic family of devices offering acoustic immittance measurements.
- *NICU*: Neonatal Intensive Care Unit.
- *Optimal power transference*: The term is used to indicate that the sound stimulus from the stapes enters (i.e., propagates) the inner ear structures with very little energy losses.
- *Otoacoustic emissions* (*OAEs*): Responses elicited from the inner ear, after its stimulation with a transient or continuous stimulus. TEOAEs are evoked by acoustic click stimuli and they are the most used protocol in Neonatal Hearing Screening (NHS). DPOAEs are evoked by two frequency tones, having a specific frequency ratio between them.
- *Static immittance*: Measurement of acoustic immittance at ambient (i.e., normal pressure conditions).
- *WAI*: Wideband acoustic immitance, according to a consensus in 2012 [39] this is the proper term to use. The term WBT (see below) belongs to the family of measurements under WAI.
- *WBT*: Wideband tympanometry.

Author details

Thais Antonelli Diniz Hein[1], Stavros Hatzopoulos[2]*, Piotr Henryk Skarzynski[3, 4, 5] and Maria Francisca Colella-Santos[1]

*Address all correspondence to: sdh1@unife.it

1 Child and Adolescent Heath Program, Faculty of Medical Sciences, State University of Campinas, Campinas, São Paulo, Brazil

2 Audiology & ENT clinic, University of Ferrara, Ferrara, Italy

3 World Hearing Center, Warsaw, Poland

4 Department of Heart Failure and Cardiac Rehabilitation, Medical University of Warsaw, Warsaw, Poland

5 Institute of Sensory Organs, Kajetany, Poland

References

[1] Shanks JE, Lilly DJ. An evaluation of tympanometric estimates of ear canal volume. J Speech Hear Res. 1981;24(4):557–66.

[2] Durrant JD, Lovrinic JH. Bases of Hearing Science. 3rd Edition. Williams & Wilikins, Baltimore; 1995.

[3] Tharpe AM, Seewald R. The Comprehensive Handbook of Pediatric Audiology. 2nd Edition. Plural Publishing; San Diego; 2011.

[4] Block MG, Wiley TL. Overview and basic principles of Acoustic Immitance measurements. Handbook of Clinical Audiology. 4th Edition. Baltimore: Williams & Wilkins; 1994.

[5] James W Hall III and David Chandler. Tympanometry in Clinical Audiology. In: Katz J, Gabbay WL, editors. Handbook of clinical audiology. 4th ed. Baltimore: Williams & Wilkins; 1994:283–99.

[6] Alaerts J, Luts H, Wouters J. Evaluation of middle ear function in young children: clinical guidelines for the use of 226- and 1,000-Hz tympanometry. Otol Neurotol. 2007;28(6):727–32.

[7] Hunter LL, Margolis RH. Multifrequency tympanometry: current clinical application. Am J Audiol. 1992;1(3):33–43.

[8] Tazinazzio TG, Diniz TA, Marba STM, Colella-Santos MF. Otoacoustic emissions and measurements of acoustic immitance with probe tones of 226 and 1000 Hz in infants (text in Portuguese). Rev CEFAC. 2011:479–88.

[9] Li M, Zheng Y, Li G, Wang K. Investigation of tympanogram in newborns with 226 hz and 1000 hz probe tones. Lin Chung Er Bi Yan Hou Tou Jing Wai Ke Za Zhi. 2012;26(22):1009–13.

[10] Baldwin M. Choice of probe tone and classification of trace patterns in tympanometry undertaken in early infancy. Int J Audiol. 2006;45(7):417–27.

[11] Campos UEP, Hatzopoulos S, Śliwa LK, Skarżyński PH, Jędrzejczak WW, Skarżyński H, et al. Relationship between distortion product—otoacoustic emissions (DPOAEs) and high-frequency acoustic immittance measures. Med Sci Monit. 2016;22:2028–34.

[12] Ratynska J, Grzanka A, Mueller-Malesinska M, Skarzynski H, Hatzopoulos S. Correlations between risk factors for hearing impairment and TEOAE screening test outcome in neonates at risk for hearing loss. Scand Audiol. 2001;30:15–7.

[13] Hatzopoulos S, Tsakanikos M, Grzanka A, Ratynska J, Martini A. Comparison of neonatal transient evoked otoacoustic emission responses recorded with linear and QuickScreen protocols. Audiology. 2000;39(2):70–9.

[14] Zimatore G, Hatzopoulos S, Giuliani A, Martini A, Colosimo A. Comparison of transient otoacoustic emission responses from neonatal and adult ears. J Appl Physiol (1985). 2002;92(6):2521–8.

[15] Koike KJ, Wetmore SJ. Interactive effects of the middle ear pathology and the associated hearing loss on transient-evoked otoacoustic emission measures. Otolaryngol Head Neck Surg. 1999;121(3):238–44.

[16] Prieve BA, Vander Werff KR, Preston JL, Georgantas L. Identification of conductive hearing loss in young infants using tympanometry and wideband reflectance. Ear Hear. 2013;34(2):168–78.

[17] Frade C, Lechuga R, Castro C, Labella T. Analysis of the resonant frequency of the middle ear in otosclerosis. Acta Otorrinolaringol Esp. 2000;51(4):309–13.

[18] Shahnaz N, Longridge N, Bell D. Wideband energy reflectance patterns in preoperative and post-operative otosclerotic ears. Int J Audiol. 2009;48(5):240–7.

[19] Feeney MP, Grant IL, Mills DM. Wideband energy reflectance measurements of ossicular chain discontinuity and repair in human temporal bone. Ear Hear. 2009;30(4):391–400.

[20] Aithal S, Kei J, Driscoll C, Khan A, Swanston A. Wideband absorbance outcomes in newborns: a comparison with high-frequency tympanometry, automated brainstem response, and transient evoked and distortion product otoacoustic emissions. Ear Hearing. 2015;36(5):e237–50.

[21] Mazlan R, Kei J, Ya CL, Yusof WN, Saim L, Zhao F. Age and gender effects on wideband absorbance in adults with normal outer and middle ear function. J Speech Lang Hear Res. 2015;58(4):1377–86.

[22] Stinson MR. Revision of estimates of acoustic energy reflectance at the human eardrum. J Acoust Soc Am. 1990;88(4):1773–8.

[23] Kei J, Sanford CA, Prieve BA, Hunter LL. Wideband acoustic immittance measures: developmental characteristics (0 to 12 Months). Ear Hearing. 2013;34:S17–26.

[24] Hunter LL, Keefe DH, Feeney MP, Fitzpatrick DF, Lin L. Longitudinal development ofwideband reflectance tympanometry in normal and at-risk infants. Hear Res 2016; 340:3–14.

[25] Groon KA, Rasetshwane DM, Kopun JG, Gorga MP, Neely ST. Air-leak effects on ear-canal acoustic absorbance. Ear Hearing. 2015;36(1):155–63.

[26] Keefe DH, Simmons JL. Energy transmittance predicts conductive hearing loss in older children and adults. J Acoust Soc Am. 2003;114(6 Pt 1):3217–38.

[27] Shahnaz N, Polka L. Standard and multifrequency tympanometry in normal and otosclerotic ears. Ear Hear. 1997;18(4):326–41.

[28] Aithal S, Kei J, Driscoll C. Wideband absorbance in young infants (0-6 months): a cross-sectional study. J Am Acad Audiol. 2014;25(5):471–81.

[29] Jaisinghani VJ, Paparella MM, Schachern PA, Schneider DS, Le CT. Residual mesenchyme persisting into adulthood. Am J Otolaryngol. 1999;20(6):363–70.

[30] Miura T, Suzuki C, Otani I, Omori K. Marrow-tympanum connections in fetuses and infants. Nihon Jibiinkoka Gakkai Kaiho. 2008;111(1):14–20.

[31] McLellan MS, Webb CH. Ear studies in the newborn infant: natural appearance and incidence of obscuring by vernix, cleansing of vernix, and description of drum and canal after cleansing. J Pediatr. 1957;51(6):672–7.

[32] Proctor B. Embryology and anatomy of the Eustachian tube. Arch Otolaryngol. 1967;86(5):503–14.

[33] Holborow C. Eustachian tubal function. Changes in anatomy and function with age and the relationship of these changes to aural pathology. Arch Otolaryngol. 1970;92(6):624–6.

[34] Holborow C. Eustachian tubal function: changes throughout childhood and neuro-muscular control. J Laryngol Otol. 1975;89(1):47–55.

[35] Aithal V, Kei J, Driscoll C, Swanston A, Roberts K, Murakoshi M, et al. Normative sweep frequency impedance measures in healthy neonates. J Am Acad Audiol. 2014;25(4):343–54.

[36] Hunter LL, Feeney MP, Lapsley Miller JA, Jeng PS, Bohning S. Wideband reflectance in newborns: normative regions and relationship to hearing-screening results. Ear Hear. 2010;31(5):599–610.

[37] Silva KA, Urosas JG, Sanches SG, Carvallo RM. Wideband reflectance in newborns with present transient-evoked otoacoustic emissions. Codas. 2013;25(1):29–33.

[38] Santos PPD, Araújo ES, Costa Filho OA, Piza MDT, Alvarenga KDF. Wideband acoustic immittance measures using chirp and pure tone stimuli in infants with middle ear integrity. Medidas de imitância acústica de banda larga com estímulo chirp e tom puro em lactentes com normalidade de orelha média. Audiol Commun Res. 2015;20(4):300–4.

[39] Feeney MP, Hunter LL, Kei J, Lilly DJ, Margolis RH, Nakajima HH, et al. Consensus statement: Eriksholm workshop on wideband absorbance measures of the middle ear. Ear Hear. 2013;34 Suppl 1:78S–9S.

Chapter 4

Suppression of Otoacoustic Emissions Evoked by White Noise and Speech Stimuli

Kelly C.L. Andrade, Gabriella O. Peixoto,
Aline T.L. Carnaúba, Klinger V.T. Costa and
Pedro L. Menezes

Additional information is available at the end of the chapter

http://dx.doi.org/10.5772/66700

Abstract

Introduction: Suppressing otoacoustic emissions is one of the objectives, noninvasive methods that can be used to assess the efferent auditory system. When the ascending reticular activating system is stimulated, the cortex becomes more alert. The system reacts better to an important stimulus than an unimportant one.

Objective: Assess the effect of suppressing otoacoustic emissions by transitory stimulus in the presence of different auditory stimuli in normal listeners.

Methods: This cross-sectional, observational analytical study. The sample was composed of eight participants. The following procedures were adopted: recording otoacoustic emissions, suppression with white noise, suppression with white noise and pure tone, auditory training, new recording of suppression with white noise and pure tone, suppression using a speech pattern, suppression using a reversed speech pattern, suppression using familiar speech, and suppression using reversed familiar speech and suppression singing "happy birthday" in a familiar voice.

Results: There was a significant difference between the otoacoustic emission values, mainly at frequencies of 1000 and 1500 Hz.

Conclusion: Individuals submitted to the effects of suppression exhibit more effective results at frequencies of 1000 and 1500 Hz. Furthermore, it was found that the efferent activity of the auditory system is more efficient when it involves the use of the speech spectrum.

Keywords: audiology, suppression, efferent pathways, noise, speech perception

1. Introduction

Noise is defined as an undesirable sound, characterized by multiple amplitudes and frequencies that occur simultaneously in a nonharmonic fashion. It is increasingly common in several environments and often not considered harmful to hearing, but interferes directly in word comprehension and communication.

Speech recognition occurs in conjunction with acoustic, linguistic, semantic, and circumstantial cues. However, under favorable conditions, some of these cues may be disregarded. For the message to be transmitted efficiently, acoustic cues vary according to the situation and context of communication, such as in conversation and noisy environments [1, 2].

Speech comprehension is an important point to observe during audiological assessment, since it provides data on how individuals understand a spoken message in daily situations [3], which are generally associated with the presence of competitive noise. When presented with speech and competitive noise at the same time, even normal listeners often have greater difficulty hearing and understanding it [4]. These difficulties arise because several auditory channels are required to obtain speech recognition during the assessment process with noise, suggesting that more detailed sensory information is necessary in difficult-to-hear situations [5].

Assessment of speech perception is important in establishing the relationship between hearing ranges, using information obtained from audiological diagnostic procedures, and hearing performance, which is related to how the individual is developing functionally. For good speech perception, joint action of the auditory system is required. This involves the outer, middle, and inner ear, cranial nerve VIII, the retrocochlear portion, and the central nervous system [6].

During audiological assessment, speech comprehension difficulties can only really be observed with speech stimuli that represent a communicative situation [7], thereby providing important information on the capacity of the individual to recognize words in noisy environments [3, 8].

The conventional tests used to assess language comprehension are a microscopic view of auditory function [2, 9], and speech recognition evaluation in the presence of noise would be a more realistic way of assessing hearing [10, 11].

Otoacoustic emission (OAE) testing is a relatively simple, fast and noninvasive objective method. OAEs are defined as the release of sound energy from the inner ear when the cochlea is stimulated, reaching the external auditory canal. Sound waves are captured by a small probe introduced into this canal.

Their discovery contributed substantially to the creation of a new concept regarding the function of the cochlea, demonstrating that they are able not only to receive sounds, but also to produce acoustic energy [12]. This phenomenon is related to cochlear micromechanics, and it is suggested that when OAEs are generated in the cochlea, there is a mechanically active component coupled to the basilar membrane through which the reverse process of sound energy transduction occurs [13]. This property has recently been attributed to outer hair cells (OHC) and is controlled by efferent auditory pathways.

Suppression is characterized by a decrease in both the amplitude and peak phase of the emission. Test-retest comparison shows that the suppressive effects are repetitive and that suppressing OAEs is clinically useful in assessing and managing peripheral and central hearing loss [14].

Medial efferent fibers may inhibit this active contractile component of OHC, regulating low contractions with attenuation of rapid contractions, thereby decreasing the amplitude of OAEs, when they are affected by electrical, chemical, or noise stimulation [15].

The frequent complaints of speech recognition difficulties, primarily in noisy environments, even in those considered normal listeners from the quantitative standpoint, as well as discoveries of the active role of the cochlea, specifically OHC, are sufficient to prompt the investigation of new methods that can be used to help stimulate the structures responsible for speech recognition in situations of competitive noise.

2. Otoacoustic emissions, suppression and auditory pathways

Auditory perception occurs in three stages: a physical stimulus; a set of events through which a stimulus is transduced into a message of nerve impulses and a response to the message, frequently as perception or internal representation of sensations [16].

Sound is perceived through pressure waves, where this physical stimulus is transformed into an electrochemical stimulus, making it possible to convert auditory information into meaning. Part of our ability to make all this coherent owes to the fact that we develop models of what we expect to hear: phonemes, words, music, etc. [17].

Otoacoustic emissions (OAEs) are sounds created within the cochlea, spontaneously or as a response to acoustic stimulation [18]. OAE tests are used as an objective, noninvasive assessment of the first stages of sound processing, at the biomechanical activity level of the OHC [19, 20].

The olivocochlear bundle, the best known circuit in the efferent system, includes the medial and lateral tracts [21]. The lateral tract is composed of nonmyelinated fibers that terminate at the inner hair cells (IHC), located in the cochlea; and the medial tract consists of myelinated fibers that originate in the area around the medial superior olive connected to the OHC.

Although the role of the olivocochlear bundle in hearing performance has not been fully explained, some functions have been attributed to the medial efferent system: location of the sound source, auditory attention, improved hearing sensitivity, enhanced acoustic signal detection in the presence of noise, and a protective function [22]. Moreover, stimulating the efferent olivocochlear bundle decreases the neural response of the cochlea and auditory nerve [23].

Objective noninvasive methods can be used to assess the efferent auditory system, such as OAE suppression and obtaining an acoustic reflex [24]. OAE suppression occurs when noise is applied contralaterally, ipsilaterally, or bilaterally to the examined ear, assessing the activity of the medial olivocochlear efferent system [25].

Attenuating OAE responses in the presence of contralateral, ipsilateral, or binaural noise occur due to the action of medial olivocochlear tract fibers, via synapses in the ECC [26]. Competitive noise has an inhibitory effect on the functioning of the ECC of the cochlea, resulting in decreased OAE levels. The presence of this effect, called OAE suppression, in normal listeners shows the involvement of the medial olivocochlear system in the suppression of emissions [27, 28] and is not related to the presence of artifacts, interaural attenuation, or the effect of the middle ear [27].

Studies demonstrate a relationship between the population with speech recognition difficulties in noisy environments and the action of the medial olivocochlear efferent system. It has also been reported that this population exhibits less or no OAE suppression, suggesting a decline in the inhibitory effect of the efferent system [29, 30].

The cerebral cortex can exert a direct or indirect effect on sound processing, primarily via the superior olivary complex, thereby contributing to central auditory skills, such as speech recognition in noise [31].

With respect to the study of acoustic reflex, a number of investigations have found that the acoustic reflex threshold, captured at between 70 and 90 dB SL, can be reduced by a high-frequency facilitating stimulus presented before or simultaneously to a pure-tone activator of the reflex, characterizing a sensitization process [32]. This process is similar to the effect of OAE suppression, given that a suppressor stimulus reduces the range of responses.

Electrical stimulus of the olivocochlear efferent tract is capable of attenuating afferent auditory activity in the cochlea. Some efferent fibers exert spontaneous activity while others enter into activity after sound stimulation, suggesting a feedback system. This mechanism suggests that the olivocochlear efferent pathway plays an important role in discriminating messages in the presence of competitive noise [23].

2.1. Speech discrimination in noise X familiar speech

Although the ability to understand speech in noise is one of the functions attributed to the efferent auditory system, other anatomic structures are also involved, such as reticular formation. Evidence suggests that when the ascending reticular activating system is stimulated, the cortex becomes more alert and attentive. Thus, the system reacts better to an important stimulus than a nonimportant one. This may be one of the mechanisms involved in selective attention and the ability to hear in the presence of noise [33].

Studies describe the central auditory pathway as a flexible processing structure in which the descending feedback pathways play an important short- and long-term role in adaptive plasticity. These findings confirm the relationship between the efferent auditory system and auditory training in the presence of speech in noise [34].

Efferent auditory system activity, in terms of the medial olivocochlear system, has been implicated in the perception of speech in noise, in both children [35] and adults [36]. Therefore, it is necessary to investigate whether this system also plays a role in a training-induced improvement of speech perception in noise.

According to a cognitive model of voice perception in the analysis of the primary auditory cortex, vocal information is processed in three pathways that partially interact: (1) discourse analysis, preferentially in the left hemisphere, (2) vocal analysis of affective information, predominantly in the right hemisphere, (3) vocal identity analysis, involving voice recognition and semantic knowledge related to the individual, also predominant in the right hemisphere [37]. From this standpoint, different levels of cognition and awareness contribute to the analysis of auditory stimulus.

For familiar voice stimuli, there is strong desynchronization in the right hemisphere [38]. In line with this viewpoint, the study demonstrated that because of their biographic and emotional relevance, familiar voices are able to increase the level of cortical responses.

2.2. New findings

In order to assess the effect of transient evoked otoacoustic emission (TEOAE) suppression in normal listeners in the presence of different suppressor stimuli, a pilot study was conducted assessing eight individuals with no auditory complaints: five women (62.5%) and three men (37.5%), aged between 22 and 26 years (mean = 24.12). A total of 16 ears were analyzed [39].

TEOAEs were measured by an ILO apparatus, whereas suppressor stimuli, pure tones, and speech stimuli were emitted by a duly calibrated AC 40 audiometer. All the measurements were made three consecutive times, in order to calculate the average of the three, thereby increasing the reliability of the results.

TEOAEs were initially measured bilaterally. TEOAE suppression measures were recorded using white noise as a suppressor stimulus with an intensity of 60 dB above the speech recognition threshold (SRT) of the individual. The same measurement was taken, using a pure tone modulated at a frequency of 1000 Hz at 65 dB in the ear contralateral to the suppressor noise. Auditory training, consisting of three stages, was then conducted, as follows:

1. Presentation of stimuli emitted at a fixed intensity of 50 dB SL, at 500 and 1000 Hz and 1000 and 4000 Hz, without the presence of noise, with the aim of instructing the participant on identifying the reference stimulus at a frequency of 1000 Hz. The participant was asked to state whether the stimuli were equal or different.
2. Presentation of the same pairs of stimuli, at a fixed intensity of 60 dB SL, in the presence of white noise at an intensity of 30 above the SRT. The participant stated whether the stimuli were equal or different.
3. The stimulus at a frequency of 1000 Hz was randomly presented three times in a short period of time, at a fixed intensity of 75 dB SL, in the presence of white noise at an intensity of 55 dB SL. The participants were instructed to identify each stimulus by raising their hand.

After auditory training, three measurements were taken to determine the effect of suppression using white noise at 60 dB above the SRT simultaneously to present the pure tone at 65 dB also in the contralateral ear, in order to analyze the amplitude of TEOAEs with a pure tone stimulus at 1000 Hz after training.

The effect of suppression was measured in the presence of balanced sentences from the HINT protocol, emitted by standard speech as suppressor noise. The effect of suppression was then measured in the presence of reverse sentences from the HINT protocol as suppressor noise.

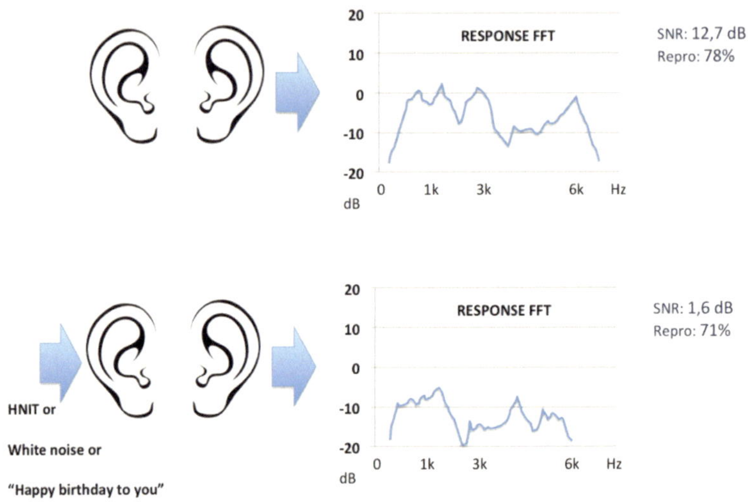

Figure 1. The effect of suppressing TEOAEs using 1 kHz stimuli (above) and using speech as suppressor noise (below).

The effect of suppression was measured in the presence of white noise and the same balanced sentence from the HINT protocol was presented using speech familiar to the subject. The sentence was presented orally by the subject's mother or sister using an AC 40 audiometer. The same occurred with the ensuing measurements, where the reverse sentence from the HINT protocol was presented using familiar speech.

Finally, the effect of suppressing TEOAEs was measured, using the "Happy Birthday" song emitted, using familiar speech as suppressor noise, as shown in **Figure 1**. All the speech stimuli as suppressor noise were emitted at an intensity of 60 dB above the speech reception threshold (SRT) of each participant.

TEOE*	Mean (dB)	Standard deviations (dB)	*p*-Values
1000 Hz	12.72	6.84	0.000*
1000 Hz + white noise	0.14	7.49	
1500 Hz	15.30	6.02	0.000*
1500 Hz + white noise	4.50	9.30	
2000 Hz	9.92	5.25	0.392
2000 Hz + white noise	9.04	5.99	
3000 Hz	7.70	6.04	0.468
3000 Hz + white noise	7.31	6.23	
4000 Hz	6.82	5.48	0.182
4000 Hz + white noise	6.18	5.51	

*Siginificance.

Table 1. Transient-evoked otoacoustic emissions and the effects of suppressing these emissions in the presence of white noise.

TEOE*	Mean (dB)	Standard deviations (dB)	*P*-values
1000 Hz	12.72	6.84	0.000*
1000 Hz + white noise+ 1000 Hz	-1.07	6.16	
1500 Hz	15.30	6.02	0.000*
1500 Hz + white noise+ 1000 Hz	5.61	5.86	
2000 Hz	9.92	5.25	0.316
2000 Hz + white noise+ 1000 Hz	9.30	5.63	
3000 Hz	7.70	6.04	0.742
3000 Hz + white noise+ 1000 Hz	7.84	6.51	
4000 Hz	6.82	5.48	0.379
4000 Hz + white noise+ 1000 Hz	6.43	5.52	

*Siginificance.

Table 2. Transient evoked otoacoustic emissions and the effects of suppressing these emissions in the presence of white noise and pure tone at a frequency of 1000 Hz before auditory training.

According to the analyses, the *t*-test showed a suppression effect at all the frequencies tested in all the individuals. However, when TEOAEs and suppression values were compared, a statistically significant difference was observed only for frequencies of 1000 and 1500 Hz ($p < 0.01$), as shown in **Table 1**.

Comparison between TEOAEs and the effect of suppression using a pure tone at 1000 Hz shows a statistical significance also for frequencies of 1000 and 1500 Hz ($p < 0.01$), as demonstrated in **Table 2**.

When the mean suppression values were compared using the balanced HINT sentence, the *t*-test showed a statistically significant decline in the amplitude of TEOAEs at frequencies of 1000 and 1500 Hz (**Table 3**).

It was also found that the suppression amplitude, using the normal balanced HINT sentence, was much greater than the mean suppression values using white noise. There was a statistically significant difference for the frequencies of 1000 and 1500 Hz (**Table 4**).

There was also a decrease in the suppressor effect of the "happy birthday" song compared to the normal balanced HINT sentence using standard speech. In this case, a statistically significant difference was observed only at a frequency of 1000 Hz (**Table 5**).

The present study showed that all the statistically significant suppression results occurred at frequencies of 1000 and 1500 Hz. Other studies have demonstrated that the suppression effect occurs at specific frequencies [28, 40]. A study that conducted in adults with normal hearing thresholds and no auditory complaints found that frequencies of 1000–2000 Hz exhibited a greater suppression effect [41]. Another study analyzed the effect of contralateral noise and a complete lesion of the olivocochlear system on the action potentials of the auditory nerve in cats, showing that contralateral noise decreased the action potential of the auditory nerve,

TEOE*	Mean (dB)	Standard deviations (dB)	*P*-values
1000 Hz	12.72	6.84	0.004*
1000 Hz + standard speech_HINT	7.40	6.45	
1500 Hz	15.30	6.02	0.007*
1500 Hz + standard speech_HINT	11.12	6.88	
2000 Hz	9.92	5.25	0.105
2000 Hz + standard speech_HINT	8.06	6.09	
3000 Hz	7.70	6.04	0.824
3000 Hz + standard speech_HINT	7.56	6.14	
4000 Hz	6.82	5.50	0.340
4000 Hz + standard speech_HINT	6.30	5.92	

*Siginificance.

Table 3. Transient evoked otoacoustic emissions compared to the effect of suppressing these emissions in the presence of the normal balanced HINT sentence emitted in standard speech.

TEOE*	Mean (dB)	Standard deviations (dB)	*P*-values
1000 Hz + white noise	0.13	7.48	0.008*
1000 Hz + standard speech_HINT	7.40	6.45	
1500 Hz + white noise	4.50	9.30	0.017*
1500 Hz + standard speech_HINT	11.12	6.88	
2000 Hz + white noise	9.04	5.98	0.278
2000 Hz + standard speech_HINT	8.06	6.09	
3000 Hz + white noise	7.31	6.23	0.542
3000 Hz + standard speech_HINT	7.56	6.14	
4000 Hz + white noise	6.18	5.51	0.815
4000 Hz + standard speech_HINT	6.30	5.92	

*Siginificance.

Table 4. Effect of suppressing otoacoustic emissions by transient stimulus in the presence of white noise compared to suppression using the normal balanced HINT sentence emitted with standard speech as suppressor noise.

and that the section of this system overrides the inhibitory effect of the nerve [42]. In this study, the highest inhibition values were found at frequencies of 1000–2000 Hz. Other studies have confirmed that the suppression effect is more effective at low frequencies, despite the fact that the olivocochlear bundle is thicker in the basal portion of the cochlea [43, 44].

http://dx.doi.org/10.5772/66700

TEOE*	Mean (dB)	Standard deviations (dB)	*P*-values
1000 Hz + standard speech_HINT	7.40	6.45	0.038*
1000 Hz + happy birthday	4.13	7.92	
1500 Hz + standard speech_HINT	11.12	6.88	0.489
1500 Hz + happy birthday	9.87	8.27	
2000 Hz + standard speech_HINT	8.06	6.09	0.579
2000 Hz + happy birthday	7.17	7.22	
3000 Hz + standard speech_HINT	8.14	6.34	0.285
3000 Hz + happy birthday	7.13	6.37	
4000 Hz + standard speech_HINT	6.53	6.11	0.781
4000 Hz + happy birthday	6.65	5.40	

*Siginificance.

Table 5. Effect of suppressing otoacoustic emissions by transient stimulus in the presence of standard speech compared to using the "happy birthday" song as suppressor noise.

The results of stimuli before and after auditory training show no statistically significant differences for the frequencies tested. However, a study that investigated the involvement of the medial olivocochlear system in perceptual learning found a significant improvement in responses and olivocochlear system activity after 5-day auditory training with 16 normal listeners, using a phonemic discrimination task, when compared to a control group [34]. Other studies demonstrated growing evidence that the adult auditory cortex is a dynamic and adaptive processing center. This has been shown in auditory perceptual learning studies, in which long-lasting neuronal changes were observed in the auditory cortex of animals [45, 46] and human beings [47, 48] after intensive auditory training.

Comparison between the suppression effect using white noise and that using a normal-balanced HINT sentence demonstrated that suppression amplitude using the spoken sentence in the contralateral ear was far greater than the mean suppression values using white noise. This finding is possibly explained by the fact that speech demands more attention, albeit unconsciously, from the individual. This corroborates a study conducted with normal listeners, who were asked to detect sounds at a particular frequency in the contralateral ear simultaneous in the presence of background noise [49]. It was concluded that contralateral suppression of OAEs was greater when attention was directed to the contralateral ear. Another study analyzed the suppression effect in adult women in four situations: (1) with no contralateral stimulation; (2) with contralateral stimulation at 60 dB SPL; (3) with contralateral stimulation at 60 dB SPL and words simultaneously emitted in the test ear, and the patient required to recognize the semantic field of these words; and (4), identical to situation (3), without having to recognize the words. The authors observed that the effect of suppression was higher in situations 3 and 4, in which more attention to speech was required, concluding that the cortical structures controlled efferent activity in the auditory system, primarily in situations involving the use of the speech spectrum [50]. A comparison between speech suppression using a standard sentence and the "happy birthday" song revealed that the suppression effect was lower with the song, possibly because it involved automatic predictable speech, given that the song is universally known. In this case, attention to the suppressor stimulus was lower, causing fewer changes in cochlear activity and a smaller reduction in OAEs amplitude. However, to confirm this hypothesis, more research using speech as suppressor stimulus is needed, since we found no studies along these lines. Another study aimed at determining the best conditions to assess the efferent auditory system. The authors assessed 11 adults with normal thresholds, using three suppressor stimuli: clicks, narrow band noise, and pure tones. It was found that the click and pure-tone stimuli were the most and least effective suppressors, respectively [47]. Speech, however, was not considered.

The authors concluded that suppressing TEOAEs in normal listeners is more effective at low frequencies, specifically at 1000–1500 Hz. Moreover, the efferent activity of the auditory system is more efficient when suppression involves a speech stimulus, compared to white noise, which has no significant effect. The efferent auditory system is more alert and attentive to standard speech stimuli, but less efficient when this speech is automatic [39].

2.2.1. Personal experience regarding the present study

The experience of conducting this study was very rewarding and indeed resulted in important findings for a more detailed investigation. For example, a reasonable variability was observed in TEOAE amplitudes, regardless of the presence of a suppressor stimulus using the same testing standards (same ear, same professional, same acoustic environment, etc.). This variability was observed when the tests were repeated. To minimize this problem, the tests were repeated three times and the average computed. However, future studies will involve five repetitions to decrease variability and provide even more consistency. Furthermore, posttraining results were not statistically significant, possibly due to the short duration. Data in the literature suggest the need for more robust training that can guarantee better learning on the test, in order to be able to observe differences [34, 45–48].

3. Final considerations

Given that the ability to recognize speech is one of the most important measurable aspects of auditory function, the tests used in clinical practice are of the utmost importance for audiological diagnosis.

Studies that allow more thorough assessment of individuals with speech comprehension difficulties in noise should be encouraged, since understanding the entire mechanism involved in this dynamic, from sound detection to comprehension, will make it possible to standardize auditory tests and design therapies for specific stimulations.

http://dx.doi.org/10.5772/66700

Glossary

dB—decibels

dB SPL—decibels sound pressure level

dB SL—decibels sensation level. The amount in decibels by which a stimulus exceeds the hearing threshold

OHC—outer hair cells

HINT—hearing in test noise

Hz—Hertz

IHC—inner hair cells

OAEs—otoacoustic emissions

TEOAEs—transient evoked otoacoustic emissions

Author details

Kelly C.L. Andrade[1]*, Gabriella O. Peixoto[1], Aline T.L. Carnaúba[1], Klinger V.T. Costa[2] and Pedro L. Menezes[1, 2]

*Address all correspondence to: kellyclandrade@gmail.com

1 State University of Health Sciences of Alagoas, Maceió, Alagoas, Brazil

2 University Center CESMAC, Maceió, Alagoas, Brazil

References

[1] Gama MR. Speech perception: a qualitative evaluation proposal. 1st ed. São Paulo: Pancast; 1994.

[2] Caporali SA, Silva JA da. Speech recognition in noise: young and old with hearing loss. Rev Bras Otorrinolaringol. 2004;**70**(1):525–32.

[3] Theunissen M, Swanepoel DW, Hanekom J. Sentence recognition in noise: variables in compilation and interpretation of tests. Int J Audiol. 2009;**48**:743–57.

[4] Cóser PL, Costa MJ, Cóser MJS, Fukuda Y. Recognition of sentences in silence and noise in individuals with hearing loss. Rev Bras Otorrinolaringol. 2000;**66**(4):362–70.

[5] Ziegler JC, Catherine P, George F, Lorenzi C. Speech perception in noise deficits in dyslexia. Dev Sci. 2009;**12**(5):732–45.

[6] Danieli F, Bevilacqua MC. Speech recognition in children using cochlear implants using two different speech processors [thesis]. São Paulo: Audiology Communication Research; 2010. 7 p.

[7] Freitas CD, Lopes LF, Costa MJ. Reliability of sentence recognition thresholds in silence and noise. Rev Bras Otorrinolaringol. 2005;**71**(5):624–30.

[8] Grose JH, Mamo SK, Hall JW. Age effects in temporal envelope processing: speech unmasking and auditory steady state responses. Ear Hear. 2009;**30**(5):568–75.

[9] Corrêa GF, Russo ICP. Self-perception of the handicap in adults and elderly hearing impaired. Rev Cefac. 1999;**1**(1):54–63.

[10] Duarte VG. The effect of noise on the perception of speech of young and elderly normal-hearing individuals [thesis]. São Paulo: PontíficaUniversidadeCatólica de São Paulo; 1998.

[11] Pichora-Fuller MK, Souza PE. Effects of aging on auditory processing of speech. Int J Audiol. 2003;**42**(Suppl 2):11–6.

[12] Castor X, Veuillet E, Morgon A, Collet L. Influence of aging on active cochlear micromechanical properties and on the medial olivocochlear system in humans. Hear Res. 1994; 77(1–2):1–8.

[13] Lim DJ. Functional structure of the organ of Corti: a review. Hear Res. 1986;22:117–46.

[14] Hood LJ, Berlin CI, Hurley A, Cecola RP, Bell B. Contralateral suppression of transient-evoked otoacoustic emissions in humans: intensity effects. Hear Res. 1996; 101(1–2):113–8.

[15] Berlin CI, Hood LJ, Wen H, Szabo P, Cecola RP, Rigby P, Jackson DF. Contralateral suppression of non-linear click-evoked otoacoustic emissions. Hear Res. 1993;71(1–2):1–11.

[16] Kandel ER, Schwartz JH, Jessel TM. Fundamentals of Neuroscience and Behavior. Rio de Janeiro: Guanabara Koogan; 1997.

[17] Ratey JJ. How to increase the health, agility and longevity of our brains through the latest scientific discoveries. In: O cérebro - um guia para o usuário. 1st ed. Rio de Janeiro: Objetiva; 2002.

[18] Norton SJ, Stover LJ. Otoacoustic emissions: an emerging tool. In: Katz J (Ed.). Handbook of clinical audiology. 4th ed. Baltimore: William and Williams; 1994.

[19] Lonsbury-Martin BL, Martin GK, Mccoy MJ, Whitehead ML. New approaches to the evaluation of the auditory system and a current analysis of otoacoustic emissions. Otolaryngol Neck Surg. 1995;**112**(1):50–63.

[20] Campos U de P, Sanches SG, Hatzopoulos S, Carvalho RMM, Kochanek K, Skarzynski H. Alteration of distortion product otoacoustic emission input-output functions in subjects with a previous history of middle ear dysfunction. Med Sci. 2012;**18**(4):27–31.

[21] Warr WB. Efferent components of the auditory system. Ann Otorhinolaryngol. 1980;**89** (5 Pt 2):114–20.

[22] Bruel MLF, Sanches TG, Bento R. Efferent auditory pathways and their role in the auditory system. ArqOtorrinolaringol. 2001;**5**(2):62–7.

[23] Galambos R. Suppression of auditory nerve activity by stimulation of efferent fibers to cochlea. J Neurophysiol. 1955;**19**(5):424–37.

[24] Burguetti FAR. Suppression of otoacoustic emissions and sensitization of acoustic reflex in auditory processing disorders [thesis]. Universidade de São Paulo; 2006.

[25] Grataloup C, Hoen M, Veuillet E, Collet L, Pellegrino F, Meunier F. Speech restoration: an interactive process. J Speech Lang Hear Res. 2009;**52**(4):827–38.

[26] Guinan JJ, Backus BC, Lilaonitkul W, Aharonson V. Medial olivocochlear efferent reflex in humans: otoacoustic emission (OAE) measurement issues and the advantages of stimulus frequency OAEs. J Assoc Res Otoralyngol. 2003;**4**(4):521–40.

[27] Collet L, Kemp DT,Veuillet E, Duclaux R, Moulin A, Morgon A. Effect of contralateral auditory stimuli on active cochlear micromechanical properties in human subjects. Hear Res. 1990;**43**(2–3):251–61.

[28] Veuillet E, Collet L, Duclaux R. Effect of contralateral acoustic stimulation on active cochlear micromechanical properties in humans subjects: dependence on stimulus variables. J Neurophysiol. 1991;**65**(3):724–35.

[29] Muchnika C, Roth DAE, Othman-Jebara R, Putter-Katz H, Shabtai EL, Hildesheimer M. Reduced medial olivocochlear bundle system function in children whit auditory processing disorders. AudiolNeuro-Otology. 2004;**9**(2):107–14.

[30] Sanches SGG, Carvalho RM. Contralateral suppression of transient evoked otoacoustic emissions in children whit auditory processing disorder. Audiol Neurotol. 2006;**11**(6):366–72.

[31] Khalfa S, Bougeard R, Morand N, Veuillet E, Isnard J, Guenot M, et al. Evidence of peripheral auditory activity modulation by the auditory cortex in humans. Neuroscience. 2001;**104**(2):347–58.

[32] Kumar A, Barman A. Effect of efferent-induced changes on acoustical reflex. J Audiol. 2002;**41**(2):144–7.

[33] Musiek FE, Oxholm VB. Anatomy and physiology of the central auditory nervous system: a clinical perspective. In: Audiology: diagnosis. New York: Thieme Medical Publishers; 2000. pp. 47–71.

[34] Boer J de, Thornton ARD. Neural correlates of perceptual learning in the auditory brainstem: efferent activity predicts and reflects improvement at a speech-in-noise discrimination task. J Neurosci. 2008;**28**(19):4929–37.

[35] Kumar UA, Vanaja CS. Functioning of olivocochlear bundle and speech perception in noise. Ear Hear. 2004;**25**(2):142–6.

[36] Giraud AL, Garnier S, Micheyl C, Lina G, Chays A, Chéry-Croze S. Auditory efferents involved in speech-in-noise intelligibility. Neuroreport. 1997;**8**(7):1779–83.

[37] Samson F, Zeffiro TA, Toussaint A, Belin P. Stimulus complexity and categorical effects in human auditory cortex: an activation likelihood estimation meta-analysis. Front Psychol. 2011;**JAN**(1):241.

[38] Giudice R, Lechinger J, Wislowska M, Heib DPJ, Hoedlmoser K, Schabus M. Oscillatory brain responses to own names uttered by unfamiliar and familiar voices. Brain Res. 2014;**DEC 3**(1591):63–73.

[39] Peixoto GO, Menezes PL, Oliveira MFF, Andrade KCL. The effect of suppression of otoacoustic emissions in the presence of pure tone stimuli before and after auditory training and speech stimuli. In: Boechat E et al. International Meeting of Audiology; São Paulo; 2016. p. 3630.

[40] Collet L, Moulin A, Morlet T, Giraud AL, Micheyl C, Chery-Croze S. Contralateral auditory stimulation and otoacoustic emissions: a review of basic data in humans. Br J Audiol. 1994;**28**:213–8.

[41] Lautenschlager L, Tochetto T, Costa MJ. Reconhecimento de fala em presença de ruído e suas relações com a supressão das emissões otoacústicas e o reflexo acústico. Brazilian J Otorhinolaryngol. 2011;**77**(1):115–20.

[42] Warren EH, Liberman MC. Effects os contralateral sound on auditory-nerve responses. I. Contributions of cochlear efferents. Hear Res. 1989;**37**(2):89–104.

[43] Gorga MP, Neely ST, Dorn PA, Konrad-Martin D. The use of distortion product otoacoustic emission suppression as an estimate of response growth. J AcoustSoc Am. 2002;**111**(1):271–84.

[44] Gorga MP, Neely ST, Dierking DM, Kopun J, Jolkowski K, Groenenboom K, et al. Low-frequency and high-frequency distortion product otoacoustic emission suppression in humans. J Acoust Soc Am. 2008;**123**(4):2172–90.

[45] Bao S, Chang EF, Woods J, Merzenich MM. Temporal plasticity in the primary auditory cortex induced by operant perceptual learning. Nat Neurosci. 2004;**7**(9):974–81.

[46] Polley DB, Steinberg EE, Merzenich MM. Perceptual learning directs auditory cortical map reorganization through top-down influences. J Neurosci. 2006;**26**(18):4970–82.

[47] Alain C, Snyder JS, He Y, Reinke KS. Changes in auditory cortex parallel rapid perceptual learning. Cereb Cortex. 2007;**17**(5):1074–84.

[48] Wassenhove V Van, Nagarajan SS. Auditory cortical plasticity in learning to discriminate modulation rate. J Neurosci. 2007;**27**(10):2663–72.

[49] Maison S, Micheyl C, Collet L. Influence of focused auditory attention on cochlear activity in humans. Psychophysiology. 2001;**38**(1):35–40.

[50] Garinis AC, Glattke T, Cone BK. The MOC reflex during active listening to speech. J Speech Lang Hear Res. 2011;**54**(5):1464–76.

Section 3

Advances in Cochlear modeling

Chapter 5

Power Amplification and Frequency Selectivity in the Inner Ear: A New Physical Model

Piotr Kiełczyński

Additional information is available at the end of the chapter

http://dx.doi.org/10.5772/66542

Abstract

This Chapter presents a new physical model for signal processing phenomena (power amplification and frequency selectivity) occurring in the inner ear (Cochlea). It is generally accepted that Outer Hair Cells (OHCs) play a pivotal role in the Cochlear signal processing. In the proposed new model we postulate that all signal processing phenomena in the Cochlea are due to electrical currents flowing in the Cochlea structure. Three crucial characteristics of the OHCs are: 1) a forward mechanoelectrical transduction, 2) a strong piezoelectric effect (direct and inverse), and 3) a transmembrane nonlinear capacitance. The new model postulates existence of a biological electromechanical transistor (EMT) in each of the OHCs (based on a forward mechanoelectrical transduction phenomenon), which enhances the power of an incoming acoustic signal. Consequently, the nonlinear capacitance of the appropriate OHCs is charged (pumped) by an AC current source generated at the output of the proposed EMT transistor. Power amplification and frequency selectivity are realized on the nonlinear capacitance, which constitutes an essential part of a parametric amplifier circuit. The amplified and sharpened in frequency electric signal is then converted to a mechanical signal by the OHCs (inverse piezoelectric effect) and transferred to the Inner Hair Cells that transform this mechanical signal into an output electrical signal supplied to the afferent nerves.

Keywords: mechanism of hearing, cochlear amplifier, equivalent circuits, nonlinear capacitance, electromechanical transistor, parametric-piezoelectric amplifier, piezoelectric effect, power amplification, selectivity

1. Introduction

Acoustic signals, which can be detected by human auditory organ, are acoustic (pressure) waves propagating in a material medium, such as gas, liquid, or solid. Acoustic waves cannot propagate in vacuum, contrary to light waves. Acoustic waves are in fact pressure disturbances that propagate in air and are characterized by longitudinal (compressional) particle movements. Initially, acoustic waves enter the ear pinna and ear canal (outer ear). Then, acoustic waves travel through a sequence of elements in the auditory pathway, such as middle ear and inner ear, where they are converted into electrical impulses transmitted directly into the central nervous system. The most important element in the auditory pathway is the inner ear with the cochlea. In turn, the main constituent of the cochlea is the organ of Corti located between the basilar membrane (BM) and tectorial membrane (TM). The organ of Corti contains a large number of sensory cells such as the outer hair cells (OHCs) and inner hair cells (IHCs). It is generally assumed that the process of power amplification of input acoustic signals occurs in the cochlea and is accompanied by sharpening of its frequency selectivity. High sensitivity of the cochlea enables hearing of low-level acoustic signals. On the other hand, high selectivity allows for frequency discrimination between two tones with nearly the same frequency.

The inner ear is one of the most complex sensory elements of the human body. It receives acoustic stimuli of various amplitudes and frequencies, carrying information from the external world. It is a highly nonlinear element presenting remarkable properties, such as:

1. Ultra-low power consumption (14 μW = 14×10^{-6} W) [1].

2. Possibility to amplify power of very weak input acoustic signals. The human ear can receive and distinguish acoustic signals with power slightly above the power of thermal noise in air (1.9×10^{-18} W). Power density (intensity) of these acoustic signals equals 10^{-12} W/m^2 at a frequency of 1000 Hz [2].

3. Very high dynamic range (120 dB). The power level of a very loud sound (1 W/m^2), such as roaring of jumbo-jet engines, can exceeds trillion times the threshold of human hearing (10^{-12} W/m^2). Thus, the dynamic range of reception amounts to (1 W/10^{-12} W = 10^{12}), 12 orders of magnitude, i.e., 120 dB [3].

4. Very high frequency selectivity. Humans (who have perfect pitch) are able to distinguish between musical sounds differing only by 0.2%, e.g., 1000 cycles per second (Hz) and 1002 Hz. It is noteworthy that the frequency difference between the tones generated by any two adjacent keys (semitone), in the contemporary piano tuned to an equal (well) tempered scale, equals ~6%, or exactly $\left(\sqrt[12]{2} - 1\right) \times 100\%$ [4]. The frequency range of the human ear spans approximately 10 octaves, i.e., from ~20 to ~20,000 Hz.

None of the technical devices built up to date by humans can even approach the above characteristics. This would be impossible if an input acoustic signal were processed in a passive manner. Achievement of such an amazing performance requires that some active processes take place in the cochlea, i.e., an extra energy has to be added to the input acoustic signal, in order to amplify the power of the received acoustic signal and enhance the frequency selectivity (narrow bandwidth) of the cochlea characteristics.

For nearly 2000 years humans tried to elucidate the nature of the physical processes occurring in the human hearing organ (cochlea). So far, there is no complete theory and understanding of the physical phenomena occurring in the cochlea.

Modeling of physical processes occurring in the cochlea is indeed a very complex task. There are still many exciting and unresolved research problems related to the complicated electrical

http://dx.doi.org/10.5772/66542

and mechanical phenomena responsible for the mechanism of hearing. For example, a fascinating area of research is reception and perception of acoustic signals generated by musical instruments. Do aesthetic impressions, offered by music, depend on proper operation of the human auditory organ (cochlea)? Does music have healing properties for autistic children with a perfect pitch?

Accurate knowledge of the mechanism of hearing may allow construction of an artificial cochlea and determination of a possible correlation between the cochlea characteristics and musical skills. Is the construction of the human hearing organ (cochlea) significantly different for musical geniuses (Bach, Mozart, Chopin, etc.) and those individuals only moderately gifted in music?

The mechanism of hearing is not yet fully understood, even though it was, and is the subject of intense research activities in many renowned scientific centers around the world (in USA, Japan, France, Germany, Switzerland, etc.). In particular, the following features of the cochlea are not yet explained:

1. power amplification,
2. high sensitivity in reception of faint (low-level) acoustic signals,
3. high frequency selectivity of acoustic signals (narrow bandwidth analyzer),
4. nonlinear phenomena, and
5. emphasis of weak acoustic signals and compression of large acoustic signals.

A complete and accurate model of the physical processes occurring in the cochlear amplifier (CA) should explain the course of these aforementioned processes.

Full understanding of the physical mechanism of hearing may be of paramount importance for:

a. automation of the speech recognition processes,
b. investigation of emotional behavior of human by using speech analysis,
c. explanation of how the speech perception depends on the cochlea,
d. explanation of how the perception of musical sounds occurs (why some individuals are musical geniuses, e.g., Chopin, and the others are tone-deaf),
e. construction of effective tools for man-computer communication,
f. invention of new and more effective methods for digital coding of sound signals, and
g. construction of new hearing aids.

1.1. What is the sensitivity?

The sensitivity of a given device or system is defined as the lowest amplitude of the signal, which can be detected by the system. In case of the human auditory organ (cochlea) sensitivity is defined as the lowest level of the input acoustic signal, for which the cochlear amplifier, treated as a receiver, produces an output electrical signal of an appropriate level, i.e., the signal with a satisfactory signal to noise ratio. In other words, sensitivity of the human hearing organ (cochlea) corresponds to a threshold acoustic signal, for which one can still hear with an acceptable quality and perception.

1.2. Active processes in the cochlea

Postmortem measurements of BM motion in the cochlea (passive cochlea) show that increase of the amplitude of sound gives rise to a linear increase in the amplitude of BM mechanical vibrations. However, passive cochlea is not able to explain the amazing amplitude sensitivity and frequency selectivity of the human hearing organ. It was found that with a passive cochlea only very loud sound could be heard (low sensitivity) with a poor frequency selectivity.

1.2.1. What are the active processes?

In order to explain the fabulous properties of the human hearing organ (sensitivity and selectivity), the concept of the active element and the cochlear amplifier were introduced as early as in 1948 by Gold [5] and later extended by many researchers (e.g., Davis in [6]). The introduction of the active element served to explain the phenomenon of power amplification and sharpening the frequency characteristics that occur in the cochlea, see Refs. [5, 6]. In general, power amplification process requires that some extra energy is delivered from an external source to the system. The system with power amplification capability is called active in contrast to a passive system, which can only dissipate (lose) the energy.

Properties of active elements (where active processes can occur) allow in a natural way to explain such features of human hearing organ as high sensitivity and selectivity (narrow bandwidth). An example of active elements found in classical electronics can be transistors, bipolar, as well as unipolar (field effect transistors). These elements operating in the amplifier circuit can amplify the power of the electrical input signals.

At present the existence of the cochlear amplifier is widely accepted in the literature, see Ref. [7]. However, the exact mechanism of the power amplification in the cochlea is still the subject of extensive research. It is also generally accepted that OHCs play a key role in the cochlear power amplification process [8]. Power amplification and sharpening of the frequency response occurs in the OHCs, see Ref. [6], that are located in the Cochlea. In fact, loss of the OHCs causes that the cochlear amplifier is not operating, and as a consequence hearing capabilities are lost.

1.2.2. IHC operates as sensors

Another type of sensing element is inner hair cells (IHCs) that are also located in the cochlea, between the BM and TM. The inner hair cells (IHCs) detect the mechanical signal, which was previously amplified by the OHCs. The IHC plays the role of sensor [9]. The IHC converts the input mechanical signal into an electrical signal and transmits the latter to the central nervous system via the afferent innervation. In this case the afferent innervation of the IHCs may be called an output circuit of the entire cochlear amplifier.

1.2.3. OHC can operate as sensor and actuator

The OHC is not only the mechano-mechanical transducer. The OHC is both the mechano-electrical transducer and the electromechanical transducer. This can be attributed to two phenomena, i.e., the "forward mechano-electrical transduction" and the inverse piezoelectric effect (electromotility), which play an essential role in the operation of the OHC and the cochlear amplifier as a whole [10]. An input acoustic signal entering the OHC is transferred to the electric side through the direct piezoelectric effect. There, on the electric side the signal is amplified.

1.2.4. What is the piezoelectric effect (direct and inverse)?

The direct piezoelectric effect is the ability of certain materials to generate an electric charge (voltage) in response to applied mechanical stress [11]. The inverse piezoelectric effect in turn is responsible for generating of mechanical deformations (stresses) induced by voltage applied to the material. Piezoelectric properties were found in certain solid media and biological materials, such as bones, ligaments, OHCs, and selected proteins. The piezoelectric effect, which is present in OHCs, is also termed in the literature as the electromotility or somatic motility. The piezoelectric effect is reversible, i.e., if the direct piezoelectric effect occurs in a material then the inverse piezoelectric effect will be present as well.

1.2.5. Electric side and mechanical side

A rectangular plate cut-off from the piezoelectric material, with two parallel electrodes attached to the plate, forms the simplest piezoelectric transducer used in practice. The transducer is in fact a three-port device with one electrical and two mechanical ports. Application of an electrical signal to the electric port (two parallel electrodes) of the transducer will force the two parallel surfaces of the plate (two mechanical ports) to vibrate with the frequency equal to that of the electrical excitation. Conversely, application of a mechanical signal (force) to the mechanical port(s) will generate voltage in the electrical port with the frequency equal to that of the mechanical driving force. In this way, mechanical and electrical quantities are mutually interrelated and can be transformed one to each other via the piezoelectric effect.

1.2.6. Importance of the electrical phenomena in the OHC

The role of electrical phenomena occurring in the OHC is not merely auxiliary, but in the contrary, is essential. According to the author's analysis, the process of power amplification of the input acoustic signal (applied to one mechanical port of the OHC), as well as the process of sharpening the frequency characteristics (increased frequency selectivity), is carried out on the electrical side of the OHC. Consequently, sharpened electrical signal with amplified power is transferred back to both ports of the mechanical side of the OHC, through the inverse piezoelectric effect. Therefore, the OHC performs mechanical work on its both mechanical ports, i.e., on the BM and on TM. The mechanical energy supplied by the OHC to the TM is transferred to the corresponding IHC by the movement of its stereocilia. The IHC processes its input (in relation to the IHC) mechanical signal into an output electrical signal by opening ion channels (mechano-electric transduction effect). These ionic currents affect the afferent nerve endings, where they are transformed into a series of electrical impulses that are transmitted into the central nervous system. It is assumed that there is no phenomenon of the power amplification in the IHC, which works as a passive sensor. Effectively, the IHC is a mechano-electrical transducer that converts the mechanical signal received from the OHC, into a useful electrical signal, which is an "electrical image" of the received acoustic waves that we can hear.

In this chapter, the author emphasizes the crucial role of the electrical phenomena in the processes of power amplification of input acoustic signals and sharpening of the frequency characteristics of the cochlea. In the second part of this chapter (Sections 9–13), the results of the original author's research, i.e., new model and concept of the cochlear amplifier are presented.

2. Role of the outer hair cells in the cochlear amplification

It is generally accepted that most important processes governing the selectivity and sensitivity of the human ear occur in the organ of Corti located in the cochlea. The cochlea contains about 20,000 outer hair cells (OHCs) spanned between the basilar membrane (BM) and the tectorial membrane (TM). The outer hair cells (OHCs) are nonlinear electro-mechanosensory cells and are critically important for the high sensitivity and frequency selectivity of the human ear. The electromechanical properties of the outer hair cells (OHCs) are believed to be the critical component of the cochlear Amplifier (CA) concept, but its internal "circuitry" still remains unknown. Mode of operation of this amplifier still arouses controversy and it is still unclear.

The OHC is a layered piezoelectric cylinder, with a diameter of about 9 μm and length that varies from 15 to 90 μm, depending on their location in the cochlea. The OHC wall thickness is equal to 100 nm. The membrane capacitance of the OHC comprises a linear component and nonlinear component. The most striking feature of the OHC is its giant piezoelectric effect, which is four order of magnitude higher than that in the best known piezoelectric materials. Therefore, piezoelectric phenomena have been included in the modeling of the OHC operation. Other observations provide also an evidence that movements of electrical charges within the OHC walls are directly coupled with mechanical elongation and shortening of the OHC structure. At the top of sensory cells (OHCs and IHCs) a tuft (called hair bundle–HB) of a few tens to a few hundreds of stereocilia is located.

Existing so far theories of the amplification in a single OHC and in the entire cochlea do not describe all the phenomena experimentally observed, or they are entirely phenomenological theories, not related to actual physical (physiological) processes occurring in a single OHC and in the entire inner ear. Similarly, the previously published electromechanical models of a single OHC and the whole cochlea only reflect their external characteristics and not the physical processes in them.

A characteristic feature of the OHC is the presence of the piezoelectric effect. Electric voltage applied across the walls of the cell membrane of the OHC results in a change (increase

http://dx.doi.org/10.5772/66542

or decrease) of its length (inverse piezoelectric effect). Similarly, change in the length of the OHC generates electrical voltage across the walls of the cell membrane of the OHC (direct piezoelectric effect). Thanks to the piezoelectric effect, amplified in the OHC (on the electric side) acoustic signal is transferred to the tectorial membrane (TM) and subsequently to the inner hair cells (IHCs).

In summary, OHCs as elements of the cochlear amplifier provide:

1. power amplification,
2. frequency selectivity,
3. dynamics, and
4. generation of otoacoustic emissions.

2.1. What is the power amplification?

In order to verify whether a given system or device, such as the cochlea, is passive or active it is necessary to determine the balance of power flowing in and out of the device. To this end, the device should be surrounded by a closed surface with its normal vector $\vec{n}$ pointing outwards. Then, one has to identify all power components (electrical and mechanical) flowing through the surface and calculate the corresponding fluxes of the power density. A negative value of the total flux (power) is the signature of the fact that the system is a passive one, in which the power is dissipated (more power is flowing into the system than outflows from it). An example of such a system can be an electrical network consisting of resistors, inductors, and capacitors. A positive value of the total flux (power) indicates that the device is an active element, i.e., more power is flowing out of the device than flowing into the device. An example of such a system (device) can be either a bipolar transistor or a field effect transistor (MOS) operating in the amplifier circuit.

Simply speaking, if the output useful power exceeds the input signal power, then the device amplifies the power.

2.2. What is the frequency selectivity?

The frequency selectivity of the system is its ability to unambiguously discriminate between two signals with very close frequencies. This property occurs, for example, in narrow band resonant circuits with quartz resonators. High frequency selectivity of the cochlear amplifier is an evidence that the frequency characteristics of the cochlea can be tuned to a narrow frequency band, e.g., from 1000 to 1002 Hz. This frequency selectivity is essential for comprehension of speech and music perception.

2.3. What is the dynamics?

The dynamic range (dynamics) of the device is the ratio P_2/P_1 of the maximum P_2 and minimum power P_1 of the input signal, which can be handled properly by the device (cochlea). For convenience, the dynamics is represented in a logarithmic scale, i.e., $Dynamics = 10 \log$

(P_2/P_1), measured in decibels (dB). Here, the symbol "log" stands for the logarithm to base 10. For example, if power density $P_2 = 1\ W/m^2$ and $P_1 = 10^{-6}\ W/m^2$, then the dynamics equals $10\log(1/10^{-6}) = 60$ dB. The dynamics of the cochlear amplifier can reach 120 dB. Colloquially speaking, the dynamics tells us about the difference between the loudest and the weakest sound that we can still hear.

3. Role of the electric currents flowing in the structure of the cochlea

It is generally accepted that most important processes of acoustic signal processing (power amplification and frequency selectivity) occur in the inner ear. In the outer ear and the middle ear, the power of the received sound is not amplified, since the outer and middle ears are passive devices. In the middle ear there is only a mechanical impedance matching, whereas the power of travelling sound is not amplified.

3.1. What is the impedance?

In general, the impedance is a measure of opposition displayed by mechanical (damper, spring, mass) or electrical (resistor, capacitor, inductor) elements to external driving forces (mechanical stresses or electrical voltage, respectively). In case of an electrical excitation the electrical impedance is defined as the ratio of voltage applied to the electrical element to the current flowing through the element. On the other hand, the mechanical impedance is defined as the ratio of force applied to the mechanical element to the velocity at which the element moves. For harmonic (sinusoidal) excitations, the electrical and mechanical impedances can be conveniently described by complex number quantities. The above definitions for mechanical and electrical impedances are valid only for so-called lumped elements, i.e., the elements without spatial dimensions. Lumped elements are subject of the circuit theory. Somewhat different definitions of the impedance are introduced for acoustic and electromagnetic waves propagating in the three-dimensional media. However, in case of the cochlear amplifier the wavelength of the acoustic waves reaching the OHC (1.5 m at a frequency of 1000 Hz) is much higher than physical dimensions of the OHC (90 μm). Therefore, the circuit theory description holds [12].

The incoming acoustic wave passes through the outer ear to the middle ear, where it causes vibrations of the bones (hammer an anvil and stapes). Vibrations of the stapes through the oval window excite acoustic waves in liquids contained in the cochlea of the inner ear. This acoustic wave motion generates a transverse acoustic wave propagating along the basilar membrane. This mechanical wave travelling in the BM excites to vibration OHCs that are located between the BM and TM, see **Figure 1**.

Mechanical displacement of stereocilia, located on top of the OHCs, opens ion channels which provokes the flow of ionic current (K+ cations) in a closed circuit starting from the stria vascularis (DC voltage source) to the body of the OHC and then back to the stria vascularis. Sinusoidal deflection of stereocilia produces a sinusoidal in time flow of electric current (ions K^+) in this circuit. Produced in this way (AC) current source pumps energy into the

http://dx.doi.org/10.5772/66542

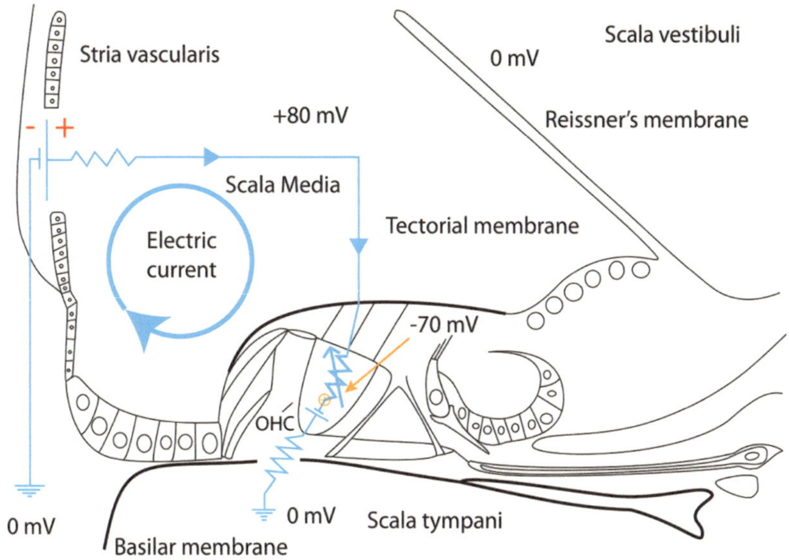

Figure 1. The flow of ionic currents (K+) in a closed circuit including a DC voltage source (stria vascularis), scala media (+80 mV), OHC (-70 mV), and scala tympani (0 mV). Demonstratively, only one OHC is shown in the figure. Stria vascularis powers the activity of the cochlear amplifier.

nonlinear capacitance, which constitutes a part of the cochlear parametric amplifier. The existence of this nonlinear capacitance was confirmed experimentally [13]. This parametric amplifier provides the necessary selectivity of the frequency characteristics of the cochlear amplifier that is based on a single OHC. The above mentioned problems will be explained in more detail in Sections 9–11.

3.2. Electric currents in the cochlea

Presence of natural (physiological) sources of a DC voltage (stria vascularis) and conductive liquids (electrolytes) in the cochlea creates favorable conditions for flow of electrical currents. It should be emphasized that ionic currents in the cochlea must flow in a closed circuit, according to the classical circuit theory. **Figure 1** shows an example of an ionic current flowing through one of the 20,000 OHCs in the cochlea. This ionic current (K^+ cations) flows from the positive pole of the stria vascularis voltage source (battery), through the scala media (SM; +80 mV) and ion channels at the top (apical) part of the OHC, into the bulk of the OHC (-70 mV). Then, through channels in the lower (basolateral) part of the OHC to perilymph, which has a zero (0 mV) electric potential (right grounding in **Figure 1**). The current loop closes in the negative pole of the stria vascularis battery (grounding in the left side of **Figure 1**).

3.3. Zero of electric potential

It should be remembered that the value of an electric potential at any point is measured with respect to the potential at a reference point, assumed to be zero. As a result, we can only measure the potential difference (voltage). In the cochlear structure in **Figure 1** we assume as zero potential (grounding), the potential of perilymph in scala vestibuli and scala tympani (0 mV). With respect to this reference point, the potential in scala media (SM) is +80 mV and the potential inside the OHC is equal to -70 mV. As it will be shown later in this chapter, the flow of electric currents in the cochlea plays a primary role in the phenomena of power amplification and frequency selectivity, which occur in the cochlea.

4. Stria vascularis

4.1. Direct current (DC) voltage source in the cochlea

A fundamental role in the cochlear amplifier, besides the OHCs, is played by the stria vascularis, which produces a source of DC voltage between endolymph and perilymph. This potential difference, resulting from difference in ion concentrations in endolymph and perilymph, is sustained by metabolic processes occurring in the cochlea. This source of a DC voltage stores energy in the form of an electrical (potential) energy. In fact, the cochlear amplifier draws energy from the stria vascularis battery to amplify power of an incoming acoustic wave. The stria vascularis battery will play a key role in the generation of electrical signals and currents (both direct and alternating) flowing in the cochlear amplifier. In the circuit model of physical phenomena in the cochlea, the stria vascularis is represented by a (DC) voltage source, see the upper left part of **Figure 1**.

5. The cochlea as a set of nonlinear oscillators

The cochlea is characterized by tonotopic organization, i.e., its resonant properties are a function of the longitudinal position (a given stimulus frequency corresponds to a given location) and vary along the cochlea from base to apex. Structurally, the cochlea can be modeled as a series of radial sections [cochlear partitions (CPs)] starting at the base and ending at the apex. Each section of the CP is considered to be a highly resonant structure, which can vibrate preferably at only one frequency named as characteristic frequency (CF). The resonant frequency of each section of the CP is governed by the average mass, stiffness, and damping of the corresponding elements, e.g., basilar membrane, OHCs, and tectorial membrane constituting this section.

The elements responsible for the active processes occurring in the cochlea are OHCs. Manifestations of this active process are high sensitivity and frequency selectivity with respect to week stimuli, nonlinear compression of input stimuli with small and large amplitudes, and spontaneous otoacoustic emissions [14].

From a mathematical point of view, all this features are consistent with the operation of a set of nonlinear oscillators within the inner ear that are tuned to different frequencies [15].

In other words, the cochlear amplifier can be treated as a set of nonlinear electromechanical oscillators, represented by CPs with the corresponding OHCs, with the fundamental

http://dx.doi.org/10.5772/66542

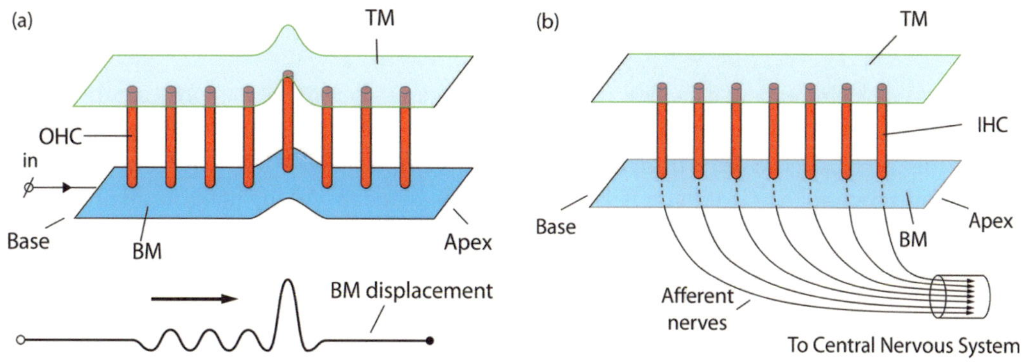

Figure 2. (a) Cochlea as a set of nonlinear oscillators (represented by OHCs), (b) a set of IHCs in the cochlea acts as a sensor. It should be noted that the OHCs and IHCs operate in a liquid environment, not air.

frequencies of vibrations extending approximately from 20 Hz to 20 kHz. The nonlinear electromechanical oscillators are stimulated to vibrations by transverse acoustic waves traveling along the basilar membrane, see **Figure 2a** and **b**.

Mechanical input signal that stimulates the wave traveling in the BM (see **Figure 2a**) represents the input acoustic signal, which reaches the inner ear through the oval window. Vibrations of the oval window excite acoustic waves in liquids (perilymph, endolymph) filling the cochlea. This wave motion in turn generates a pressure distribution that induces mechanical transverse waves propagating along the BM. This transverse acoustic (mechanical) wave traveling in the BM, when moving from base to apex, stimulates to vibrations OHCs, which rest on the BM. The OHCs which are located in the vicinity of the partition with CF (characteristic frequency) that corresponds to the frequency of the input acoustic signal are excited to oscillate.

In **Figure 2a** we can see the OHC, which is located at the area where the BM displacement is maximal. It is this OHC (with a natural frequency of, e.g., 1000 Hz) which will be excited to vibration. The vibrations of this OHC amplify deflection of BM and TM. Mechanical energy forwarded by this OHC to TM is transferred through TM to the stereocilia of the IHC (see **Figure 2b**) with a proper frequency (i.e., 1000 Hz). In this IHC, transformation of mechanical energy into electrical energy occurs, which stimulates afferent nerve endings that produce a series of electrical impulses transmitted to the central nervous system.

If the frequency of the input acoustic signal is, for example, 1000 Hz, then this wave stimulates vibrations of the oscillator with a natural frequency equaled also to 1000 Hz. These vibrations are further amplified actively in this resonant circuit, see **Figure 2a**. The resonant curve of the nonlinear oscillator can be quite narrow (high selectivity) and can be therefore characterized by a high quality factor. For weak acoustic signals, the electrical and mechanical power at the output of the oscillator may exceed many times (e.g., 500 times) the power of the input acoustic wave. In this manner, in the nonlinear (active) electromechanical oscillator (represented by the OHC), phenomena of power amplification and frequency discrimination occur.

6. State of the art

Hermann von Helmholtz was the first who created mechanical model of the cochlea in 1863 [16]. In his model the BM is represented as a system of harmonic oscillators tuned to different frequencies. In this model, the cochlea is treated as a kind of a spectrum analyzer. Next significant cochlear model was proposed by Georg von Békésy in 1928 [17]. In his model the mechanism of hearing is described in terms of the traveling wave propagating in the passive BM (*in vitro*). Position of the maximum of the wave depends on the frequency. In other words, the basilar membrane was found to be tonotopically organized: a given stimulus frequency corresponds to a given location. However, the theory of Bekesy was not able to explain the phenomenon of power amplification and frequency selectivity as well as other actual properties of the cochlea in living humans.

In 1948, Gold [5] concluded that the inner ear cannot act only passively. Only the active element can provide amplification and experimentally observed selectivity. As a model of such an element Gold introduced a valve regenerative amplifier. But these were suggestions, purely hypothetical, and not supported by any physical and physiological data. Therefore, they were not accepted at that time. Thirty years later Kemp experiments [18] concerning otoacoustic emissions and works of Davis [6] confirmed the existence of active processes in the organ of Corti. For many years, discussions continued on what is the physical mechanism of this phenomenon. It is now widely accepted that the active component is the cochlear amplifier. Still, the controversy raises a mechanism of action of this amplifier [19, 20].

7. Deficiencies of the existing models of the OHC and whole cochlea

So far the existing models (theories) of the amplification in a single outer hair cell (OHC) and the entire cochlea do not take into account all the physical phenomena experimentally observed. They are phenomenological theories, not related to actual physical (physiological) processes occurring in a single OHC and in the entire inner ear. In recent years a theory has gained popularity, which attributed the phenomenon of the cochlear amplification to Hopf bifurcations [21]. This theory, however, raised many doubts among others concerning the problem of stability [22]. Many authors of papers published very recently stated that in the theory of the cochlear amplification many unresolved problems still exist and work on it must be continued [14, 23–27].

A similar discussion applies considering electronic models of a single OHC and the entire cochlea. These models to a greater or lesser extent, describe the characteristics of a single OHC and the whole cochlea, but do not reflect their physical structure.

In conclusion, one can state that none of the existing theories of hearing explains satisfactorily the mechanism of the signal processing phenomena occurring in the cochlea.

8. Contemporary models of the cochlear amplifier

Below, we present an overview of recently developed models of operation of the OHC and the entire Cochlea.

http://dx.doi.org/10.5772/66542

(1) Model presented in Ref. [21]

In this model the operation of an individual OHC is described in terms of a Hopf bifurcation. The cochlear amplifier (based on an individual OHC) has the dynamical characteristics of a Hopf bifurcation. This model can explain the nonlinear effects, selectivity, and resonance phenomena.

Critique: there is no description of power amplification, it is a purely phenomenological model, not a physical one. Electrical phenomena are not taken into account. There is no explanation of the role of ionic currents in the processes of power amplification and sharpening of the frequency characteristics.

(2) Model introduced in Ref. [28]

This model describes the resonant effects in a single OHC and the entire cochlea. The phenomenological parameters are introduced to match the theoretical and experimental curves.

Critique: there is no description of power amplification, it is a phenomenological model.

(3) Model presented in [29]

This model describes the behavior of a single OHC and the entire cochlea. The mechanical aspects of the model are characterized by using the concepts from hydrodynamics. Resonant characteristics of the cochlea are obtained by superposition of acoustic waves propagating in fluids inside the organ of Corti.

Critique: there is no description of power amplification, it is a phenomenological and a purely mechanical model. Electrical phenomena are not considered. The explanation of resonant phenomena is very complicated. To this end, an exotic concept of so-called squirting waves is employed. There is no explanation of the role of ionic currents in the processes of power amplification and sharpening of the frequency characteristics.

(4) Model introduced in Ref. [30]

This model interprets the nonlinear resonant phenomena in a single OHC in terms of a Hopf bifurcation. To obtain proper resonant curves two phenomenological parameters are introduced.

Critique: There is no description of the power amplification, this is a purely phenomenological model. There is no analysis of electrical phenomena.

(5) Model presented in Ref. [31]

This model describes acoustic, mechanical, and electrical phenomena in a single OHC and the entire cochlea. The phenomenological parameter is introduced to match the experimental and theoretical curves. Some nonlinear effects are discussed.

Critique: there is no description of power amplification. The presence of nonlinear capacitance is ignored.

(6) Model introduced in Ref. [32]

This model gives an electrical equivalent circuit of an individual OHC. Elements of an equivalent circuit have their counterparts in the actual structure of the cochlea. The model is a physical model. Nonlinear phenomena are modeled by the nonlinear stiffness and capacitance.

Critique: there is no description of power amplification. The theory is incomplete.

(7) Model presented in Ref. [33]

The model analyses the electromechanical phenomena in a single OHC using black boxes and flow chart diagrams. Amplitude responses to sine wave and random noise excitations are given.

Critique: there is no description of power amplification, this is a purely phenomenological model. No correspondence between physical elements in an actual OHC and model elements.

(8) Model introduced in Ref. [34]

This is an experimental, piezoelectric, and hydrodynamic model of the cochlea operation. Theoretical analysis is performed for motion of BM along with surrounding liquids. Resonant characteristics of the cochlea are obtained.

Critique: there is no description of power amplification, it is a phenomenological model. There is no description of ion currents flow. Nonlinear analysis is not carried out.

(9) Model presented in Ref. [35]

In this model the role of HB motility and electromotility is presented. Resonant characteristic of the cochlea are given.

Critique: there is no description of power amplification, incomplete theory.

(10) Model introduced in Ref. [36]

The model comprises finite element method analysis of the mechanical part of the cochlear partition. Electrical representation of the OHC is given. Responses of an isolated OHC to electrical stimuli are analyzed.

Critique: there is no description of power amplification, it is an incomplete theory. The presence of nonlinear capacitance is ignored.

(11) Model presented in Ref. [37]

Time domain and resonant characteristics of the cochlea are obtained by solving a set of nonlinear partial differential equations.

Critique: there is no description of power amplification, it is a phenomenological model, a purely mechanical model. Electrical phenomena are not considered.

(12) Model published in Ref. [38]

The macromechanical and micromechanical model of the cochlea is presented. Electrical model of a single OHC and the organ of Corti is given. Time domain and frequency domain analysis of electric signals in the cochlea structure is performed.

Critique: in the model there is no description of power amplification. The theory is incomplete.

http://dx.doi.org/10.5772/66542

(13) Model published in [39]

The author formulated an original theory of cochlea functioning using a concept of a laser. The theory is interesting; however, it seems to be rather nonphysical.

Critique: there is no description of power amplification, incomplete theory, theory is rather qualitative.

(14) Model published in Ref. [3]

The macromechanical and micromechanical model of the cochlea is presented.

Critique: the theory is only mechanical. There is no description of power amplification. The theory is incomplete.

In summary, it is evident that the existing models of hearing processes exhibit numerous deficiencies. The physical (mechanical and electrical) processes occurring in the cochlear amplifier are not well understood.

In the following of this chapter, the author presents his new and original concepts and physical models for the phenomena of power amplification and sharp frequency tuning occurring in the cochlea.

9. Power flow in the OHC

9.1. Introduction of the concept of an electromechanical transistor

A single OHC element represents one of 20,000 active elements in the cochlear amplifier. The most important feature of the active element is its ability to amplify the power of an input acoustical signal. It is amazing that by analyzing power flow in the OHC, the author arrived to the new concept of an electromechanical transistor.

The analysis performed in this section is based on the phenomenon of forward mechano-electric transduction that occurs in the apical part of the OHC.

9.1.1. Power amplifier

Here, we will present the conditions which must be fulfilled by the system (device) to be a power amplifier. Such a system must include the following components:

1. a source of potential energy
2. a valve that controls the flow of the power from the source to the load (controlled element)
3. input circuit
4. output circuit

The principle of operation of the amplifier is based on the control of a higher output power by a lower input power. In our case, see **Figure 3a** and **b**, the low power P_{in} in the mechanical

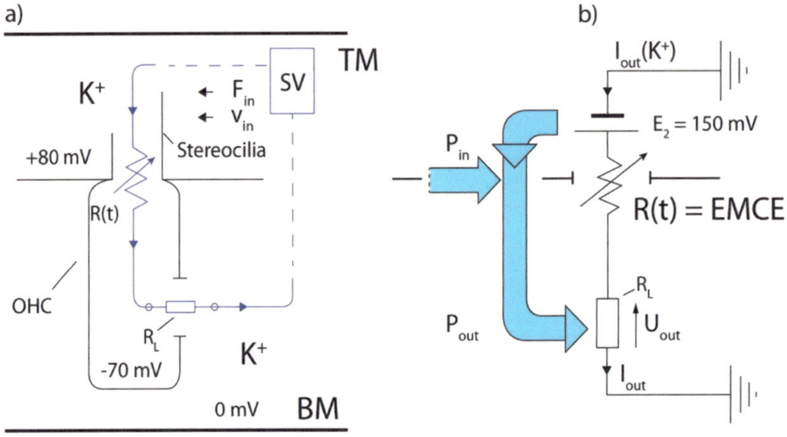

Figure 3. (a) Structure of the proposed electromechanical biological transistor, built around a single OHC. Arrows indicate the flow of K^+ ionic electric current in the electromechanical transistor (amplifier), $R(t)$ is a time-varying channel resistance, which represents the electromechanical control element (EMCE), and R_L is a load resistor. BM is the basilar membrane, TM is the tectorial membrane, and SV denotes the stria vascularis, (b) electrical equivalent circuit of the OHC's electromechanical transistor, electromotive force E_2 = 150 mV represents the difference of an endocochlear potential and intracellular potential inside the OHC.

input circuit (stereocilia of the OHC) controls the high power flow from the stria vascularis battery to the output electrical circuit, P_{out}. As it will be seen later, all of the above conditions are satisfied by the system composed of the following elements:

1. Stria vascularis

2. Stereocilia + ionic channels located in the apical part of the OHC

3. Ionic channels located in the basolateral part of the OHC

9.1.2. Electromechanical amplifier

The active electromechanical device, presented in **Figure 3a**, is composed of the initial part of the OHC and the entire amplifying tract of the cochlear amplifier that begins with BM deflection and terminates in IHC, where the amplified mechanical signal is transformed into an electrical signal stimulating the afferent nerves.

Figure 3a presents schematic view of the proposed electromechanical (biological) transistor, built around a single OHC. To illustrate the principle of operation of the new amplifying device, dimensions of channels at the upper (apical) part and in the lower (basolateral) part of the OHC in **Figure 3a** are greatly exaggerated. Operation of the channels at the apical part and at the basolateral part of the OHC is modeled by one resultant (effective) channel, i.e., one effective channel for the apical part and one effective channel for the basolateral part. The flow of potassium ions K^+ is of crucial importance for electrical phenomena occurring in the OHC. The current of potassium ions K^+, see **Figure 3a**, flows in a closed circuit starting from the stria vascularis (DC voltage source) to the body of the OHC and then back to the stria vascularis. The top apical channels play a role of a controlled (time-varying) resistance $R(t)$.

9.1.3. Electromechanical control element (EMCE)

The time-variable resistance $R(t)$ in **Figure 3a** and **b** is controlled by a time-varying input acoustic signal, i.e., particle velocity $v(t)$ and/or mechanical force $F(t)$. As a consequence, the current flowing through the load resistance R_L varies in time unison with the changes of the input acoustic signal. This time-variable resistance $R(t)$ can be identified as an electromechanical controlled element (EMCE), see Ref. [40].

9.1.4. Load resistance

The basolateral channels in **Figure 3a** are modeled by a load resistance R_L, which represents the output power receiver. The power dissipated on the load resistance R_L is not a lost power, but in contrary constitutes a useful power, which pumps energy into the parametric electromechanical amplifier, based on the nonlinear capacitance of the OHC. This will be shown in more details in Sections 11–13 of this chapter.

Figure 3b shows an equivalent circuit model of the amplifying electromechanical device presented in **Figure 3a**. In this circuit model we can identify a source of potential energy (DC battery), an active control element (electromechanical transistor) represented by a controlled (time-varying) resistance $R(t)$, and finally a load resistance R_L.

9.1.5. Power flow in the electromechanical amplifier

Power flow in the electromechanical amplifier, based on the phenomenon of the forward mechano-electrical transduction, which is triggered by the movement of the OHC stereocilia, is as follows:

1. The electric power from the stria vascularis battery flows through ion channels in the apical part of the OHC to the body of the OHC. Then, through the interior of the OHC the electric power flows into the output circuit, where it is dissipated on the load resistance R_L.
2. The power of the input signal is transmitted to the control circuit formed by the stereocilia of the OHC. The amount of power from the stria vascularis battery, which flows to the output circuit, depends on the power level of the input control signal.
3. The signal in the output electric circuit varies in time synchronously with changes of the input acoustic signal in the control circuit. The signal in the output circuit reproduces the characteristics of the input signal. However, the power of the signal in the output circuit can surpass many times the power of the input control signal. Thus, power amplification phenomenon takes place.

The physical foundation of operation of the proposed electromechanical transistor is the phenomenon of forward mechano-electrical transduction, taking place in the apical part of the OHCs (stereocilia + ion channels).

9.1.6. Input and output circuits

The input circuit of the proposed electromechanical transistor is a mechanical circuit consisting of the OHC's stereocilia. Input control signal is the particle velocity and/or the mechanical force exerted on the stereocilia. The output circuit is an electrical circuit, see **Figure 3a** and **b**. Electrical output controlled signal is the current and/or the voltage across the load resistance R_L. The electric circuit in **Figure 3a** and **b** closes through the structures lying outside the OHC (back to the stria vascularis).

9.1.7. Electromechanical transistor (EMT)

The electromechanical amplifying system in **Figure 3a** and **b** satisfies four necessary conditions for power gain to occur, namely:

1. There is a source of potential energy (voltage source E_2).
2. There is a device (electromechanical controlled element – electromechanical transistor) to control the flow of energy from the voltage source E_2 to the load resistance R_L, i.e., $EMCE = R(t)$. The value of the resistance $R(t)$ is controlled by the input mechanical (acoustical) signal (velocity and/or force). Ion channels in the apical part of the OHC play the role of the controlled resistance $R(t)$.
3. There is a mechanical control input circuit (stereocilia of the OHC).
4. There is an electric controlled output circuit (ion channels in the basolateral part of the OHC).

Thus, this electromechanical controlled element $EMCE = R(t)$ represents an electromechanical transistor. This transistor is a close analog of the electronic unipolar field effect transistor (FET), see **Figure 4a** and **b**.

9.2. Analogy between the proposed EMT type transistor and the FET type transistor

The proposed electromechanical transistor is analogous to the classical field effect transistor (FET). Certainly, the proposed electromechanical transistor resembles also a vacuum tube or a bipolar transistor, but according to the author, similarity in this case is less direct (explicit). This is due to the following reasons:

a. In the proposed electromechanical transistor, similarly as in the field effect transistor (FET), the process of electric current conduction involves only monopolar carriers of the same sign. Therefore, like in case of the classical FET electronic transistor, the electromechanical transistor is a "unipolar" transistor, since the process of current conduction in the electromechanical transistor employs only positive potassium cations K^+.

b. In the proposed electromechanical transistor, similarly as in the FET transistor, channel resistance is modulated. These channels exist physically in the structure of the OHC, i.e., they have definite dimensions, spatial positions, and play the role of the controlled resistor $R(t)$.

c. In case of the FET transistor, the channel is formed in the semiconductor material, which is sandwiched between two electrodes (source and drain). Resistance of this channel is modulated by changing voltage applied to the gate. This results in a change of channel's cross-section and its conductivity.

d. In case of the electromechanical transistor (EMT), the role of the channel is played by ion channels existing in the apical part of the OHC. Their resistance $R(t)$ varies depending on the degree of opening or closing of the channels (deviation of stereocilia). This resistance exists physically and could be measured using an ohmmeter. The resistance $R(t)$ is modulated by an input acoustic (mechanical) signal reaching OHC.

e. By contrast, the resistance which is modulated in the vacuum tube or in the bipolar transistor is rather an effective resistance (a phenomenological concept). This resistance is not located in a definite site. For example, in the vacuum tube (triode), the resistance which is modulated by the grid voltage is an apparent resistance of the region distributed between the cathode and anode.

Therefore, we can state that the proposed electromechanical transistor is a close analog of the classical electronic field effect transistor (FET), see **Table 1**.

The principle of operation of the proposed EMT transistor and the classical FET transistor is presented below in **Figure 4**.

Transistor type	**EMT**	**FET**
Carrier type	K^+ ions	Electrons or holes
Input circuit	Stereocilia (mechanical circuit)	Gate + input source (electrical circuit)
Output circuit	OHC walls + ionic channels in the basolateral part of the OHC	Drain + load resistance R_L
Channel type	Ionic channels in the apical part of the OHC	Semiconductor channel
Controlled element	Variable resistance $R(t)$ of the ion channels in the apical part of the OHC	Variable resistance $R(t)$ of a semiconductor channel
Mechanism changing channel resistance	Deflection of stereocilia	Change of the gate voltage
Power amplification	Yes	Yes

Table 1. Comparison of the features of the electromechanical transistor (EMT) and the field effect transistor (FET).

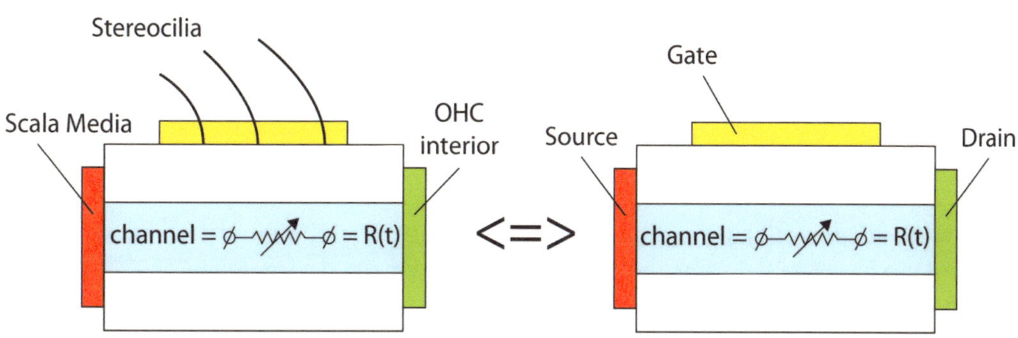

Figure 4. Physical models of (a) proposed electromechanical transistor EMT, and (b) classical field effect transistor FET.

It is not surprising that the structures of both transistors presented in **Figure 4a** and **b** are almost identical. In case of the proposed EMT transistor, movement of the stereocilia modulates the conductivity of ion channels. On the other hand, in the classical FET transistor, the voltage applied to the gate modulates the conductivity of the semiconductor channel. Thus, the proposed EMT transistor and classical FET transistors are controlled, correspondingly, by mechanical and electrical signals.

The channels in the EMT and FET transistors exist physically and can be modeled by a time-varying resistance $R(t)$. It is worth noticing that the transistor itself does not generate any energy. In fact, its essential function is to control (according to changes in the input modulating signal) the flow of energy from an external "high" energy source (such as a DC voltage battery) into the output circuit (load resistance).

9.3. Small signal linearized electric equivalent circuit of the EMT

Operation of the proposed EMT transistor can be presented in the form of an equivalent electrical circuit.

9.3.1. Small-signal electrical equivalent circuit

The input circuit of the proposed electromechanical transistor EMT is represented by two mechanical quantities, i.e., the velocity v_1 and mechanical force F_1 on the cilia. The output circuit of the proposed electromechanical transistor EMT is represented by two electrical quantities, i.e., output voltage U_2 and current I_2. In general, the relationships between (F_1, v_1) and (U_2, I_2) are described by complex nonlinear functions. However, for small signal amplitudes, the link between (F_1, v_1) and (U_2, I_2) can be linearized, i.e., described by linear functions framed in a matrix form.

Classical circuit theory allows modeling of the transistor in the form of an equivalent circuit composed of passive admittances and active current sources. In this way, instead of investigating a large number of complex 3D physical phenomena occurring in the actual spatial structure of the transistor, operation of the transistor can be satisfactorily described using a combinations of lumped circuit elements, such as admittances and controlled sources. The resulting circuit constitutes a small-signal equivalent circuit of the transistor. Influence of these elements on the operation of the transistor can be calculated by applying the laws of the current flow, known from the classical circuit theory [12].

Figure 5 shows small signal equivalent circuit of the proposed electromechanical transistor for small values of the output AC electric signals (voltage and current) and input mechanical signals (velocity and force on stereocilia).

The matrix equation linking together the input mechanical and output electrical signals in **Figure 5** can be presented using the concept of a hybrid matrix $[h]$, as follows:

$$\begin{bmatrix} F_1 \\ I_2 \end{bmatrix} = \begin{bmatrix} h_{11} & h_{12} \\ h_{21} & h_{22} \end{bmatrix} \cdot \begin{bmatrix} v_1 \\ U_2 \end{bmatrix} = \begin{bmatrix} Z_{in} & 0 \\ g_{em} & g_{22} \end{bmatrix} \cdot \begin{bmatrix} v_1 \\ U_2 \end{bmatrix} \quad (1)$$

http://dx.doi.org/10.5772/66542

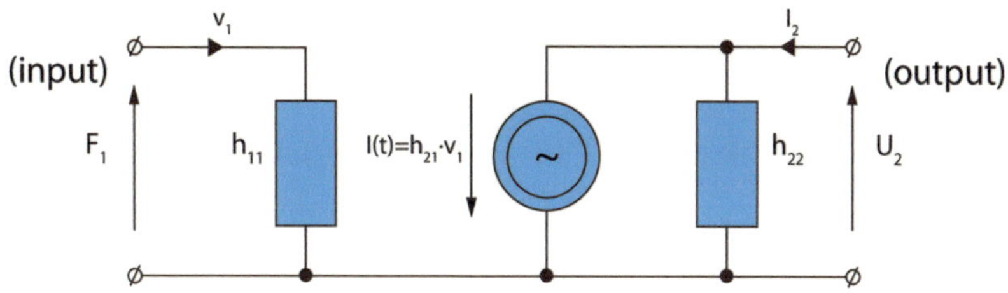

Figure 5. Linearized electromechanical equivalent circuit of the electromechanical transistor that uses a phenomenon of forward mechano-electric transduction occurring in the apical part of an OHC (hair bundles + ionic channels).

The elements of the matrix [h] have the following physical interpretation:

$h_{11} = Z_{in}$ is a mechanical input impedance,

$h_{22} = g_{22}$ is an electrical output conductance, and

$h_{21} = g_{em}$ is a coefficient of electromechanical transduction.

9.3.2. Occurrence of the alternating currents (AC) in the cochlea

In Sections 3 and 4 of this chapter, we found that (DC) voltages and currents are present in the cochlear structure. In the following, the problem of occurrence in the structure of the cochlea (AC) voltages and currents will be analyzed in more detail.

From the analysis presented formerly by the author it follows that the transistor effect (based on the phenomenon of forward mechano-electric transduction) generates alternating electric current (AC) in the cochlea. This current is represented in **Figure 5** by an active current source.

This analysis can serve as a theoretical description of the (AC) voltages and currents in the structure of the cochlea. These (AC) voltage and current sources are produced in the circuit: DC voltage source + time variable resistance $R(t)$, see **Figure 3b**.

The output circuit has the properties of the controlled current source. Output current I_2 is generated by the controlled current source $I(t) = h_{21} v_1(t)$, which depends linearly on the input velocity $v_1(t)$. This is a characteristic feature of active elements (in this case electromechanical transistors).

As it will be presented later, the controlled (AC) current source, shown in **Figure 5**, will act as the electrical signal that pumps energy into the parametric amplifier established on the basis of the nonlinear capacitance of the OHC, see **Figure 7**. More details concerning the operation of this electromechanical transistor can be found in the work of the author [40].

9.3.3. Otoacoustic emission

Discovered in 1978, phenomenon of otoacoustic emission (OAE) relies on the generation of sound waves in the inner ear. Acoustic waves generated in this way travel into the middle and outer ear [41, 42]. To explain the phenomenon of the OAE, we can examine the properties of the active elements constituting the cochlear amplifier, which in certain conditions can produce sustained "undamped" vibrations. The active elements in the cochlear amplifier, such as the proposed electromechanical transistors and parametric amplifiers based on the nonlinear capacitance of the OHC, can be responsible for the generation of periodic self-sustaining vibrations in the inner ear. Under certain conditions any amplifying element can become a generator.

Generation of the OAE signals in the OHCs occurs on the electric side. Subsequently, these signals through the inverse piezoelectric effect are transformed on the mechanical side. These mechanical (acoustic) signals leave the inner ear and can be received in the outer ear. The occurrence of the OAE phenomenon is an evidence that active processes in the cochlea do exist. The measurement of the OAE is now routinely employed for the detection of hearing impairment in newborns (in newborn hearing screening).

The phenomenon of the OAE can be treated as a side effect of operation of the cochlear amplifier.

10. Nonlinear capacitance of the OHC

Between the inner and outer cell membrane of the OHC, there is a linear (static) capacitance and nonlinear capacitance. The linear capacitance has a constant value (~30 pF), which does not depend on the applied voltage u. The nonlinear capacitance $C(u)$ depends on the voltage applied between the inner and outer wall of the OHC. The shape of this function resembles a bell curve, with a maximum value of approximately 25 pF. It is assumed that the nonlinear capacitance $C(u)$ is produced by the movement of confined charges in walls of the OHC.

This nonlinear capacitance of the OHC $C(u)$ will be used as an active element in the proposed parametric cochlear amplifier based on a single OHC. In classical electronics, nonlinear voltage-dependent capacitance is called "varactor." By driving a nonlinear capacitance $C(u)$ with a the time-dependent voltage $u(t)$, we obtain the capacitance $C(t)$ which is a function of time.

11. Parametric-piezoelectric model of the cochlear amplifier

In general, parametric amplification can be achieved in a resonant circuit, when one of its reactive elements (capacitance $C(t)$ or inductance $L(t)$, see **Figure 6**) changes in time. The variations of $C(t)$ and $L(t)$ will supply energy to the resonant circuit.

Figure 6 shows the layout of a serial (electrical) resonance circuit whose capacitance $C(t)$, formed by two parallel plates, varies sinusoidally in time. The capacitance of this planar capacitor is modulated by moving up and down the upper plate of the capacitor. Here, the lower plate of the capacitor is fixed. Setting the upper plate of the capacitor into motion requires an additional external source of energy, which is called the pumping source (pump).

In the circuit of the electronic parametric amplifier (where the variable in time capacitance $C(t)$ is the varactor), this external energy is delivered from an electrical (AC) pumping signal

http://dx.doi.org/10.5772/66542

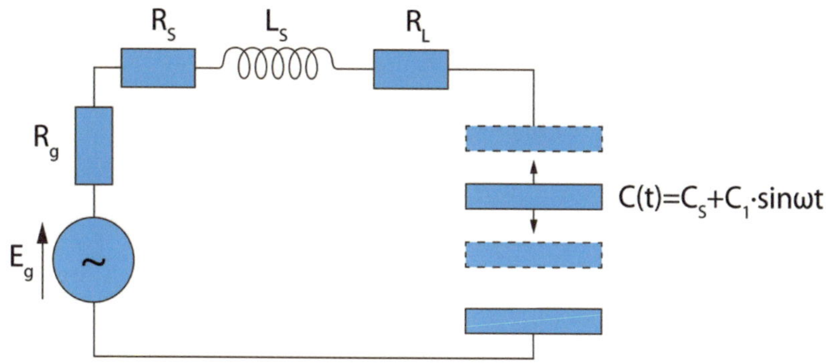

Figure 6. Illustration of the idea of a parametric amplifier that uses a time-variable capacitance $C(t)$. The inductor L_s = const.

source of appropriate frequency, in relation to the frequency of the input signal E_g. Nonlinear (variable in time) capacitance (varactor) transfers energy from the pump circuit into the input signal circuit (R_s, L_s, C_s). In this way the energy (power) of the input signal (represented by E_g) is amplified and dissipated on the load resistance R_L. At the same time, sharpening of the frequency characteristics (resonance curve) of the parametric amplifier occurs. These are characteristic features of the parametric amplifier.

11.1. Proposed parametric: piezoelectric model of the OHC

A new physical (parametric-piezoelectric) model of the OHC cochlear amplifier was proposed by the author in 2013 [43]. This model explains the mechanisms of power amplification and frequency selectivity that occur in the cochlear amplifier. The proposed model is a direct consequence of the idea of Gold. In the following a physical interpretation of the active element is given. The active element is related to specific physical (physiological) components of the cochlea. The model proposed by the author removes most of the deficiencies of the existing models, presented in Sections 6–8.

Below, the proposed parametric amplifier model of the cochlea will be briefly described.

One OHC element is represented by a piezoelectric tube, see **Figure 7**. The left side of the OHC shown in **Figure 7** is the region of the OHC adjacent to the basilar membrane (BM). The right side of the OHC in **Figure 7** displays the apical part of the OHC in the vicinity of tectorial membrane (TM). Nonlinear capacitance $C(u)$ between the inner and the outer wall of the OHC is a key component of the proposed cochlear parametric amplifier.

11.2. Operation of the proposed OHC parametric-piezoelectric amplifier

Force source $F(t)$, on the left side of **Figure 7**, represents an input acoustic signal, which acts on the OHC from the BM side. Through the direct piezoelectric effect this force source $F(t)$ is transformed into the electric side as an alternating current (AC) voltage or current source. The cylinder, which represents the structure of the OHC exhibits piezoelectric properties. On the right side of **Figure 7**, one can see OHC stereocilia located at the apical part of the

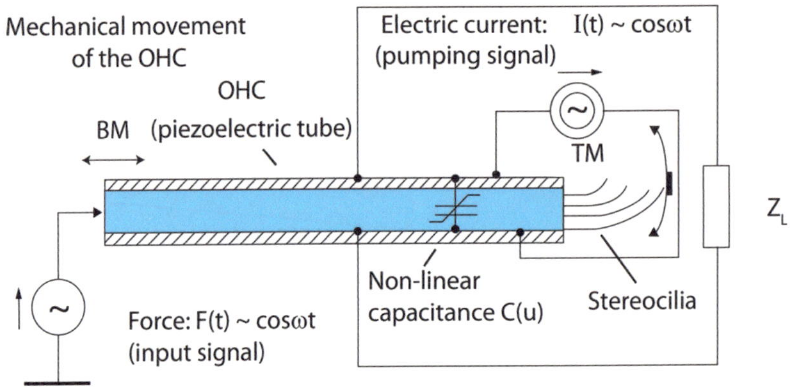

Figure 7. Simplified electromechanical diagram of a single OHC operating as a parametric amplifier. $F(t)$ represents the input acoustic signal, Z_L is the electrical load impedance, $C(u)$ is the nonlinear capacitance of the OHC, and u is the voltage between the inner and outer walls of the OHC.

OHC. Movement of stereocilia causes the flow of ionic currents (through the ion channels) into the bulk of the OHC. Taking place here, the phenomenon of forward mechano-electric transduction produces a transistor effect. As shown in **Figure 5**, the operation of the electromechanical transistor generates an alternating current source (AC). This variable current source $I(t)$, which is also visible at the top right in **Figure 7**, acts as a pumping signal that pumps power to the nonlinear capacitance of the OHC $C(u)$, which is visible on the right side of **Figure 7**.

This nonlinear capacitance $C(u)$ operates in a parametric amplifier circuit. Transformed, on the electric side, the input acoustic signal is amplified in this parametric amplifier circuit. Apart from the power amplification, the phenomenon of the sound sharpening (sharp tuning) occurs here. This enhanced (on the electrical side) acoustic input signal is subsequently transformed into the mechanical side (inverse piezoelectric effect), where it performs useful work on the TM and BM. The work carried out on the mechanical side represents, on the electrical side, the power that dissipates in the output circuit on the load resistance R_L. The electric power which is dissipated on the resistance R_L is not a lost power, i.e., it is not transformed to heat. On the contrary, this is the useful power that represents the amplified (on the electrical side) power of the input acoustic signal.

Sequence of the physical phenomena that occur in an individual OHC is as follows:

1. The incoming acoustic signal sets in motion the BM and TM membranes.

2. The movement of BM acts on a corresponding OHC and causes its motion with respect to TM. As a consequence, deflection of the OHC stereocilia occurs, which triggers operation of the proposed electromechanical transistor. In this stage, the transformation of mechanical energy into electric energy occurs.

3. Subsequently, nonlinear capacitance of the OHC is charged (pumped) by an AC current source $I(t) \sim \cos\omega t$, generated at the output of the proposed electromechanical amplifier

http://dx.doi.org/10.5772/66542

(EMT transistor). In fact, in the EMT transistor, the changes in the mechanical deflection of stereocilia are transformed to changes in the channel conductance and consequently to changes in the ion channel current (K^+ ions) flow, see **Figures 3a, b** and **4**. Power to the nonlinear capacitance $C(u)$ is supplied by an AC electric pump signal represented by the variable current source $I(t)$. The mechanism of power gain in the EMT transistor is similar to that occurring in the electronic field effect transistor, with a modulated channel conductance [40].

4. The input driving signal is an acoustic (mechanical) signal (represented by the force $F(t)$ and/or velocity $v(t)$) acting on the piezoelectric tube (OHC) from the basilar membrane (BM) side (see left side of **Figure 7**). Through the direct piezoelectric effect, this input (acoustic) mechanical signal is transferred to the electrical side as a voltage source $E(t)$ and then is amplified in the parametric amplifier based on a nonlinear capacitance $C(u)$. Power to the nonlinear capacitance is supplied by an AC electric pump signal represented by a variable current source $I(t)$.

5. The electric signal amplified at the output of the proposed parametric amplifier is dissipated (performs useful work) at the electrical load impedance Z_L. The output electrical signal is then transferred to the mechanical side by an inverse piezoelectric effect.

6. The output useful signal from the OHC amplifier is therefore a mechanical signal (force, velocity, or displacement) acting on the basilar membrane (BM) and tectorial membrane (TM) and as a consequence on stereocilia of the inner hair cells (IHCs). Finally, IHCs sensors transform mechanical signals into electrical signals (electric pulse trains) in afferent nerves connected to the central nervous system.

The power of the output mechanical signal in the OHC amplifier can surpass many times the power of an input acoustic signal. Since the parametric amplifier is a highly selective system, it can get a very narrow frequency characteristic (sharp tuning). More details concerning the operation of the proposed cochlear parametric amplifier can be found in the author's paper [43].

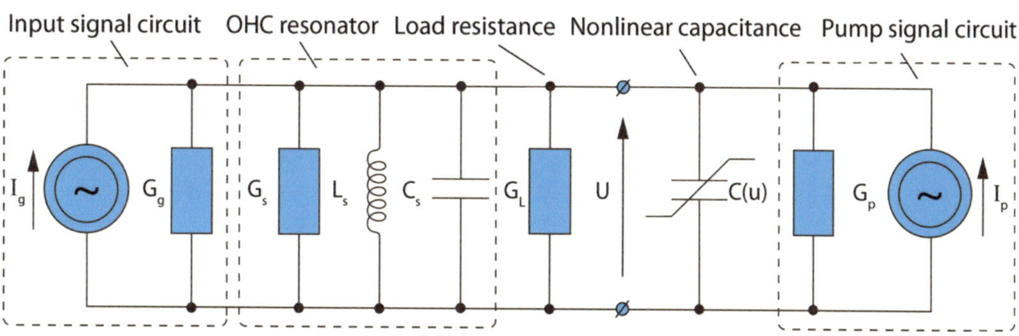

Figure 8. Nonlinear electrical equivalent (Norton) circuit of the proposed parametric cochlear amplifier built around a single OHC. I_g is the input signal current source, G_g is the source conductance, G_L is the load conductance, G_S is the loss conductance, L_s is the inductance of the OHC's resonator, $C(u)$ is the nonlinear capacitance, I_p is the pumping current source, and G_p is the pumping source conductance.

11.3. Nonlinear Norton equivalent circuit of the proposed parametric cochlear amplifier

The operation of a nonlinear oscillator resulting from the proposed model of the parametric cochlear amplifier can be described using the concept of a parallel (Norton) electrical equivalent circuit, see **Figure 8**.

The input electric signal, represented by the current source I_g with an admittance G_g (see left side of **Figure 8**), corresponds to the input acoustic signal transformed into electrical side by the direct piezoelectric effect. The input electrical signal I_g is subsequently amplified in the proposed parametric amplifier (formed with the nonlinear capacitance $C(u)$). The electric power is supplied to the circuit by the pumping current source I_p, which is generated by the forward mechano-electric transduction effect (see right side of **Figure 8**). After amplification, the electric signal is dissipated at the output load conductance G_L. The dissipated power is a useful output power of the proposed parametric amplifier.

It is noteworthy that mathematical description of the operation of the electrical circuit presented in **Figure 8** is a nonlinear ordinary differential equation of the second order. This equation results from Kirchhoff's laws applied to the circuit in **Figure 8**. The solution of this nonlinear equation describes nonlinear properties of the OHC amplifier for an arbitrary level of signals (small and large). For low-level signals, the solution of this equation should display an enhanced value of the quality factor and therefore higher value of amplification of the input signal.

11.4. Negative conductance

To explain the power amplification phenomenon in the parametric amplifier the concept of negative conductance was introduced. Negative conductance $-G_a$ occurs in parallel to the nonlinear capacitance $C(u)$ that represents an active element in the parametric amplifier. Positive conductance (resistance) dissipates electric power. By contrast, negative conductance supplies energy to the circuit. The negative conductance represents energy transfer from an external source to the circuit of the resonator, thereby the reduction of attenuation (undamping) of the resonant circuit occurs. In this way, the negative conductance characterizes an active element in the parametric amplifier circuit (e.g., the nonlinear capacitance of the OHC). The resultant conductance of the parallel OHC resonant circuit decreases ($G = G_s - G_a$) which increases the quality factor of the resonant circuit, see right side of **Figure 9**. As a result, a sharpening of the resonance curve of the resonant circuit occurs. This leads to higher sensitivity and selectivity

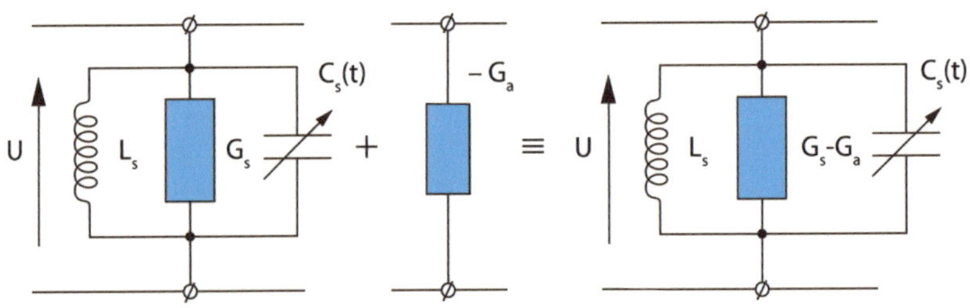

Figure 9. Operation of the active element, based on the nonlinear (time-varying) capacitance of an OHC, produces a negative conductance $-G_a$, which reduces the loss of the OHC resonant circuit and increases its quality factor.

(i.e., the ability to distinguish two tones with nearly the same frequencies, e.g., 1000 and 1005 Hz) of the proposed cochlear amplifier, as well as its power gain.

It is known from the classical circuit theory that parametric effect introduces an effective negative conductance (resistance) to the resonant parametric circuit, see **Figure 9**.

In summary, electromechanical parametric amplifier built with a single OHC performs the following functions:

1. amplifies the power of the input acoustical (electrical) signal,
2. increases the amplitude of the input acoustical (electrical) signal,
3. enhances the selectivity of the OHC's cochlear amplifier (larger quality factor Q), and
4. improves the sensitivity of the OHC's cochlear amplifier.

12. Interplay between HB motility and electromotility in the OHC

In previous theories of the cochlear amplification and selectivity sharpening the following hypotheses, about which type of motility is the prime mechanism of operation, were considered:

1. In active processes of power gain and sharpening of frequency selectivity involved is only HB motility.
2. In active processes of power gain and sharpening of frequency selectivity involved is only electromotility.
3. Both HB motility and electromotility are necessary for the operation the cochlear amplifier.

From the theoretical analysis performed by the author it follows that the correct choice is the third hypothesis, i.e., both mechanisms (HB motility and electromotility) are necessary to provide high sensitivity and sharp frequency selectivity in the mammalian cochlea. HB motility and electromotility in isolation cannot provide simultaneously power amplification and selectivity sharpening.

13. Role of the electrical phenomena

Remarkable properties of the hearing human organ (cochlea) are due to the presence in the cochlea of the sensory hair cells, i.e., OHCs and IHCs.

Electrical and mechanical phenomena occurring in the cochlea are mutually coupled. It is amazing that the flow of ionic currents (e.g., K^+ ions) in the cochlea is governed by the same laws as the flow of electric currents in conventional electronic circuits (i.e., Ohm's and the Kirchhoff's laws). Therefore, it was possible to establish an equivalent electrical circuit for the cochlear amplifier. Moreover, to model the operation of the cochlea (cochlear amplifier) we can employ elements well-known in the classical circuit theory, such as resistors, capacitors, inductors, voltage sources, and current sources both direct current (DC) and also alternating current (AC). In fact, the capacitors, inductors, and resistors in the equivalent electrical circuit of the cochlear amplifier are built of biological materials. In addition, these elements in the electrical equivalent circuit of the cochlear amplifier are lumped elements.

As it was shown in previous sections the role of electrical phenomena in the hearing process is enormous, since signal processing, power amplification, and frequency selectivity takes place on the electric side of the cochlear amplifier. The energy necessary to amplify the power of an input acoustic signal is drawn from the stria vascularis (DC voltage battery). Power amplification occurs in a circuit that consists of the following elements: input electromechanical transistor (formed by hair bundle stereocilia and ion channels), body of the OHC, and stria vascularis.

The fundamental element of the proposed cochlear amplifier is a parametric amplifier using the nonlinear capacitance of the OHC and its piezoelectric effect. The cochlear parametric amplifier is pumped by an electrical current source formed by ionic currents triggered by deflection of stereocilia (input electromechanical transistor). In the cochlear amplifier, a DC electric power is converted to an AC electric power. Moreover, the transformation of electrical to mechanical energy and vice versa occurs due to direct and inverse piezoelectric effect. In this parametric amplifier the sharpening of frequency selectivity occurs.

Operation of the cochlear amplifier can be compared to the operation of an "old fashioned" analog "straight" radio receiver (i.e., a receiver with a direct amplification, without frequency mixing). In a classical analog transistor, "straight" radio receiver, one can enumerate the following elements:

1. antenna,

2. selective amplifier,

3. detector,

4. power amplifier, and

5. loudspeaker.

Similar elements and associated processes can be found in the human cochlea. Namely, the role of the antenna in the cochlea is played by the outer ear and middle ear, the role of the selective and power amplifier is played by the cochlear amplifier, and the main components of the cochlear amplifier are OHCs. The role of loudspeaker is played by afferent nerves endings.

13.1. Novelty of the proposed parametric-piezoelectric model

Novelty of the model proposed by the author relies on the use of well-known electronics idea of parametric amplification. Exploration of this concept was motivated by the existence in the actual structure of the cochlea and the nonlinear electrical capacitance of the OHC. It is worth noticing that in existing models of the cochlear amplifier, the presence of nonlinear capacitance is ignored.

The model proposed by the author is able to explain in a logical, natural, and complete way the following so far unresolved physical processes occurring in the cochlear amplifier: (1) power amplification, (2) selectivity of acoustic signals reception, and (3) nonlinear phenomena.

13.2. Physical (physiological) model

The model proposed by the author is a physical and a not phenomenological model. The main element of the model is the parametric amplifier providing adequate gain, sensitivity, frequency selectivity, and dynamics. Elements of the model are uniquely linked to the actual physical (physiological) components that are present in a single OHC and in the entire cochlea. Moreover, these elements are directly related to the physical phenomena occurring in a single OHC and in the inner ear (electromotility, the flow of ionic currents, piezoelectricity, nonlinear capacitance, stereocilia movements, movements of the basilar membrane, nonlinear effects, generation of electrical potentials by metabolic processes in the stria vascularis, etc.). The model is internally coherent, consistent with experimental data published in the literature and it describes comprehensibly (qualitatively and quantitatively) the phenomena of the cochlear amplification.

13.3. Results of numerical simulations with the new model

The results of numerical calculations (simulations) with the new model have been presented previously by the author in his two former papers [40, 43]. Here, we will repeat briefly some results showing increased frequency selectivity due to the parametric effect occurring in the OHC parametric amplifier.

Applying the Kirchhoff's laws to the linearized equivalent circuits (series and parallel), describing the operation of the parametric amplifier built around a single OHC, gives rise to linear ordinary differential equations of the Mathieu and Ince types [43]. The resulting differential equations of the second order with variable in time coefficients were solved numerically (for various values of frequency) using a Scilab software package. In the numerical simulations the resonant frequency of the resonant circuit (OHC oscillator) was assumed as $f_0 = 1000$ Hz.

The following values of the parameters of the equivalent (parallel Norton) circuit were applied:

1. Conductance of the input signal source G_g, conductance of the resonant circuit G_s, and the load conductance G_L are in the range from 7.5 to 23 nS.
2. The linear capacitance of the OHC is about 30 pF. Maximum of the nonlinear capacitance is 25 pF.
3. The value of the input signal current source is $I_g = 30$ pA.

The above numerical values of the elements of the equivalent circuit are compatible with the physiological data [8, 24, 35, 44–46].

The results of numerical calculations with the Scilab package show that using the above parameters, the parametric effect increases the quality factor of the OHC resonator from $Q = 12$ to $Q = 120$ (10 times). It is noteworthy that the passive OHC resonator with the quality factor 12 has an effective frequency bandwidth of 80 Hz (8%), for example, from 960 to 1040 Hz. On the other hand, the active OHC resonator with the quality factor 120 has an effective frequency bandwidth of 8 Hz (0.8%), for example, from 996 to 1004 Hz. The latter case represents a remarkable frequency selectivity (0.8%) enabling for frequency discrimination much narrower than one semitone in modern musical scales (6%).

13.4. Consequences resulting from the author's model

1. Power amplification of the acoustic signal occurs in the circuit of the input electromechanical transistor formed by stereocilia of an outer hair cell (OHC), ion channels, bulk of the OHC, and the stria vascularis. Selectivity of the reception of acoustic signals is realized by a parametric amplifier based on the nonlinear capacitance of the OHC and the piezoelectric phenomenon.

2. Electromechanical transistor (based on the forward mechano-electric transduction) supplies (pumps) the power to the nonlinear capacitance (parametric amplifier), producing a negative resistance in the resonant circuit.

3. The parametric amplifier is realized with a reactive element (nonlinear capacitance), not on a resistive element (like laser amplifier or tunnel diode amplifier). It is worth noticing that a source of noise is mostly resistive elements. From that reason, the parametric amplifier exhibits a very good noise characteristics.

4. By the inverse piezoelectric effect (electromotility), amplified acoustic (on electric side) signal is transformed into the mechanical side where it stimulates the tectorial membrane (TM).

5. Both mechanisms (HB-motility and electromotility) must operate simultaneously in order to achieve the power amplification and selectivity in the cochlear amplifier.

6. TM stimulates mechanically stereocilia of the IHC. Thus, the mechanical energy from the TM is delivered to the IHC stereocilia and transformed by the IHC into electrical ion currents. These currents excite the afferent nerves, which generate a series of electrical impulses that are transmitted into the central nervous system.

14. Conclusions

The new theory of the hearing processes, proposed by the author, links together the concepts emerged in former theories of hearing, such as a resonant theory, travelling wave theory, and Gold's theory of active amplification (cochlear amplifier). The new model of the phenomena occurring in the cochlea is a physical (physiological) model (not phenomenological), in which the role and operation of individual elements of the actual cochlea are explained qualitatively and quantitatively.

To initiate the research on the mechanism of hearing the author was motivated by incompleteness of the existing models of the hearing process. In fact, the existing theories of hearing are phenomenological in nature and do not directly correspond to the physical components in the

http://dx.doi.org/10.5772/66542

cochlea. Another stimulus was a potential importance for various possible applications, such as hearing aids, digital sound coding, perception of music, etc.

Full physical model of the cochlea is described mathematically by nonlinear ordinary differential equations (ODE). Linearized physical model of the cochlea is described by linear ODE of Mathieu and Ince's type. In the established model of the cochlea new concepts from electronics (e.g., parametric amplification and electromechanical transistor) are applied. This goes significantly beyond the range of methods and concepts used so far in the existing theories of the hearing.

The model proposed by the author explains the process of power amplification and frequency selectivity that take place in the cochlear amplifier. By contrast, existing models of the cochlear amplifier are incomplete and do not describe satisfactorily the physical processes that occur in the organ of Corti. Furthermore, in scope of the author's model, the phenomenon of an otoacoustic emission can be described.

The new model of a single OHC, developed by the author, conforms qualitatively to the existing experimental data. A novel refined theory of the hearing processes, based on the piezoelectricity and parametric amplification, can open new horizons for research including deeper understanding of the physical phenomena underlying auditory processes, new phenomena in musical and speech acoustics, etc. This may create a possibility to design new musical instruments as well as new audio codecs that could outperform the existing MP3 codecs.

The author hopes that the results of this study (which relate to the validity of crucial electrical phenomena occurring in the cochlea) can also be useful in the construction and design of a new generation of hearing aids. Today, most hearing aids are based on power amplification of the input audio signals at specific frequencies without increasing the selectivity (the ability to distinguish between signals of different frequencies).

Therefore, the future hearing aids should be more closely based on the knowledge of complicated electrical and mechanical phenomena occurring in the cochlea. In these devices, in addition to the power amplification of the input acoustic signal, adequate selectivity of acoustic signal reception (sharpening of the receiving characteristics of the receiver—the cochlear amplifier) should also be ensured.

Glossary of technical terms	
Acoustic waves	Pressure disturbances propagating in gases, liquids, and solids. Acoustic waves rarely propagate along straight lines, but can be easily reflected, refracted, diffracted, or guided
AC signal	A signal which is variable in time
Active element	An element, which can deliver more (useful) active energy than it consumes
Admittance	An element, defined as the inverse of impedance. Electrical admittance is a measure of how readily the circuit or device allows a current to flow
Actuator	A component of a device which is responsible for moving or controlling a mechanism or system

Glossary of technical terms	
Ampere (A)	The SI unit of electric current intensity. If the current flowing through a cross-section of a conductor has intensity of 1 A, then within 1 s the charge of 1 C flows through this cross-section, namely: 1 A = 1 C/s, where C stands for the coulomb and s for the second
Anions	Negatively charged ions
Bandwidth	A difference between the maximum and minimum frequencies handled by a device
Bipolar transistor	A transistor that uses both negative electrons and positive holes, in contrast to unipolar FET transistors
Capacitor	A passive electrical element, which can store electrical energy. Capacitance of the capacitor is measured in farads (F) to honor English scientist M. Faraday (1791–1867). 1 F = 1 C/1 V, where C stands for the coulomb and V for the volt. Typical capacitance may vary from about 1 pF (10^{-12} F) to about 1 mF (10^{-3} F)
Cations	Positively charged ions
Charge	A measure of the amount of electricity. The electric charge is measured in coulombs to honor French physicist C.A. Coulomb (1736–1806). 1 C = 1 As, where A stands for the ampere and s is the second. There are positive and negative charges. The electric charge is a discrete quantity. The smallest electric charge is carried by the electron. An electron has a charge equal $1e = 1.602 \times 10^{-19}$ coulombs
Circuit theory	A set of techniques, definitions, and mathematical tools used to describe the flow of currents and voltage distribution in electrical networks composed of lumped passive and active elements. The theory includes Ohm's law, Kirchhoff's laws, and theorems (Thévenin, Norton), which are based on first physical principles, such as conservation of energy, conservation of electrical charge, etc.
Conductance	A resistive electrical element defined as an inverse to the electrical resistance
Coulomb (C)	The SI unit of electric charge, defined as the charge carried by a constant current of intensity of 1 A that passes through a cross-section of a conductor in one second. Therefore, charge $Q = It$, where I is the current and t is time
Current source	An active electrical element providing DC or AC electric current on its terminals
DC battery	A source of potential electrical energy
DC signal	A signal, which is constant in time
Decibel (dB)	A logarithmic unit used to express the ratio of two values of a physical quantity. For example, the device dynamics, measured in dB, equals 10 $\log_{10}(P_2/P_1)$, where P_2 and P_1 correspond, respectively, to the maximum and minimum input power, which can be properly handled by the device
Differential equation	An equation for an unknown function, e.g., $y(t)$ containing sum of derivatives up to a certain order. For example, a differential equation describing harmonic oscillations contains derivatives up to order two

http://dx.doi.org/10.5772/66542

Glossary of technical terms	
Direct piezoelectric effect	A generation of net electrical charges (voltage) in the material subjected to a mechanical stress (direct piezoelectric effect). Direct piezoelectric effect was discovered in 1880 by French physicists brothers Jacques (1855–1941) and Pierre (1859–1906) Currie
Dynamic range (dynamics)	The ratio P_2/P_1 of the maximum P_2 and minimum power P_1 of the input signal, which can be handled properly by the device. Dynamics is often expressed in a logarithmic scale in dB as $10\log(P_2/P_1)$. If power density $P_2 = 1\ \mathrm{W/m^2}$ and $P_1 = 10^{-6}\ \mathrm{W/m^2}$ then the dynamics equals $10\log(1/10^{-6}) = 60$ dB
Equivalent circuit	An electrical circuit with lumped elements, providing precise, but often simplified description of complex phenomena occurring in a physical device or system
Electric current	A stream of electrically charged particles flowing in a medium. The intensity of the electric current is measured in amperes (A) to honor French physicist A.M. Ampère (1775–1836). 1 A = 1 C/s, where C stands for the coulomb and s for the second
Electrical impedance	The ratio of the voltage applied to an electrical element (capacitor, resistor, inductor) to the electrical current flowing through the element. Electrical impedance is measured in Ohms (Ω) to honor German physicist G.S. Ohm (1789–1854). 1 Ω = 1 V/1 A, where V stands for the volt and A for the ampere
Electrical side	The electrical port of a multiport electromechanical device + an electric circuit connected to this port
Electrolyte	A substance that produces an electrically conducting solution, when dissolved in a polar solvent, such as water. The dissolved electrolyte separates into positively charged cations and negative anions
Electromechanical control element (EMCE)	A time variable electrical resistance $R(t)$ controlled by a time-varying input mechanical (e.g., acoustic) signals
Electromechanical transistor	A device to control mechanically the flow of electrical energy from a DC voltage source to the load resistance. This device can amplify an input acoustic signal and transform it into the output electrical signal with enhanced power
Energy	The ability of a system to perform work. Energy is measured in joules (J) to honor English physicist J.P. Joule (1818–1889). 1 J = 1 Ws, where W stands for the watt and s for the second
Field effect transistor (FET)	A transistor that uses an electric field to control the shape and hence the electrical conductivity of a channel with one type of charge carriers (electrons or holes) in a semiconductor material. FETs are also known as unipolar transistors as they involve a single carrier (negative or positive) type operation
Frequency selectivity	An ability of the device (system) to discriminate between two signals with close frequencies. It is an analogue of spatial resolution in optical devices
Hopf bifurcation	An advanced mathematical concept from the theory of nonlinear differential equations, gained popularity in some mathematical models of the cochlea

Glossary of technical terms	
Inductor	A passive electrical element, which can store magnetic energy. Inductance of the inductor is measured in henrys (H) to honor American scientist J. Henry (1797–1878). 1 H = 1 Wb/1 A, where Wb stands for the weber and A for the ampere
Inverse piezoelectric effect	An occurrence of a mechanical stress or deformation in the material subjected to the electrical voltage. Inverse piezoelectric effect was predicted from thermodynamic considerations in 1881 by French scientist and inventor G. Lippmann (1845–1921)
Joule (J)	The SI unit of energy. 1 J = 1 Ws, where W stands for the watt and s for the second
Kirchhoff's voltage law	It states that, an algebraic sum of all voltages on lumped elements in an arbitrary closed loop in a circuit is always zero. The law was discovered in 1845 by German physicist G. Kirchhoff (1824–1887). Kirchhoff's Voltage Law is a direct consequence of the principle of conservation of energy
Kirchhoff's current law	It states that, an algebraic sum of all electric currents flowing into and out of a node in an electric circuit equals zero. Kirchhoff's Current Law is a direct consequence of the principle of conservation of charge
Longitudinal waves	Acoustic waves with particle vibrations parallel to the direction of propagation (called sometimes compressional waves)
Lumped element	A mechanical (spring, dashpot, mass) or electrical (capacitor, resistor, inductor) element with no spatial dimensions. Lumped elements are adequately described by circuit theory
Mechanical displacement	A difference in the positions of a mechanical particle e.g., a particle that is stimulated to vibrations by an acoustic wave
Mechanical impedance	The ratio of the force applied to a mechanical element (spring, dashpot, mass) to the velocity at which the element moves. Mechanical impedance is measured in Ns/m, where N stands for Newton, m for meter, and s for the second
Mechanical side	The mechanical port of a multiport electromechanical device + mechanic elements connected to this port
Mechanical stress	The force per unit area. Mechanical stress is measured in pascals (Pa) to honor French scientist, mathematician and philosopher B. Pascal (1623–1662). 1 Pa = 1 N/m^2, where N stands for Newton and m for the meter
Micrometer (μm)	One millionth part of the meter (10^{-6} m)
Millivolt (mV)	One thousandth part of the volt (10^{-3} V)
Noise	Any unwanted signal, random or coherent
Nonlinear capacitance	An electrical capacitance, which value depends on voltage on its terminals. The constitutive equation for the nonlinear capacitance $C(u)$ is given by $Q = C(u)u$, where Q stands for the electrical charge and u for the electric voltage on the nonlinear capacitance
Nonlinear oscillators	An oscillator containing at least one nonlinear element
Nanometer (nm)	One billionth part of the meter (1 nm = 10^{-9} m)
Nanosiemens (nS)	One billionth part of the siemens (1 nS = 10^{-9} S)

http://dx.doi.org/10.5772/66542

Glossary of technical terms	
Norton equivalent circuit	Any network of linear sources and impedances at a given frequency can be presented as an equivalent current source connected in parallel with an equivalent admittance. This equivalent circuit was proposed in 1926 by Bell Labs Engineer E. L. Norton (1898–1983)
Negative conductance	A resistive electric element supplying energy to the circuit, by contrast to a positive resistance (conductance) which dissipates energy into heat
Ohm's law	It states that, the current flowing through a conductor is directly proportional to the voltage across the conductor terminals. Therefore, the current $I = U/R$, where U is the electric voltage and R is the resistance of the conductor
Picoampere (pA)	One trillionth part of the ampere (1 pA = 10^{-12} A)
Parametric oscillator	A harmonic oscillator containing at least one reactive element with a value varying in time
Parametric-piezoelectric amplifier	A parametric amplifier employing the nonlinear OHC capacitance to achieve power amplification and frequency selectivity. Direct piezoelectric effect transforms an input acoustic signal into the electrical side (sensor). Subsequently, an inverse piezoelectric effect transforms the enhanced output electrical signal on the mechanical side (actuator)
Passive element	An element, which can only store or dissipate energy, but cannot generate energy
Picofarad (pF)	One trillionth part of the farad (1 pF = 10^{-12} F)
Phenomenological model	A set of mathematical expressions that relate several different empirical observations of phenomena to each other, in a way which is consistent with fundamental theory, but is not directly derived from theory. In other words, a phenomenological model is not derived from first principles
Potential energy	An energy stored in the system. The notion of potential energy was introduced by Scottish engineer W. Rankine (1820–1872). Potential energy is measured in joules (J) to honor English physicist J.P. Joule (1818–1889). 1 J = 1 Ws, where W stands for the watt and s for the second
Power	The rate at which energy is generated or consumed. Power is measured in watts (W) to honor Scottish engineer and inventor J. Watt (1736–1819). 1 W = 1 J/s, where J stands for the joule and s stands for the second
Power amplification	Property of the device (system), in which more (useful) power is flowing out of the device than into the device
Pressure	The force applied perpendicular to the surface of a medium per unit area. Pressure is measured in pascals (Pa) to honor French scientist, mathematician and philosopher B. Pascal (1623–1662). 1 Pa = 1 N/m^2, where N stands for Newton and m for the meter
Quality factor	A quantity characterizing sharpness of the resonant circuit. It is defined as the ratio of the resonant frequency to the bandwidth of the resonant circuit
Resistor	A passive electrical element, which dissipates energy. Resistance of the resistor is measured in Ohms (Ω) to honor German physicist G.S. Ohm (1789–1854). 1 Ω = 1 V/1 A, where V stands for the volt and A for the ampere

Glossary of technical terms	
Resonant circuit	A passive electrical or mechanical circuit with two different type of reactive elements (capacitor and inductor or spring and mass), connected in series or in parallel. It displays a natural, preferred frequency of oscillations
Sensitivity	The lowest level of the input signal, applied to the device, resulting in an output signal of an acceptable quality (signal-to-noise ratio)
Sensor	A device which provides a usable output in response to a specified physical stimulus. Sensors are more general than transducers, since their input and output energies may be different, like in transducers, or the same
Siemens (S)	The SI unit of the electrical conductance. $1\ S = 1/\Omega$, where Ω stands for the ohm. Siemens was introduced to honor German inventor and industrialist E.W. von Siemens (1816–1892)
Signal frequency	Number of cycles per second for a sinusoidal signal. Frequency is measured in hertz (Hz) to honor German physicist H. R. Hertz (1857–1894). $1\ Hz = 1/s$, where s stands for the second
Tonotopy	A property of the device (system) in which different signal frequencies are processes in different locations within the device. Tonotopy was introduced by German physicist and physician H. von Helmholtz (1821–1894)
Transducer	A device which converts one form of energy to another. For example, piezoelectric transducer converts mechanical signals to electrical signals (sensor) and vice versa (actuator)
Transverse waves	Acoustic waves with particle vibrations perpendicular to the direction of propagation (called sometimes shear waves)
Vacuum tubes	Electronic devices used to process and amplify electric signals, before appearance of transistors
Varactor	A nonlinear (time-varying) capacitor which capacitance depends on voltage applied to its terminals. By contrast, capacitance of a linear capacitor is constant and does not depend on voltage across its terminals. Varactor constitutes the main component of the parametric amplifier
Volt (V)	The SI unit of voltage. $1\ V = 1\ W/1\ A$, where W stands for the watt and A for the ampere
Voltage	The difference between an electrical potential at two points. Voltage is measured in volts (V) to honor Italian physicist A. Volta (1745–1827).
Voltage source	An active electrical element providing DC or AC electric voltage on its terminals
Watt (W)	The SI unit of power. $1\ W = 1\ J/s$, where J stands for the joule s for the second

Author details

Piotr Kiełczyński

Address all correspondence to: pkielczy@ippt.gov.pl

Laboratory of Acoustoelectronics, Institute of Fundamental Technological Research, Polish Academy of Sciences, Warsaw, Poland

References

[1] Elliott S.J., Shera C.A., (2012), The cochlea as a smart structure, Smart Materials and Structures, vol. 21, 064001 (11 pp). DOI:10.1088/0964-1726/21/6/064001

[2] van der Heijden M., Versteegh C.P.C., (2015), Questioning cochlear amplification, AIP Conference Proceedings 1703, 050002; DOI: 10.1063/1.4939347

[3] Allen J.B., Neely S.T., (1992) Micromechanical models of the cochlea, Physics Today, vol. 45, 40–47. DOI: 10.1063/1.881349

[4] Benson D.J., (2006), Music: A Mathematical Offering, Cambridge University Press, Cambridge, UK, Chapter 5.14, p. 190, ISBN: 0521853877

[5] Gold T., (1948), The physical basis of action in the cochlea, Proceedings of the Royal Society London, Biological Sciences, vol. 135, 492–498.

[6] Davis H., (1983), An active process in cochlear mechanics, Hearing Research, vol. 9, no 1, 79–90.

[7] Ashmore J., Avan P., Brownell W.E., Dallos P., Dierkes K., Fettiplace R., Grosh K., Hackney C.M., Hudspeth A.J., Jülicher F., Lindner B., Martin P., Meaud J., Petit C., Santos Sacchi J.R., Canlon B., (2010), The remarkable cochlear amplifier, Hearing Research, vol. 266, no 1, 1–17. DOI: 10.1016/j.heares.2009.12.005

[8] Ospeck M., Dong X., Iwasa K.H., (2003), Limiting frequency of the cochlear amplifier based on electromotility of outer hair cells, Biophysical Journal, vol. 84, 739–749. DOI: 10.1016/S0006-3495(03)74893-0

[9] Fridberger A., Tomo I., Ulfendahl M., Boutet de Monvel J., (2006), Imaging hair cell transduction at the speed of sound: Dynamic behavior of mammalian stereocilia, PNAS, vol. 103, 1918–1923. DOI: 10.1073_pnas.0507231103

[10] Spector A., Jean R.P., (2004), Modes and balance of energy in the piezoelectric cochlear outer hair cell wall, Journal of Biomechanical Engineering, vol. 126, 17–25. DOI: 10.1073_pnas.0507231103

[11] Royer D., Dieulesaint E., (2000), Elastic Waves in Solids I, Chapter 3.3, p. 147, Springer, Berlin, ISBN 3-540-65931-5

[12] Van Valkenburg M.E., (1974), Network Analysis, Prentice-Hall, Englewood Cliff, NJ.

[13] Wang X., Guo W.W., Yang S.M., (2012), Quantitative relations between outer hair cell electromotility and nonlinear capacitance, Journal of Otology, vol. 7, no 1, 45–53. DOI: 10.1016/S1672-2930(12)50010-3

[14] Reichenbach T., Hudspeth A.J., (2014), The physics of hearing: fluid mechanics and the active process of the inner ear, Reports on Progress in Physics, vol. 77, 076601 (45 pp). DOI: 10.1088/0034-4885/77/7/076601

[15] Zweig G., (2016), Nonlinear cochlear mechanics, Journal of the Acoustical Society of America, vol. 139, no 5, 2561–2578. DOI: 10.1121/1.4941249

[16] Helmholtz H.L.F., (1954), On the Sensation of Tone as a Physiological Basis for the Theory of Music, Dover Publications Inc., New York.

[17] Bekesy G., (1960), Experiments in Hearing, McGrow-Hill, New York.

[18] Kemp D.T., (1978), Stimulated acoustic emissions from within the human auditory system, Journal of the Acoustical Society of America, vol. 64, no 5, 1386–1391. DOI: 10.1121/1.382104

[19] Ni G., Elliott S.J., Baumgart J., (2016), Finite-element model of the active organ of Corti, Journal of the Royal Society Interface, vol. 13, 20150913. DOI: 10.1098/rsif.2015.0913

[20] Nin F., Yoshida T., Sawamura S., Ogata G., Ota T., Higuchi T., Murakami S., Doi K., Kurachi Y., Hibino H., (2016), The unique electrical properties in an extracellular fluid of the mammalian cochlea; their functional roles, homeostatic processes, and pathological significance, Pflügers Archiv – European Journal of Physiology, vol. 468, no 10, 1637–1649. DOI 10.1007/s00424-016-1871-0

[21] Eguiluz V.M., Ospeck M., Choe Y., Hudspeth A.J., Magnasco M.O., (2000), Essential nonlinearities in hearing, Physical Review Letters, vol. 84, no 22, 5232–5235. DOI: 10.1103/PhysRevLett.84.5232

[22] Hudspeth A.J., Jülicher F., Martin P., (2010), A critique of the critical cochlea: Hopf – a bifurcation – is better than none, Journal of Neurophysiology, vol. 104, no 3, 1219–1229. DOI:10.1152/jn.00437.2010

[23] Hudde H., (2011), The Corti resonator – an actively driven system underlying the cochlear amplifier, Forum Acusticum, Aalborg, Denmark, pp. 1085–1089. ISBN: 978-84-694-1520-7

[24] Ramamoorthy S., Nuttall A.L., (2012), Outer hair cell somatic electromotility in vivo and power transfer to the organ of Corti, Biophysical Journal, vol. 102, no 2, 388–398. DOI: 10.1016/j.bpj.2011.12.040

[25] Szalai R., Champneys A., Homer M., (2013), Comparison of nonlinear mammalian cochlear-partition models, Journal of the Acoustical Society of America, vol. 133, no 1, 323–336. doi: 10.1121/1.4768868

[26] Liu Y., Gracewski S.M., Nam J.H., (2015), Consequences of location-dependent organ of Corti micro-mechanics, PLoS ONE, vol. 10, no 8, e0133284 (25 pp). DOI: 10.1371/journal.pone.0133284

[27] Iwasa K.H., (2016), Energy output from a single outer hair cell, arXiv.1601.01643v1 [phys-bio-physics] 7 Jan., 1–21.

[28] Cohen A., Furst M., (2004), Integration of outer hair cell activity in a one-dimensional cochlear model, Journal of the Acoustical Society of America, vol. 115, no 5, 2185–2192. DOI: 10.1121/1.1699391

[29] Bell J.A., (2005), The underwater piano: A resonance theory of cochlear mechanics, PhD thesis, Research School of Biological Sciences, The Australian National University, Canberra, Australia.

[30] Martignoli S., van der Vywer J.J., Kern A., Uwate Y., Stoop R., (2007), Analog electronic cochlea with mammalian hearing characteristics, Applied Physics Letters, vol. 91, no 6, 064108-1-3. DOI: 10.1063/1.2768204

[31] Ramamoorthy S., Deo N.V., Grosh K., (2007), A mechano-electro-acoustical model for the cochlea: Response to acoustic stimuli, Journal of the Acoustical Society of America, vol. 121, no 5, 2758–2773. DOI: 10.1121/1.2713725

[32] Liu Y.W., Neely S.T., (2009), Outer hair cell electromechanical properties in a nonlinear piezoelectric model, Journal of the Acoustical Society of America, vol. 126, no 2, 751–761. DOI: 10.1121/1.3158919

[33] Stasiunas A., Verikasa A., Miliauskas R., Stasiuniene N., (2009), An adaptive model simulating the somatic motility and the active hair bundle motion of the OHC, Computers in Biology and Medicine, vol. 39, 800–809. DOI:10.1016/j.compbiomed.2009.06.010

[34] Shintaku H., Nakagawa T., Kitagawa D., Tanujaya H., Kawano S., Ito J., (2010), Development of piezoelectric acoustic sensor with frequency selectivity for artificial cochlea, Sensors and Actuators A, vol. 158, 183–192. DOI:10.1016/j.sna.2009.12.021

[35] Reichenbach T., Hudspeth A.J., (2010), A ratchet mechanism for amplification in low-frequency mammalian hearing, Proceedings of the National Academy of Sciences U.S.A, vol. 107, no 11, 4973–4978. DOI: 10.1073/pnas.0914345107

[36] Nam J.H., Fettiplace R., (2012), Optimal electrical properties of outer hair cells ensure cochlear amplification, PLoS ONE, vol. 7, no 11, e50572 (10 pp). DOI: 10.1371/journal.pone.0050572

[37] Sabo D., Barzelay O., Weiss S., Furst M., (2014), Fast evaluation of a time-domain non-linear cochlear model, Journal of Computational Physics, vol. 265, 97–112. DOI: 10.1016/j.jcp.2014.01.044

[38] Ayat M., Teal P., McGuinness M., (2014), An integrated electromechanical model for the cochlear microphonics, Biocybernetics and Biomedical Engineering, vol. 34, no 4, 206–209. DOI: 10.1016/j.bbe.2014.06.001

[39] Shera C. A., (2007), Laser amplification with a twist: Travelling-wave propagation and gain functions from throughout the cochlea, Journal of the Acoustical Society of America, vol. 122, no 5, 2738–2758. DOI: 10.1121/1.2783205

[40] Kiełczyński P., Szalewski M., (2014), Transistor effect in the cochlear amplifier, Archives of Acoustics, vol. 39, no. 1, 117–124. DOI: 10.2478/aoa-2014-0012

[41] Shera C.A., Bergevin C., (2012), Obtaining reliable phase-gradient delays from otoacoustic emission data, Journal of the Acoustical Society of America, vol. 132, no 2, 927–943. DOI: 10.1121/1.4730916

[42] Shera C.A., Abdala C., (2016), Frequency shifts in distortion-product otoacoustic emissions evoked by swept tones, Journal of the Acoustical Society of America, vol. 140, no 2, 936. DOI: 10.1121/1.4960592

[43] Kiełczyński P., (2013), Power amplification and selectivity in the cochlear amplifier, Archives of Acoustics, vol. 38, no. 1, 83–92. DOI: 10.2478/aoa-2013-0010

[44] Weitzel E.K., Tasker R., Brownell W.E., (2003), Outer hair cell piezoelectricity: Frequency response enhancement and resonant behavior, Journal of the Acoustical Society of America, vol. 114, no 3, 1462–1466. DOI: 10.1121/1.1596172

[45] Lu T.K., Zhak S., Dallos P., Sarpeshkar R., (2006), Fast cochlear amplification with slow outer hair cells, Hearing Research, vol. 214, 45–67. DOI: 10.1016/j.heares.2006.01.018

[46] Fettiplace R., (2006), Active hair cell movement in auditory hair cells, Journal of Physiology, vol. 576,. 29–36. DOI: 10.1113/jphysiol.2006.115949

Section 4

Aging

Chapter 6

Hearing Impairment in Old Age

Gro Gade Haanes

Additional information is available at the end of the chapter

http://dx.doi.org/10.5772/66372

Abstract

Background

Age related hearing impairment is a risk factor for functional decline, reduced social participation and accidents.

Aims

To obtain knowledge about the characteristics of age related hearing impairments and to help elderly optimize their hearing function.

Design and method

Study 1; Baseline description of data on hearing impairments. Study 2; ROC curve to compare self-assessments with a gold standard test. Study 3; RCT to test whether removal of earwax, and referral to a specialist can improve functional hearing.

Results

More than 90% had hearing impairments. Mean PTAV was 40,4 dB. Self-assessment of hearing function with a single global question correlated only weakly with the PTAV measurements. Comparison yielded 18 false negatives, indicating many reported their hearing as good when the standardized test indicated that it was not.

Conclusion

Elderly people live with hearing impairments not sufficiently attended to. Asking about their hearing with a single global question will not provide accurate information. It is necessary to use standardized tests in addition. When asking more detailed questions about communication abilities, the elderly reported having difficulties. Many elderly could not be expected to do all the self-care activities necessary to improve their functional hearing. Close monitoring and assistance is recommended.

Keywords: hearing loss, hearing impairment, sensory impairment, old age, elderly

1. Introduction

The proportion of elderly aged ≥80 years of age (the 80+) is expected to increase dramatically over the next few decades and is projected to triple in Europe by 2060 [1]. Both the World Health Organization (WHO) and the European Union (EU) are concerned with programs on successful aging [2], and since hearing impairment is a known risk factor for functional decline, reduced social participation, withdrawal, and accidents [3–6], good functional hearing is therefore crucially important for elderly to be able to manage themselves and take care of their own lives and maybe also help their partner or spouse [7–10]. For patients in a home-care setting, hearing impairment can cause additional stress along with reduced capacity and other health challenges [11].

Hearing impairment is however a natural part of old age, and most people will experience increasingly impaired hearing as they grow older, but because this impairment can threaten functioning and well-being, communication, and quality of life, it is important to shed light on this issue and to help the elderly with this problem [7, 11, 12]. Age-related hearing impairments are sometimes possible to remedy or improve, but it is important to discover and tend to this issue as early as possible [6, 13].

Traditionally, hearing impairments have to a large extent been an area for the elderly themselves or their relatives have been responsible for, but it seems that there is a lack of information because many elderly never check their hearing, apply for hearing aids, or seek any other professional help for their hearing impairment [13, 14].

Hearing is connected to the memory function and there is evidence that hearing impairment can have an impact on the mental functioning [15–17]. Age-related hearing impairment is correlated with Alzheimer disease, and reduced hearing can contribute to falls and fractures [18], greater dependence on others, and loneliness [19–21]. For those who have ailments and chronic diseases, hearing impairments constitute an additional negative factor to the other problems and perhaps an unnecessary burden, which may lead to the latter part of life being more troublesome than necessary [11, 22]. Since age-related sensory impairments in general have been taken care by the elderly themselves, it has largely been overlooked by nurses in the home-care service and by health authorities in general [4, 23]. Knowledge and understanding about how to maintain the hearing function in old age seem to be crucial in order to manage every day activities, daily living, and participation in social activities, even if one has other health challenges and is receiving home care [24].

Decline in sensory abilities and their effects on physical and psychosocial capacities in older individuals have been discussed in previous studies [15–17], however, most prevalence studies of hearing impairments involve population from the general community and include people from younger age groups, so studies among older people over 80 years receiving home care are few.

Grue [11] has discussed the burden of dual sensory impairment in the elderly and also the risk of falling when hearing is impaired.

http://dx.doi.org/10.5772/66372

One would think that it is in the elderly's own interest to maintain the function of the hearing sense throughout the life course, but our randomized, controlled trial indicated that many elderly could not be expected to do all the self-care activities necessary to improve their hearing function themselves. Close monitoring and assistance is necessary.

2. Presbycusis and hearing impairment

Age-related hearing impairment (presbycusis) is characterized by reduced hearing sensitivity and speech understanding in noisy environments, and an impaired ability to localize sound sources [13, 25]. Our study indicated that more than 90% of the elderly participants 80+ were living with hearing impairments that had not been checked by specialists.

The auditory system is restricted to the outer ear, middle ear, and the inner ear and is associated with the hearing center in the brain via the hearing nerve. Sound perceived by humans range from 20 to 20,000 Hz. Common speech is often in the range of 200–800 Hz and the volumes of speech vary between 30 dB (whisper) and 80 dB (shouting).

Age-related hearing loss starts from about 40 years of age when the high tones disappear. However, for many elderly it is usually not a real problem before reaching the age of maybe 75–80 years when consonants such as s, sh, f, v, t, p, and b disappear because their energy is concentrated around the frequencies 2000–8000 Hz. Thus, with increasing age, hearing ability progressively weakens, especially the ability to hear high-frequency sounds and to distinguish one sound from another.

Hearing changes for an elderly person is related to anatomical and physiological changes in the ear, in addition to elements in the surroundings and inherited factors [25–28].

It is common in Norway and other countries to simply ask elderly patients in the home-care setting about their hearing with a global question and not use any further examinations if the elderly states that the hearing is good. Our ROC curve analysis revealed that there was a discrepancy between patient self-assessments and results obtained from standardized instruments when they answered the global question, "Do you consider your hearing to be good, not so good, poor, or very poor/deaf".

The elderly often adapt to the situation so that they do not notice themselves that the hearing has been deteriorated [9, 29]. Some elderly people may also have difficulties in admitting that they have reduced hearing. It is however more common to wear glasses than a hearing aid and many elderly people are loath to admit that they have a hearing problem in fear of the social stigma it signifies [13]. Some elderly people also underestimate their hearing loss and think that they have better hearing than they actually do.

It seems however that the elderly admit having problems when they are asked more detailed questions about their hearing and communication abilities. Results from assessing hearing and communication abilities on more detailed questions indicate, for example, that the elderly find it difficult to understand speech when several other people speak simultaneously, and that they find it difficult to understand dialects or foreign accents.

Hearing impairment can also lead to misunderstandings and suspicion in addition to the social isolation [9, 30]. The sound may be difficult to locate, especially for one who has combined visual impairment and hearing loss, who has different hearing aids in the right and left ear, or one who just uses a hearing aid in one ear [31].

3. Hearing impairment in community health care

The 80+ often have serious health issues in addition to hearing impairments that may significantly impact their independence and functioning in daily life. It is therefore necessary to have accurate information about sensory functioning in this population. Researchers in a Norwegian study initially used a checklist method to ask the participants about their hearing [32] and then used the obtained results to apply further tests and follow-up to those who described their hearing as impaired. A major problem with that study is that it did not determine objectively whether the subjects who did not rate their hearing as impaired actually had normal hearing.

We know that there is a discrepancy between patient self-assessment and results obtained from standardized tests such as pure-tone audiometry test in the 80+ [33]. In addition, there seems to be little knowledge about whether the 80+ have sufficient information to even seek help in the first place, and whether they do receive the help that is available to compensate for their impairments [34]. Communication and access to information are considered to be especially important for the 80+, since many remain at home most of the time and have limited contact with others [35]. Therefore, we cannot just hand over this responsibility to the elderly.

Studies have shown that home-care nurses appear to pay limited attention to hearing losses [11, 13], possibly resulting in the problems and difficulties related to age-related hearing loss being overlooked and underestimated. The everyday life of a nurse is busy and involves many tasks, and focusing on the senses require a little more time and consideration for the nurses than they usually spend with the patient. The nursing procedures used in home care for identifying hearing impairment among the 80+ appear to be deficient, or at best, variable so developing good procedures for detecting and tending to the elderly's hearing impairments is crucial.

In addition to risk factors for social withdrawal that can have a serious impact on a person's quality of life and result in many elderly living at home feeling lonely [35], several studies have demonstrated that hearing impairments significantly influence especially the instrumental activities of daily living (IADL), referring to activities such as using the phone, managing money, housework, and shopping [6].

Since a majority of the 80+ have severe sensory impairments [11, 13, 36], but seem to not notice it themselves [33], the most likely interpretation of this inconsistency could be that they have adapted to the situation and do not find it worth mentioning as causing difficulties in their daily life. Alternatively, they may simply be resigned to and have accepted their impairments as part

http://dx.doi.org/10.5772/66372

of the aging process, or they may think, due to a lack of appropriate knowledge, that it is not possible to correct their hearing [36]. The acceptance of an impairment situation and the willingness to report a hearing loss are associated with greater knowledge, education, and income [13].

Multimorbidity, increased risk of diseases in the sensory organs, and age-related changes in the eyes and ears not only lead to reduced hearing and vision but also make the 80+ living in a home-care setting a vulnerable group [34].

The 80+ may not have adequate information about sensory loss in old age and where to get help, treatment, and rehabilitation. It is therefore vital that health-care providers offer this information and help, particularly when the elderly person is already receiving home care. Such information may encourage the elderly to take actions to improve their situation or ask for help and support. It is likely that practical and emotional support can help the 80+ in dealing with sensory impairments.

From both preventive and health-promoting perspectives, home-care nurses can play a particularly important role by incorporating simple hearing tests in their regular procedures [34]. Examination with an otoscope to detect ear wax and check the eardrum and an examination with a portable audiometer are simple procedures that can be done by the home-care nurse.

Elderly people today might have experienced economic hardship during their childhood and upbringing, since they grew up during the recession in the 1930s and during the World War II. If they have to spend money to improve their hearing, this might affect their budget, and therefore they may not prioritize it [34]. Thus, recommendations would be to set clear goals and to closely and carefully help the elderly in every way possible to optimize their hearing function until the goals are reached [14].

It is important that nurses who work with the elderly have knowledge of age-related changes, and most importantly understand the consequences of hearing loss on certain factors of daily life: ADL/IADL, falls, loneliness, and the quality of life. It is also important that healthcare providers are aware of what can be improved, with regard to hearing impairments and are able to explain this to the elderly. When using a hearing aid, it is not the same hearing as the hearing of a 20-year-old, but it is after all much better than not hearing.

When we talk to someone who is not hearing, it is important to consider the following:

- Lowering or removing background noise such as music, radio, TV, talk, traffic, and so on.
- Have good lighting so the hearing impaired person can see the face of the person who is speaking and read the lips and facial expression.
- Ensure that the person who is listening does not see the face of the speaker "in backlight."
- Provide good information both to the elderly and to his/her family and friends.
- Do not speak until the person who is hearing is aware that you want to say something.
- Be close to the person who is hearing, but not too close and do not turn the face away from the person you are talking to.
- Speak quiet and a little slower than normal.

- Speak clearly and use the lips, but do not exaggerate.
- Use normal strength of the voice. Do not shout and certainly not against the hearing aid if the person is using one.
- Be aware of the body language of the hearing impaired person who you are talking to. There is no guaranty that the person admits he/she is not hearing.
- Do not cover the mouth with your hand when you speak.
- Do not have anything in your mouth when speaking.
- Give key words for the topics of the conversation when there are many present.
- If someone laughs, it might be good to explain what the laughing subject is.
- Hearing impaired people have difficulties to tell the difference between consonants like f and s and p or t. It is therefore important sometimes to spell out the words to avoid misunderstandings.

4. Hearing aids and advice when talking to a hearing impaired person

In addition to hearing aids, there is also optional equipment (blue tooth) that allows sound to be streamed from the TV, radio, telephone, doorbell, etc. directly into the ear through the hearing aid. This requires however some training and help to use.

One aspect that is perhaps somewhat underestimated is that some elderly who owns a hearing aid do not use them because they think that it is unattractive or a sign of old age. When this is the case, the nurses need to have enough knowledge to provide information to the elderly and explain that it is not a good idea to ignore the usage of the hearing aid. The nurse should rather find out what is the problem and help the elderly to overcome it.

Other types of hearing equipment including "flashing and vibrating lights" connected to the doorbell and alarm, inductive loop, and voice amplifier are other options.

5. Glossary

Age-related hearing impairment	Refers to the hearing progressively weakens with age, also referred to as presbycusis.
ADL	Activities of daily living (eating, bathing, dressing, toileting, etc).
Portable audiometer	Referring to a portable machine used for evaluating hearing acuity.
Baseline description	Description of the existing picture.
dB	The decibel scale measuring sound based on human hearing. Decibel provides a relative measure of sound intensity.
Cutoff points	Referring to the limit for having a hearing problem. Here it is at PTAV <35 dB.
Dual sensory impairment	Refers to both hearing and vision impairment.

Exploratory, randomized, controlled trial	Referring to a study in which participants are allocated at random to receive a clinical intervention.
False negative	Indicate a failed test. False negative is the proportion of positives which yield negative test outcomes with the gold standard test.
Functional hearing	Age-related hearing impairment is common in old age and improved functional hearing refers to an optimization of the hearing function.
Hearing function	The hearing process. How the hearing works.
Hearing impairment (hearing loss)	Occurs when you lose part or all of your ability to hear. Hearing impairment can be mild, moderate, severe, or profound.
Global question	Asking a global question as opposed to specific questions means asking one question here "Do you consider your hearing to be good, not so good, poor or very poor/deaf?"
Global self-assessments	The person is evaluating his/her hearing by one question: "Do you consider your hearing to be good, not so good, poor or very poor/deaf?"
Gold-standard	Refers to a diagnostic test or benchmark that is the best available under reasonable conditions.
Hz	Hertz, referring to the unit of frequencies in the International System of Units (SI).
Otoscope	Referring to an auroscope which is a medical device used to look into the ears.
IADL	Instrumental activities of daily living (using the phone, managing money, etc).
Multimorbidity	Referring to the co-occurrence of two or more chronic medical conditions in one person.
ROC curve analysis	Receiver operating characteristic is a diagnostic test in statistics – used for decision making in medicine.
Presbycusis	Age-related hearing impairment.
Pure-tone average (PTAV)	Refers to audiology pure-tone testing and the average of hearing threshold levels at a set of specified frequencies, here 500, 1000, 2000, and 4000 Hz which is the frequencies recommended by the World Health Organization (WHO) to check the hearing of the elderly.
Pure-tone audiometry test	Referring to a standardized hearing test which is used to determine the presence or absence of hearing loss.
Self-care activities	Referring to the tasks or actions that a person with age-related hearing impairment must perform to safeguard his/her hearing function.
Standardized test	A test that is administered and scored in a consistent or standard manner. Here it refers to pure tone audiometry.

Author details

Gro Gade Haanes

*Address all correspondence to: groh@setur.fo

Department of Nursing, Faculty of Natural and Health Sciences, University of The Faroe Islands, Tórshavn, Faroe Islands

References

[1] Eurostat Statistical Books. Eurostat yearbook 2008. Europe in Figures. Luxemburg: Eurostat Statistical Books; 2008.

[2] Moulaert T, Biggs S. International and European policy on work and retirement: reinventing critical perspectives on active ageing and mature subjectivity. Human Relations. 2013;66(1):23–43.

[3] Kvaal K, Halding AG, Kvigne K. Social provision and loneliness among older people suffering from chronic physical illness. A mixed-methods approach. Scandinavian Journal of Caring Sciences. 2014;28(1):104–111.

[4] Wallhagen M, Pettengill E. Hearing impairment: significant but underassessed in primary care settings. Journal of Gerontological Nursing. 2008;34(2):36–42.

[5] Raina P, Wong M, Massfeller H. The relationship between sensory impairment and functional independence among elderly. BMC Geriatrics. 2004;4(1):3–11.

[6] Solheim J, Kværner KJ, Falkenberg E-S. Daily life consequences of hearing loss in the elderly. Disability and Rehabilitation. 2011;33(23–24):2179–2185.

[7] Caban A, Lee D, Gomez-Marin O, Lam B, Zheng D. Prevalence of concurrent hearing and visual impairment in US adults: The National Health Interview Survey, 1997–2002. American Journal of Public Health. 2005;95(11):1940–1942.

[8] Lee V, Wong T, Lau C. Home accidents in elderly patients presenting to an emergency department. Accident and Emergency Nursing. 1999;7(2):96–102.

[9] Phil E. Sansesvikt i eldre år. [Sensory impairment in older age]. In: Kirkevold M, Brodtkorb K, Ranhoff AH, editors. Geriatrisk sykepleie: god omsorg til den gamle pasienten. Oslo: Gyldendal akademisk; 2014. pp. 286–300.

[10] Yueh B, Shapiro N, MacLean CH, Shekelle PG. Screening and management of adult hearing loss in primary care. The Journal of the American Medical Association. 2003;289(15):1976–1985.

[11] Grue EV. Vision and hearing impairment in old age [thesis]. Oslo: Unipub; 2010.

[12] Sorri M, Roine R. Age-adjusted prevalence of hearing impairment has significantly increased during the last two decades. Scandinavian Audiology Supplementum. 2000(54):5–7.

[13] Solheim J. Hearing loss in the elderly: consequences of hearing loss and considerations for audiological rehabilitation [thesis]. Oslo: Unipub; 2011.

[14] Haanes G, Kirkevold M, Hofoss D, Gunnar H. An intervention designed to improve sensory impairments in the elderly and indoor lighting in their homes: an exploratory randomized controlled trial. Journal of Multidisciplinary Healthcare. 2015;8:11–20.

[15] Chia E-M, Wang JJ, Rochtchina E, Cumming RR, Newall P, Mitchell P. Hearing impairment and health-related quality of life: the Blue Mountains Hearing Study. Ear and Hearing. 2007;28(2):187–195. 10.1097/AUD.0b013e31803126b6.

[16] Gussekloo J, De Bont L, Von Faber M, Eekhof J, De Laat J, Hulshof J, et al. Auditory rehabilitation of older people from the general population – the Leiden 85-plus study. British Journal of General Practice. 2003;53(492):536–540.

[17] Appollonio I, Carabellese C, Frattola L, Trabucchi M. Effects of sensory aids on the quality of life and mortality of elderly people: a multivariate analysis. Age and Ageing. 1996;25(2):89–96.

[18] Wood JM, Lacherez P, Black AA, Cole MH, Boon MY, Kerr GK. Risk of falls, injurious falls, and other injuries resulting from visual impairment among older adults with age-related macular degeneration. Investigative Ophthalmology and Visual Science. 2011;52(8):5088–5092.

[19] Bess F, Lichtenstein M, Logan S, Burger M, Nelson E. Hearing impairment as a determinant of function in the elderly. Journal of the American Geriatrics Society. 1989;37(2):123–128.

[20] Campbell V, Crews J, Moriarty D, Zack M, Blackman D. Surveillance for sensory impairment, activity limitation, and health-related quality of life among older adults—United States, 1993–1997. MMWR CDC Surveillance Summaries. 1999;48(8):131–156.

[21] Keller B, Morton J, Thomas V, Potter J. The effect of visual and hearing impairments on functional status. Journal of the American Geriatrics Society. 1999;47(11):1319–1325.

[22] Thygesen E. Subjective health and coping in care-dependent old persons living at home. Bergen: University of Bergen; 2010.

[23] Sharts-Hopko N. Low vision and blindness among midlife and older adults: a review of the nursing research literature. Holistic Nursing Practice. 2009;23(2):94–100.

[24] Vik K. Older adults' participation in occupation in the context of home-based rehabilitation [thesis]. Huddinge: Karolinska institutet, Division of Occupational Therapy; 2008.

[25] Gates G, Mills J. Presbycusis. The Lancet. 2005;366(9491):1111–1120.

[26] Kraner S. Bakomliggande faktorer till presbyacusis; en litteraturstudie av mindre kända faktorer [Underlying factors to presbyacusis; a litterature review]. Gøteborg: Gøteborgs Universitet; 2009.

[27] Mills J, Megerian C, Lambert P. Presbyacusis and Presbyastasis. In: Snow JB, Wackym PA, Ballenger JJ, editors. Ballenger's Otorhinolaryngology: Head and Neck Surgery. Shelton, Conn.: PC Decker; 2009. pp. 333–343.

[28] Van Eyken E, Van Camp G, Van Laer L. The complexity of age-related hearing impairment: contributing environmental and genetic factors. Audiology and Neurotology. 2007;12(6):345–358.

[29] Slagsvold B. Mål eller mening: om å måle kvalitet i aldersinstitusjoner [On measuring quality in institutions for elderly]. Oslo: Norsk Gerontologisk Institutt; 1995. 355 s. p.

[30] Divenyi P, Stark P, Haupt K. Decline of speech understanding and auditory thresholds in the elderly. The Journal of the Acoustical Society of America. 2005;118(2):1089–1100.

[31] Simon H, Levitt H. Effect of dual sensory loss on auditory localization: implications for intervention. Trends in Amplification. 2007;11(4):259.

[32] Lyng K, Svingen EM. Kartlegging av alvorlig, kombinert sansetap hos eldre [Screening of serious, combined impairment in elderly]. Oslo: NOVA; 2001.

[33] Haanes GG, Kirkevold M, Hofoss D, Eilertsen G. Discrepancy between self-assessments and standardised tests of vision and hearing abilities in older people living at home: an ROC curve analysis. Journal of Clinical Nursing. 2015;24(23–24):3380–3388.

[34] Haanes G. Hearing, vision, and lighting conditions among older recipients of home care. Oslo: Oslo University; 2016.

[35] Weinstein B, Ventry I. Hearing impairment and social isolation in the elderly. Journal of Speech and Hearing Research 1982;25:593–599.

[36] Haanes GG, Kirkevold M, Horgen G, Hofoss D, Eilertsen G. Sensory impairments in community health care: a descriptive study of hearing and vision among elderly Norwegians living at home. Journal of Multidisciplinary Healthcare. 2014;7(42):217–225.

Chapter 7

Aging Auditory System and Amplification

Christiane Marques do Couto and
Izabella dos Santos Brites

Additional information is available at the end of the chapter

http://dx.doi.org/10.5772/66935

Abstract

The aging of auditory system determines the physical, sensory, and neural changes in the peripheral and central parts and may cause changes in the reception and sound processing. Age related hearing loss, also called presbycusis, can occur in the elderly population due to aging. The difficulty for compression of speech in the elderly may be due solely to hearing loss, but may be linked to degenerative issues of the central auditory system. Age is a factor that interferes with the central auditory processing. The results of auditory processing may change and more if there is the presence of peripheral hearing loss. It should be considered that the longer an individual has hearing loss, the greater the negative effects on the perception of sound and performance in listening skills. The use of hearing aids favors amplification and modification of the sound stimulus so that it reaches the eardrum with quantity increase and quality, promoting and stimulating the auditory skills. This chapter intends to make a review of the auditory processing disorder and evidence the benefit of the use of amplification in the elderly.

Keywords: hearing aid, auditory system, presbycusis, auditory processing, elderly

1. Introduction

Advancements in health care and technological developments in the areas of preventive medicine and medical technology during the last decades have considerably extended the life expectancy of the human population. As a result, a greater number of people exceed the age of 65. This category of subjects is commonly referred to as seniors or elderly group. With the increasing age, some systems of the human body start to present functional changes such as degeneration or atrophy of neurons or tissues. People older than 65 years show an increased number of nontransmissible diseases, such as cardiac or metabolic ones [1].

Associated with the transformation of the body and with the higher incidence of health complications, the elderly may present sensory, motor, and cognitive alterations. Cellular and molecular damage may also show up due to aging, possibly resulting in sensory loss (hearing or vision) or motor disability. In addition, cognitive changes such as decreased attention and working memory may also be present [1, 2].

All these factors may compromise the quality of life and the independence of the elderly. In addition, these changes can lead this segment of the population to a social isolation and depression [1].

The aging of the auditory system leads to physical, sensory, and neural changes in the peripheral and central portion of the system, which may also cause changes in the sections which receive and process the sound stimuli.

The objective of this chapter is to make a review of hearing loss and auditory processing, while considering the use of amplification technologies (hearing aids) and their intervention in the elderly.

2. Hearing

The concept of hearing is extremely complex and goes beyond the simple act of listening to a particular sound. This is a process in which motor, electrical, and biochemical changes occur along the auditory path inside the human body, which begins in the outer ear (more specifically in the pinna), and ends in the cortex, where the sound information received is decoded [3].

Sound waves generated in the environment are captured by the pinna and driven by the external acoustic meatus to the tympanic membrane, which starts a vibration process, transforming the sound waves into mechanical waves. This vibration moves the ossicles in the middle ear until it reaches the oval window, where stimulation will reach the inner ear.

The movement that begins in the inner ear promotes movement in the liquid (endolymph) that is housed in the cochlea, as well as, a change in its structures, promoting the excitement of the outer and inner hair cells, which in turn stimulate a network of nerve endings, which leads to the stimulation of the cochlear nerve to reach the central nervous system. It will be in the cerebral cortex that the stimulus will be decoded and then spatially interpreted.

As described above, hearing is an extremely complex process. What happens when the auditory system is affected by changes due to aging and it does not work properly?

2.1. Hearing loss and its consequences

When the auditory system presents structural changes, other disorders might be observed first, depending on the location where the hearing complications were first observed. For example, if a problem is observed in the external, middle, or inner ear, it will result in a reversible (or not) hearing loss. If a problem is present in the area of the auditory cortex, it will generate a processing interference, which will affect the understanding and decoding of the incoming sound stimuli.

Aging processes can alter the structures of the auditory system, resulting in hearing loss and a compromise of hearing. This is the most significant and important sensory change in the lives of the elderly, which can generate a social limitation, minimizing the social function and the participation of the elderly in the society [4].

Hearing loss due to aging is called *"presbycusis"* or *age-related hearing loss* (ARHL) [5]. It is usually identified due to complains from the elderly subjects, referring to difficulties in understanding nearby sounds, especially in environments with poor acoustics. In these cases, an audiological assessment usually results in an identification of a mild-to-moderate symmetric sensorineural hearing loss, which worsens in the course of time [6].

It is well known that 80% of the population >85 years present some form of hearing loss [7]. The incidence of the hearing impairment also has gender effects, i.e., elderly men tend to be more affected than elderly women [8].

The data in the literature show that presbycusis can be classified into three types: the **sensory** presbycusis, the **neuronal** presbycusis, and the **metabolic** presbycusis [9, 10]. In the first case, it is possible to observe a lesion in the organ of Corti, which results in an audiogram with sloping configuration. In the **neuronal** presbycusis, there is a loss of spiral ganglion neurons, which leads to a worsening in speech discrimination, which does not seem compatible with hearing loss observed in the audiogram. The **metabolic** presbycusis is caused by a degeneration of the vascular stria, characterized by a vocal discrimination preserved, even in spite of the presence of flat or high frequency configuration [9, 10]. In all the three cases above, the elderly is considered to have a sensory neural hearing loss.

However, it is necessary to account for other factors that may have affected the hearing of the elderly throughout life and that may have worsened the hearing loss, such as exposure to noise, cardiovascular diseases (hypertension or diabetes), or extensive use of antineoplastic drugs. Very often what we call presbycusis is the cumulative effect of aging with cochlear stress caused by other etiologies [11–13].

A decline of the linguistic functions is commonly observed in the elderly presenting hearing loss. Due to this sensorial disorder, an elderly subject loses the quality of sound information in communicating with others, which may generate at first a difficulty or trouble understanding a vocal message, and eventually drives the elderly into social isolation [14]. This situation has an impact in the lives of the elderly as well as in the people who surround the elderly, their caregivers.

These communication difficulties are global and they are changing the life of the elderly, reducing their communication skills with members of the family or friends. This difficulty can even show up with normal environmental sounds such as a telephone ring or the horn of a car, situations that can even put the elderly into a safety hazard [15].

The International Classification of Disability and Health (ICF) (World Health Organization, 2001) considers that a condition of good health depends (i) on the proper functioning of the body and (ii) on social and environmental factors that allow the individual to perform his/her activities and be active socially. Thus, hearing loss should not be a limitation, since it is possible to perform an intervention (hearing aids, implantable hearing aids, and cochlear implants) and to manage positively the hearing impaired adult [16].

2.2. Hearing aids and hearing performance

When hearing loss is diagnosed, an intervention is necessary. The most immediate solution is the use of a hearing aid (**HA**) technology. The HA is a little apparatus placed in the external meatus and that can amplify the sounds that reach the auditory system. With a hearing aid, the person will regain the audibility even of low-intensity sounds, making it possible to resume the activities of daily life. The usage of a hearing aid is the primary treatment option indicated for individuals with nonreversible hearing loss [17].

Since elderly subjects present a symmetrical loss profile in most cases, it is possible to use two hearing aid devices and perform a binaural fitting. Two hearing aids favor a better understanding of the sound messages and a better localization of the sound source [17].

Currently, in the market, there is a wide variety of technologies for hearing aids and resources that can be used to improve hearing. The best hearing aid is indicated for each case, and for it, a process must be followed by the audiologist, thus favoring a better adaptation of the hearing aid.

This process to determine if a hearing aid should be used or not begins with an assessment and the planning of the intervention to be held. Usually, the individual is subjected to the common audiological tests such as tonal and speech audiometry as well as immittance tympanometry tests. However, these procedures can only assess hearing complications in the auditory periphery. The sufficiency of these tests is uncertain and will be further discussed below.

The HA is selected based on desired physical and electroacoustic characteristics. At this stage, the individual complains should be considered, their fine motor skills and even cognitive factors that may influence the use and adaptation of one or other technology.

Since individuals with sensorineural hearing loss have low speech discrimination in the presence of background noise, most hearing aid devices incorporate noise suppressors that amplify the speech signal over noise and directional microphones that capture best sounds from certain directions. Even in these conditions the hearing aid cannot simulate the cochlea function, for all audible sounds. The hearing aid will amplify certain sound frequencies, but still there will be loss of sound signal quality, and a number of individuals still tend to complain about the level of amplification.

The hearing aid should amplify the incoming sounds without being uncomfortable to the person who uses it. This situation is only possible due to the components and digital or electronic operation of the hearing aid, which will amplify the low-intensity sounds, transforming them into audible sounds, without however, causing discomfort in the listener.

Care must be taken in the entire process of fitting, such as the handling conditions of the hearing aid by the elderly, the size of the device, or the occurrence of feedback. If any of these factors were not observed, the chance of the elderly not making effective use of the hearing aid is very high.

After selecting the best hearing aid for the subject case and its characteristics, the specific device performance and the individual performance with this technology must be verified through objective and subjective tests if there was an improvement in the perception of sound stimuli. The next phase consists of providing the user with proper guidance on the usage and handling of the hearing aid, enabling, after one-time use, the validation of the treatment, in other words, the perception of the impact of the intervention in the life of the new user of hearing aids [18]. Throughout this process, the audiologist should consider two important factors: the limitations in activities and participation restriction.

For this reason, even with the existing technological advancements in the field of hearing aids, some elderly subjects still complain about the amplification, signal quality, often failing to make use of this technology. Other elderly subjects, in turn, report great improvement in their lives with the use of hearing aids, accomplishing different listening tasks. So, why does it occur?

3. Auditory processing

In some cases, even if the hearing aid provides audibility of the signal, it cannot improve the listening of the elderly, especially in acoustically unfavorable environments. This may occur because of the listening difficulty caused, including, but not exclusively, by periphery of the auditory system, but also by central portion, in the cortex, thereby generating a difficulty in auditory processing, with consequent difficulty decoding the acoustic signal. This difficulty is not only a result of the increase in hearing thresholds but also of a dysfunction of the auditory processing. This has to be taken into account when selecting hearing aids.

Hearing is a function of the peripheral portion of the auditory system. However, processing and understanding of this sound is a function of the central portion of the auditory system, and incorporates many features and neurological networks, involving aspects like hearing, language, and cognitive.

For a long time, it was believed that only the basic audiological evaluation has been sufficient for diagnosis and intervention in the elderly. Alternatively, the central auditory processing tests should were performed only in individuals with thresholds within normal standard, so that this test is widely used in children with complaints of learning disability without another diagnosis or change detected [19]. However, it is possible to use the auditory processing test with adults and elderly. Several studies [20] on the auditory processing in the elderly or people with hearing loss began to be realized and it looks for the answer of this population, in a way to create a normal answer for this population and investigate if these results can change answer or feeling of the elderly with HA.

It is necessary to consider that it is not only the peripheral portion of the auditory system that is influenced by age, but all the auditory system undergoes aging interference. There may be a drop in auditory skills not only because of a peripheral alteration, but because of a difficulty in working and operating with sounds and auditory skills [21, 22].

Besides the hearing loss, the elderly have trouble in auditory processing. This fact is proven by research showing that older adults with hearing loss perform worse than adults or young people with similar hearing loss. This occurs because there is a deterioration of the central auditory system in the elderly, which generates auditory processing disorder [20]. Especially in the elderly, the acoustic signal that enters the system is distorted due to peripheral hearing loss because of aging (presbycusis) [23], what compromised more the auditory processing. If the whole system is taken into account, only amplification of sound will not be enough, because there can be a change in the processing of this sound in the central portion of the auditory system (cortex). Therefore, this interferes with the fitting of hearing aids, reducing satisfaction and their effective use.

In 1996, the American Speech-Language-Hearing Association characterized and defined "*central auditory process are the auditory system mechanisms and process responsible for the following behavioral phenomenal: sound localization and lateralization, auditory discrimination, auditory pattern recognition, temporal aspects of audition including temporal resolution, temporal masking, temporal integration and temporal ordering, auditory performance decrements with competing acoustic signals and auditory performance decrements with degraded acoustic signals*" [24].

It is important to evaluate what these abilities mean. When someone can detect from which direction the sound is coming, the person is using the sound localization. When someone can organize or memorize auditory information according to the time, they are developing the temporal ordering ability. When someone understands the auditory information in the competitive noise, they are performing the auditory closure. When someone understands the auditory information from the junction of the information provided in each ear, they are doing binaural synthesis.

In children the auditory processing disorder justifies learning or language disorders. When the sound has not been processed properly, dealing with language issues is difficult, resulting in reading and writing problems. In adults, this change can be detected only when specific or elaborate tasks of listening are requested. In the elderly, the auditory processing difficulty is perceived when the individual does not fit to the hearing aid.

3.1. Auditory processing evaluation

Therefore, to detect the presence of auditory processing disorders, it is necessary to perform an evaluation, which is conducted in a soundproof booth, using headphones. The assessment is carried out with different tests, which evaluate the individual auditory skills, such as sound localization, temporal ordering, auditory closure, binaural synthesis, and figure background.

These skills are evaluated using different procedures (**Table 1**), which can be applied in more than one session. Moreover, these tests can be applied in monaural or binaural form, i.e., in order to evaluate just one ear or the binaural integration (both ears). Each test has a specific orientation (purpose) and a specific stimulus. It is not necessary to apply all of the tests. On

Procedure	Skill
Sound localization	Sound localization
Memory for verbal sounds	Temporal ordination
Memory for nonverbal sounds	Temporal ordination
Speech with noise	Auditory closure
Dichotic digits	Integration binaural
Staggered spondaic word (SSW)	Integration binaural
Frequency and duration standard	Temporal processing
Gaps in noise (GIN)	Temporal processing
Identification of synthetic sentences	Figure background

Table 1. Auditory processing tests and auditory abilities.

the other hand, it is necessary to focus on the hearing loss type and its configuration to decide which test is the most important to be performed or can be possibly applied. This analysis is important because the tests are applied with an audible level over the hearing threshold.

Therefore, according to the hearing loss level, one particular test may not be applied because the sound level necessary on that test cannot be reached due to the limitation of the equipment. This aspect will be discussed later on.

3.2. Auditory processing in the elderly

Research comparing young and old individuals, whose hearing level is within the normal range, observed that even with normal thresholds, there is a reduction in speech understanding with background noise with the increase of the age of the individuals for short messages (consonants) or for long messages (phrases) [25].

The main complaint of the elderly is the difficulty to understand speech. There are three hypotheses that justify the difficulty to understand speech in the elderly: peripheral hearing loss, central hearing loss, and cognitive impairment. According to studies, despite being the most accepted hypothesis, only peripheral hearing loss may not generate the difficulties to understand the speech in the elderly [26]. In contrast, it adds that changes in auditory processing could enhance the difficulty that the elderly have to identify speech [27].

It is clear that the elderly has auditory processing disorder, since it is difficult for them to decode phonemes, the perception of rapidly changing speech decoding of verbal and nonverbal sounds and a slowing in interhemispheric transmission [28]. These changes associated with the peripheral hearing loss create a difficulty to understand speech, especially if it occurs in an acoustically unfavorable environment.

In addition to the hearing impairment, either peripheral or central, a decline in cognitive function can also negatively impact the processing of sound information, impairing speech understanding [29]. With the increase of age there is a decrease in attention span and in working memory, slower brain processing, and reduction in the ability to reduce the environmental interference for speech understanding [6].

Factors such as working memory and speech processing speed influence speech recognition in noise. Studies have shown that the elderly who has a good cognitive performance obtained good results, which were better than those who had poorer performance, indicating that for processing the acoustic signal there is a cognitive interference condition [30].

These cognitive changes associated with the decline in hearing thresholds and a worsening in hearing generates a change in perception and speech understanding in noise. These factors result in a decline in the elderly quality of life and can lead to social isolation [31].

3.3. Auditory processing evaluation in the elderly

Nowadays, we have the idea that there is a correlation between auditory processing tests and hearing loss and that the elderly performs worse than adults. Because of that, recent research includes study of the auditory processing and hearing loss, and look for a way to evaluate and intervene with this population.

In the elderly, it is essential to consider the presence of peripheral hearing loss, but as it is a poor signal that reaches the cerebral cortex due to peripheral hearing loss, cognition of the elderly is fundamental for a better understanding of the message. Additionally, the auditory cortex of individuals in this portion of the population tends to atrophy, which causes a change in auditory processing, i.e., the sound that enters the system is already an altered sound, and it worsens because of the way this is processed [31].

Studies show that seniors who have changes in auditory processing tend to perform a self-assessment of the hearing handicap worse than those who have no auditory processing disorder, showing that it is necessary for a better evaluation of each individual [32].

Some researches specify types of responses that can be obtained for each case. Individuals with low- and high-frequency hearing loss show difficulty in monotonic tasks. In turn, the elderly with hearing loss in high frequency or normal hearing can perform well on these tests. Therefore, audiological characteristics of the hearing loss have to be taken into account to select the processing test and understand the results achieved [33].

Many factors have to be considered to assess auditory processing in the elderly. In addition to care in the test selection, it is important to consider the age of the assessed person. It is known that when comparing the performance of adults with the elderly performance, the elderly will have a lower performance than adults, those observed even in the presence of similar hearing loss. This occurs because there is a deterioration of the central auditory system, which generates an auditory processing disorder in the elderly. This context interferes negatively with the hearing aids' fitting, reducing the satisfaction of the elderly in relation to these devices, resulting in a noneffective use [22].

To evaluate how the elderly process this sound, or their listening skills, it can map out a more detailed and correct rehabilitation plan for each case. If there is the presence of peripheral hearing loss, hearing aids must be fitted. However, with a broader look at the elderly's auditory system and their greatest difficulties, a better hearing aid fitting is possible, as well as the indication of a therapy or auditory training.

However, still in the assessment phase, it is important that the evaluator considers the presence of peripheral hearing loss when selecting and evaluating the results of tests of auditory processing, since not all tests can be applied in cases of peripheral hearing loss. It is necessary to select tests that do not suffer interference from hearing loss. Still, there is the degree of limitation of loss, with the possible application in symmetrical hearing loss, from mild to moderate (hearing loss up to 55 dB HL) [34].

Some authors suggest that the battery used to assess auditory processing should have dichotic tests, temporal processing tests, low redundancy monaural tests, and binaural interaction tests [34, 35].

Specifically to evaluate the binaural interaction, it is suggested to use the dichotic digits test. Studies show that there is a drop in performance of the left ear in the dichotic listening in the elderly. This generates a change in interhemispheric transfer of the acoustic signal, which is due to the deterioration of the callosum corpus [36]. This change in dichotic listening can alter also in working memory and selective attention, suggesting cognitive impairment [37, 38].

It is important to explain that in the dichotic test, four numbers are introduced. First of all, two numbers will be shown, at same time, but each one in each ear. Immediately after, other two numbers are shown in the same way. The listener has to pay attention and tell which numbers he listened and/or what numbers were heard in each ear.

In this age group (elderly), more problems are observed with listening skills figure background and closing, which affect the listening speech in noise in acoustically unfavorable environments. In addition, changes in auditory temporal processing are also observed in the elderly and widely discussed in the literature [39]. It is believed that the elderly people experience changes in auditory temporal processing, which can be detected both in frequency and in test duration [6].

In the temporal tests, three stimuli in sequence are presented, and the assessed individual has to name or reproduce the sound, and thick or thin the frequency test, or long and short in duration test.

The hearing performance worsens with the presentation of a complex or an acoustically unfavorable environment stimulus. Added to this, the elderly has great difficulty with sequencing activities, which involve auditory processing and cognition [40].

4. Auditory neuronal plasticity

The elderly with hearing loss suffer from the beginning of the hearing loss installation, sensory deprivation by having hearing restricted to some sounds. Thus, the introduction of sound stimuli, through the hearing aid, even after the privation period, can cause changes in the sensory system responsible for transmitting acoustic information.

The adaptation of hearing aids promotes neuronal plasticity. Neural networks are generated and areas of the brain that were not stimulated become stimulated, favoring the adaptation of the hearing aid and social reintegration of the elderly. In addition, the adaptation of the hearing aid can contribute to the stabilization of the hearing loss, namely, the reintroduction of certain sounds by the hearing aid can promote a positive plasticity (structural and functional reorganization of the central auditory system).

The longer an individual stays with hearing loss and without the use of hearing aids, the greater the negative effects on the perception of sound and performance in listening skills. The use of hearing aids favors amplification and modification of the sound stimulus so that it reaches the eardrum with quantity increase and quality, and promotes and stimulates the auditory skills.

Due to the improvement of the quality of sound that reaches the central auditory system, it is believed that after auditory stimulation for a certain period of time, the elderly tends to improve his auditory perception because there is a greater stimulation of the auditory cortex. This theory is grounded by the theory of brain plasticity, or because of high stimulation, which happens with the use of hearing aids: the brain region responsible for the understanding of the function and process the auditory information creates new neural network (plasticity), thus, generating a better performance of the individual. When this occurs, the elderly has a better hearing performance, because in fact there were positive brain changes.

In some cases, there is indication of auditory training, so that the auditory cortex can be potentially stimulated and thus there will be an improvement in hearing. Several surveys show that the auditory training is suitable for adults and the elderly with hearing loss, since this therapeutic resource improves perception and hearing in noisy or acoustically unfavorable environments.

Even with those seniors who have mild hearing loss, satisfaction with the use of hearing aids will not be great because of auditory processing disorders. Research claim that therein lies the importance of ear training because it will occur with an improvement in electrophysiological response (latency wave III in ABR) in auditory localization and speech understanding in noise [41].

This training becomes complementary to the use of hearing aids. Thus, it will be through training that the individual with hearing loss will be able to hone your listening skills so there is a better understanding of speech [42].

The auditory training can assist in the recognition of sounds that were not already heard and others that can be modified by technology, such as the lowering frequency that seeks to dislocate a high-frequency sound to a lower one.

The professional who will make the indication of the treatment must have concepts of neuroscience and aging, which should be considered at the time of the hearing aid selection and type of auditory training. Moreover, it is necessary to consider that there is brain reorganization and acclimatization with hearing aids and that these processes are closely related to cognition [43].

All this care and to look further, beyond the peripheral hearing loss, is essential for the individual with hearing aid, and notices an improvement in his understanding of speech.

The presence of hearing loss can lead to changes in the mood of the elderly and social change, taking them into isolation. Because of this, it is important to evaluate the benefits of hearing aids and how the technology can change the life and the neurologic system of the elderly.

5. The benefit of hearing aids

Modification is generated by the use of hearing aid. Benefit is the difference in the auditory performance of the individual with and without the use of this technological resource. It is expected that whenever the benefit obtained is positive, an improvement in auditory responses occurs. This is possible, as already mentioned above, due to neuronal plasticity, with no improvement in hearing thresholds or in the response of the cochlear hair cells, but with a change in the cortex, with better auditory responses.

The modification of auditory responses does not happen only by the input of the sound stimulus of higher quality or more audible. Rather, it is this better quality signal entering the hearing system that makes possible a change in neural networks, generating a better response in auditory sensation.

However, a positive benefit is not always observed. In some cases, the benefit is negative or zero, i.e., the elderly does not perceive changes in hearing with the hearing aid or even refers to a worsening. In these cases, the adaptation of the hearing aid becomes more difficult and the elderly will not make proper use of the device.

The benefit can be measured by objective and subjective tests. Objective tests assess quantitatively the improvement in hearing performance with the use of hearing aid. Usually, speech is used in noise test, functional gain, insertion responses, among other tests [44]. Speech in noise test is conducted in a soundproof booth, with calibration and standardization. It is supposed to get better performance with hearing aid.

Alongside, there are the subjective tests, such as self-assessment questionnaire, which are answered by individuals and seek to assess the feeling the individual has about the improvement in their hearing.

For many services, the subjective test has greater influence and relevance than the objective tests, since these show that the elderly are thinking about the hearing aid, as is its performance in communication activities and may differ from the data obtained in objective tests and influence more on whether or not to use the hearing aid.

The main questionnaires are HHIE (Hearing Handicap Inventory for the Elderly) [45], the APHAB (Abbreviated Profile of Hearing Aid Benefit) [46], and the COSI (Client Oriented Scale of Improvement) [47]. These questionnaires can be used alone or in a combined form and should be applied before and after using the device for the measurement of the benefit.

The HHIE seeks to assess the psychosocial effects of hearing deficiency in the elderly. The questionnaire contains 25 questions that are divided into two scales: social and emotional.

By means of these scales it is possible to assess how much the situations of difficult listening affect the individual's behavior and emotional response front to these situations. There are three possible answers: yes, no, and sometimes.

APHAB seeks to assess the hearing disability associated with hearing loss and how it was reduced after using the hearing aid. Therefore, this questionnaire should be applied before the use of hearing aid and after adaptation.

COSI focuses on individual listening difficulties. Before the adaptation, the individual must choose five categories in which I would like to hear well. For evaluation, two scales are used, a relative scale, which assesses the degree of change, and an absolute scale, which records the individual's final skill listening situations.

It is known that even being subjective, the benefit is influenced by cognitive issues, as with cognitive issue preserved, a more effective use of hearing aid will be made, and also the understanding of the auditory information, as well as the ability to understand speech in noisy environments [48]. In others, research is possible to see that the cognitive can change with the benefit of hearing aids [49].

The modification in many categories is just possible to be measured after 1 year of the use of hearing aid [48]. After 4 months of use of the hearing aid, it is possible to see a change in the quality of life of the elderly. Nevertheless, bigger modification in other categories is just perceived after 12 months of the use of this technology [49]. Some research looks for modification in the benefit after this period, like evaluating the benefit after 24 months of use. However, no significant differences have been observed because an acclimatization had occurred [50].

Many researches look for the benefit of the use of hearing aids. All of them show that the elderly have a significant change in their life to return to social activities and trying again new communication activities. In addition, it is possible to see a reduction in the emotional problems or social isolation [51].

One study evaluated the handicap (Hearing Handicap Inventory for Elderly, HHIE) before and after 6 months of use of hearing aids. One hundred and fifteen (115) elderly were divided into two groups according to the result of the dichotic digits test (normal or abnormal result). After 6 months there was a significant improvement only in the group with normal dichotic test digits. The author also states that the differences observed between the groups are not justified by memory issues, attention, or difficulty in fine motor. However, the central auditory processing, which when altered generates negative influence on the process of adaptation in the elderly [52].

Therefore, measuring the benefit is essential for a correct assessment of the hearing aid gains possible, as well as checking how the use of this technology is favoring a new neural network.

6. Final considerations

In assessing the issue and the hearing status in the elderly, many factors have to be taken into consideration so that appropriate amplification will be proposed and so the elderly make actual use of hearing aids and have the proper advantages.

With the beginning of the use of auditory processing tests to assess the elderly with hearing loss, a new scenario in audiology was established and became an integral care for the elderly hearing.

It is not enough to just consider the degree of peripheral hearing loss but also it is necessary to consider how listening skills are changed, so that a better fitting is indicated, as well as the attempted use of complementary technologies.

That way not only searches the degree of peripheral loss, but searches around which hearing abilities are altered. So, this way it is possible to select a better technology for the elderly. Considering what skills are altered, you can check which technology or which feature of the hearing aid can be used, favoring a better listening and speech understanding by the elderly, which will generate an effective use of the device.

In addition, having a better hearing, the elderly tend to relate better with people, not isolating or minimizing their quality of life and autonomy. Rather, they can develop their daily tasks more independently, which favors their mental, cognitive, and economic conditions.

Glossary

Age-related hearing loss (ARHL)	A synonym of presbycusis
Abbreviated Profile of Hearing Aid Benefit (APHAB)	A shortened version of the Profile of Hearing Aid Benefit, self-assessment, disability-based inventory that can be used to document the outcome of a hearing aid fitting
Client Oriented Scale of Improvement (COSI)	It is a clinical tool developed by NAL (National Acoustic Laboratories) for outcomes measurement. It is an assessment questionnaire for clinicians to use which allows them to document their client's goals/needs and measures improvements in hearing ability
Dichotic digits Test	This is an auditory processing test, which evaluates the ability to reproduce four digits (numbers), which are displayed in pairs, one on each ear, simultaneously
Frequency and Duration Standard	This is an auditory processing test, which assesses the ability to distinguish and name bass and treble, long and short stimuli.
GIN (Gaps-in-Noise) Test	This is an auditory processing test that evaluates which the lowest range in which you can see the occurrence of two auditory stimuli
Hearing Aid (HA)	HA is a little apparatus placed in the external meatus and that can amplify the sounds that reach the auditory system
Hearing Handicap Inventory for the Elderly (HHIE)	Is a 25-item self-assessment scale composed of two subscales (emotional and social/situational)
Identification of Synthetic Sentences	This is a test that evaluates the ability to understand speech in environments with competitive speech noise
Memory for verbal sounds	This is an auditory processing test that evaluates the memorizing ability of verbal sounds when they are presented in a particular sequence and must be played in the same sequence

Memory for nonverbal sounds	This is an auditory processing test that evaluates the memorizing ability of nonverbal sounds when they are presented in a particular sequence and must be played in the same sequence
Speech with noise	This is an auditory processing test, which evaluates the ability to understand speech in environments with background noise
Staggered Spondee Word (SSW) test	This is auditory processing test that evaluates the individual's ability to hear four words in sequence, the first in one ear, the second and third, both simultaneously, one in each ear and the last in the contralateral ear to what the first word was presented
Presbycusis	Loss of the hearing acuity in the elderly (i.e. >65 years) subjects
Sound localization	This is an auditory processing test that evaluates the ability to localize sound stimulus

Author details

Christiane Marques do Couto* and Izabella dos Santos Brites

*Address all correspondence to: christianemcouto@hotmail.com

Department of Human Development and Rehabilitation, Faculty of Medical Sciences, University of Campinas – UNICAMP, Campinas, SP, Brazil

References

[1] WHO. World report on ageing and Health. Geneva, Who Press, 2015. 247 p. ISBN 978 92 4 069481 1.

[2] Li, K.Z.H., Lindersberger, U. Relations between sensory/sensorimotor and cognitive function. Neurosci. Biobehav. Rev. 2002;26(7);777–783. DOI: 10.1016/S0149-7634(02)00073-8

[3] Gelfand, S. A. Essentials of Audiology. 4th ed. New York, Thieme, 2015. 639 p. ISBN:9781604068627

[4] Crews, J.E., Campbell, V.A. Vision impairment and hearing loss among community – dwelling older Americans: Implications for health and functioning. Am. J. Public Health. 2004;94(5);823–829. DOI: 10.2105/AJPH.94.5.823

[5] Schmiedt, R.A. The physiology of cochlear presbycusis. In: Gordon-Salant, S. et al. (eds.), The Aging Auditory System. Springer-Verlag, New York. 2010. Vol. 34; pp. 9–38. ISBN:978-1-44190993-0. DOI 10.1007/978-1-4419-0993-0

[6] Wingfield, A., Tun, P.A., McCoy, S.L. Hearing loss in older adulthood – what is and how it interacts with cognitive performance. Curr. Directions Psychol. Sci. 2005;14(3);144–148. DOI:10.1111/j.0963-7214.2005.00356.x

[7] Parham, K. et al. Comprehensive management of presbycusis: central and peripheral. Otolaryngol. Head Neck Surg. 2013;148(4); 537–539. DOI: 10.1177/0194599813477596

[8] Gopinath, B. et al. Prevalence of age-related hearing loss in older adults: Blue Mountain Study. Arch. Intern. Med. 2009;169(4);415–416.DOI:10.1001/archinternmed.2008.597

[9] Schuknecht, H.F. Further observations on the pathology of presbycusis. Arch. Otolaryngol. 1964;80;369–382. Available from: http://dx.doi.org/10.1001/archotol.1964.00750040381003.

[10] Rizk, H.G., Linthicum Jr., F.H. Histopathologic categorization of presbycusis. Otol. Neurotol. 2012;33;23–24. DOI: 10.1097/MAO.0b013e31821f84ee

[11] Martins, K. et al. Genetic and audiologic study in elderly with sensorineural hearing loss. CoDAS. 2013;25(3);224–228. DOI:10.1590/S2317-17822013000300006

[12] Kid III, A.R., Bao, J. Recent advances in the study of age-related hearing loss – a mini review. Gerontology. 2012;58(6);490–496. DOI: 10.1159/000338588

[13] Yamasoba, T. et al. Current concepts in age-related hearing loss: epidemiology and mechanistic pathways. Hear Res. 2013;303;30–38. DOI: 10.1016/j.heares.2013.01.021.

[14] Gilad, C., Glorig, A. Presbycusis: the aging ear. Part I. J. Am. Aud. Soc. 1979;4(5);195–206.

[15] Dalton, D.S. et al. The impact of hearing loss on quality of life in older adults. The Gerontologist. 2003;43(5);661–668. DOI:10.1093/geront/43.5.661

[16] WHO. The International Classification of Disability and Health (ICF). 2001. Available from: http://psychiatr.ru/download/1313?view=name=CF_18.pdf

[17] Dillon, H. Hearing Aids. Thieme. 2014;57(7);493. Available from: http://dx.doi.org/10.3342/kjorl-hns.2014.57.7.493

[18] American Speech-Hearing-Language Association. Guidelines for hearing aid fitting for adults. ASHA. 1997;2;123–130. DOI:10.1044/policy.GL1998-00012.

[19] Moore, D.R. Auditory processing disorder (APD): definition, diagnosis, neural basis and intervention. Audiol. Med. 2006;1(1);4–11. DOI:10.1080/16513860600568573

[20] Stach, B. A. et al. Special hearing aid considerations in elderly patients with auditory processing disorders. Ear Hearing. 1991;12(6);131–138. Available from: http://dx.doi.org /10.1097/00003446-199112001-00007

[21] Humes, L. et al. Central presbycusis: a review and evaluation of the evidence. J. Am. Acad. Audiol. 2012;23;635–666. DOI: 10.3766/jaaa.23.8.5

[22] Gates, G. Central presbycusis: an emerging view. Otolaryngol. Head Neck Surg. 2012;147(1);1–2. DOI: 10.1177/0194599812446282

[23] Rosdina, A.K. et al. Self-reported hearing loss among elderly Malaysians. Malaysian Family Phys. 2010;5(2);91–94.

[24] American Speech-Hearing-Language Association. Central auditory processing: current status of research and implications for clinical practice. ASHA. 1996;5;41–54.

[25] Fullgrabe, C., Moore, B.C.J., Stone, M.A. Age-group differences in speech identification despite matched audiometrically normal hearing: contributions from auditory temporal processing and cognition. Front. Aging Neurosci. 2014;6;1–25.

[26] Humes, L.E. Speech understanding in the elderly. J. Am. Acad. Audiol. 1996;7;161–167. DOI:10.3389/fnagi.2014.00347

[27] Humes, L.E., Christopherson, L. Speech identification difficulties of hearing- impaired elderly persons the contributions of auditory processing deficits. J. Speech Language Hearing Res. 1991;34;686–693. Available from: http://dx.doi.org/10.1044/jshr.3403.686

[28] Rajan, R., Cainer, E. Ageing without hearing loss or cognitive impairment causes a decrease in speech intelligibility only in informational maskers. Neuroscience. 2008;154;784–795. DOI:10.1016/j.neuroscience.2008.03.067

[29] Moore, D.R. Relation between speech-in-noise threshold, hearing loss and cognition from 40-69 years of age. PLoS One. 2014;9(9);107720. DOI: 10.1371/journal.pone.0107720

[30] Lunner, T. Cognitive function in relation to hearing aid use. Intl. J. Audiol. 2003;42;49–58. DOI:10.3109/14992020309074624

[31] Cardin, V. Effects of aging and adult-onset of hearing loss on cortical auditory regions. Front. Neurosci. 2016;10;1–12. DOI:10.3389/fnins.2016.60199

[32] Jerger, J., Oliver, T.A., Pirozzolo, F. Impact of central auditory processing disorder and cognitive deficit on the self-assessment of hearing handicap in the elderly. J. Am. Acad. Audiol. 1990;1;75–80.

[33] Cox, L.C. et al. Monotonic auditory processing disorders testes in the older adult population. J. Am. Acad. Audiol. 2008;19(4);293–308. Available from: http://dx.doi.org/10.3766/jaaa.19.4.3

[34] American Speech-Language-Hearing Association (ASHA). (Central) Auditory Processing Disorders [Technical Report]. 2005. Available from: http:// www.asha.org/docs/html/tr2005-00043.html.

[35] Bellis, T.J. Comprehensive central auditory assessment. In: BELLIS, T.J. Assessment and Management of central auditory processing disorders in the educational setting from science to practice. 2nd ed. NY: Delmar Thompsons Learning, 2003.

[36] Idrizbegovic, E. et al. Central auditory function in early Alzheimer's disease and in mild cognitive impairment. Age Ageing. 2011;40(2);249–254. DOI: 10.1093/ageing/afq168

[37] Roup, C.M., Wiley, T.L., Wilson, R.H. Dichotic word recognition in young and older adults. J. Am. Acad. Audiol. 2007;17(4);230–240. Available from: http://dx.doi.org/10.3766/jaaa.17.4.2

[38] Stewart, R., Wingfield, A. Hearing loss and cognitive effort in older adults' report accuracy for verbal materials. J. Am. Acad. Audiol. 2009;20(2);147–154. http://dx.doi.org/10.3766/jaaa.20.2.7

[39] Fitzgibbons, P.J., Gordon-Salant, S. Age-related differences in discrimination of temporal intervals in accented tone sequences. Hearing Res. 2010;264;41–47. DOI: 10.1016/j.heares.2009.11.008 DOI:10.1016%2Fj.heares.2009.11.008

[40] Gordon-Salant, S. Auditory temporal processing in elderly listeners. J. Am. Acad. Audiol. 1996;7;183–189.

[41] Gil, D., Iorio, M.C.M. Formal auditory training in adult hearing aid users. Clin. Sci. 2010;65(2);165–174. DOI:10.1590/S1807-59322010000200008

[42] Dubno, J.R. Benefits of auditory training for aided listening by older adults. Am. J. Audiol. 2013;22(2);335–338. DOI:10.1044/1059-0889(2013/12-0080)

[43] Pichora-Fuller, M.K., Singh, G. Effects of age on auditory and cognitive processing: implications for hearing aid fitting and audiologic rehabilitation. Trend. Amplif. 2006;10(1);29–59. DOI: 10.1177/108471380601000103

[44] Weinstein, B.E. Outcome measures in the hearing aid fitting. Trend. Amplif. 1997;2(4); 117–137. DOI: 10.1177/108471389700200402

[45] Ventry I., Weinsten, B.E. The hearing handicap inventory for the elderly: a new tool. Ear Hear. 1982;3;128–134. Available from: http://dx.doi.org/10.1097/00003446-198205000-00006

[46] Cox, R.M., Alexander, G.C. The abbreviated profile of hearing aid benefit. Ear Hear. 1995;16(2);176–183. Available from: http://dx.doi.org/10.1097/00003446-199504000-00005

[47] Dillon, H., James, A., Ginis, J. Client oriented scale of improvement (COSI) and its relationship to several other measures of benefit and satisfaction provided by hearing aids. J. Am. Acad. Audiol. 1996;8;27–43.

[48] Naylor, G., Elberling, C. Benefit from hearing aids in relation to the interaction between the user and the environment. Int. J. Audiol. 2003;42. DOI: http://dx.doi.org/10.3109/14992020309074627

[49] Mukrow, C.D., Tuley, M.R., Aguilar, C. Sustained benefits of hearing aids. J. Speech Language Hearing Res. 1992;35;1402–1405. DOI: 10.1044/jshr.3506.1402

[50] Humes, L.E., Wilson, D.L., Barlow, N.N., Garner, C. Chances in hearing aid benefit following 1 or 2 years of hearing aid use by older adults. J. Speech Language Hearing Res. 2002;445;772–782. DOI:10.1044/1092-4388

[51] Newman, C.W., Weinstein, B.E. The hearing handicap inventory for the elderly as a measure: of hearing aid benefit. Ear Hearing. 1988. Available from: https://doi.org/10.1097/00003446-198804000-00006

[52] Chmiel, R, Jerger, J. Hearing aid use, central auditory disorders and hearing handicap in elderly persons. J. Am. Acad. Audiol. 1996;7;190–202.

Section 5

Cochlear Implants

Chapter 8

Temporal Filterbanks in Cochlear Implant Hearing and Deep Learning Simulations

Payton Lin

Additional information is available at the end of the chapter

http://dx.doi.org/10.5772/66627

Abstract

The masking phenomenon has been used to investigate cochlear excitation patterns and has even motivated audio coding formats for compression and speech processing. For example, cochlear implants rely on masking estimates to filter incoming sound signals onto an array. Historically, the critical band theory has been the mainstay of psychoacoustic theory. However, masked threshold shifts in cochlear implant users show a discrepancy between the observed critical bandwidths, suggesting separate roles for place location and temporal firing patterns. In this chapter, we will compare discrimination tasks in the spectral domain (e.g., power spectrum models) and the temporal domain (e.g., temporal envelope) to introduce new concepts such as profile analysis, temporal critical bands, and transition bandwidths. These recent findings violate the fundamental assumptions of the critical band theory and could explain why the masking curves of cochlear implant users display spatial and temporal characteristics that are quite unlike that of acoustic stimulation. To provide further insight, we also describe a novel analytic tool based on deep neural networks. This deep learning system can simulate many aspects of the auditory system, and will be used to compute the efficiency of spectral filterbanks (referred to as "FBANK") and temporal filterbanks (referred to as "TBANK").

Keywords: auditory masking, cochlear implants, filter bandwidths, filterbanks, deep neural networks, deep learning, machine learning, compression, audio coding, speech pattern recognition, profile analysis, temporal critical bands, transition bandwidths

1. Introduction

The transformation of sound into a representation within the auditory system involves many layers of information analysis and processing. Sound is first converted into nervous impulses by cochlear hair cells, which are mechanically organized to distribute the spectral energy of their excitation along the length of the basilar membrane (**Figure 1**). The connecting nerve fibers show a bandpass response to the input signal, where the density of firings for a particular fiber varies with the stimulus intensity over a certain range. Basic information from a sound is then extracted and passed to subsequent stages for perceptual machinery to present its own construction of reality. Noninvasive methods are needed to investigate the influence of these higher-level perceptual processes on the properties of the cochlea. For example, the method of psychophysical inference is often used to fill in the gaps of physiological knowledge.

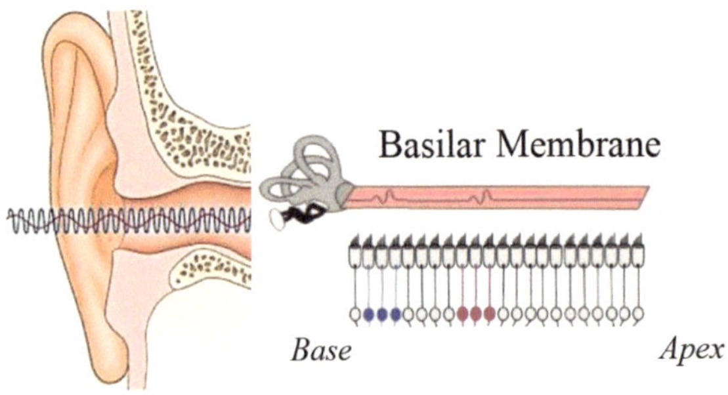

Figure 1. Spatial arrangement of cochlear hair cells along the basilar membrane (base to apex).

This chapter will be divided into two sections. In the section on human hearing research, we will predict neural firing characteristics from the perspective of psychoacoustic "*masking*" experiments. In the section on machine hearing research, we will compare artificial neural network input from the perspective of machine learning experiments. Experimental data is presented in both human hearing and machine hearing to supplement the incompleteness of current neurophysical methods by providing new insight into the stages of processing.

2. Human hearing research

2.1. Auditory masking

2.1.1. Spectral masking

The masking phenomenon of one tone by another provides quantitative data on frequency selectivity and the dynamical theory of the cochlea [1]. In a psychoacoustic experiment, the testing stimulus is called the probe, the sound that interferes with the detection of the probe is called the masker, and the amount of masking refers to the amount by which the hearing threshold of the probe is raised in the presence of the masker. The method of measuring a threshold shift is straightforward. First, the detection threshold of the probe is determined. Next, the threshold shift of the probe is determined in the presence of the masker. Auditory masking curves have established wide-ranging mathematical relationships between sensory behavioral responses and even the activity of single neurons [2]. In general, the probe is most easily masked by sounds with frequency components that are close to the probe.

http://dx.doi.org/10.5772/66627

2.1.2. *Critical band theory*

The "*critical band theory*" [3] has played an important role in hypothesizing how the auditory system resolves the components of complex sound. In classic band-widening experiments, the threshold of a sinusoidal probe is measured as a function of the bandwidth of a noise masker. First, a noise with a constant power density is centered at the probe frequency. As the bandwidth increases, the total noise power increases (which presumably has effects on the threshold for detecting the probe).

Masking curves have shown that the threshold of the probe increases at first, but flattens off as the addition of more noise (at a greater distance from the probe frequency) produces no additional masking. The bandwidth at which the probe threshold ceases to increase is called the "*critical bandwidth*." To account for these observations, the listener is assumed to make use of a filter with a center frequency close to the probe when detecting the probe in noise. According to this critical bandwidth theory, the noises outside the range of the filter should presumably have no effect on detection. If this filter passes the signal and removes much of the noise, then only the components of the noise that passes through the filter should have any effect in masking the probe. Therefore, thresholds should correspond to a certain signal-to-noise ratio at the output of the auditory filter.

According to this *power spectrum model* of masking, all stimuli are represented by their long-term power spectra (or the relative phases of the components) while short-term fluctuations in the masker are ignored. **Figure 2** shows the typical estimates of energy detection. Although *energy detection models* remain fundamental to theories of auditory perception, the axiom that energy only passes by a single auditory filter has been contradicted multiple times [4–7]. These findings violate the fundamental assumption of critical band theory and therefore challenge previous estimates of peripheral filtering.

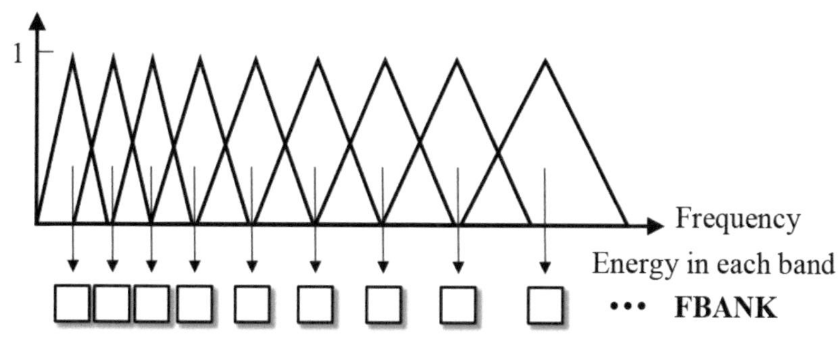

Figure 2. Energy detector model where the basilar membrane behaves as if it contains a bank of bandpass filters with overlapping passbands, where each point along the basilar membrane corresponds to a filter with a different center frequency. This Fourier-transform-based log filterbank with spectral coefficients distributed on a mel-scale is often referred to as "FBANK" in audio-coding applications involving machine learning. In the section on machine hearing research, the computational efficiency of FBANK will be evaluated in deep learning systems.

2.1.3. *Profile analysis*

According to the critical bandwidth theory, a tone added to noise should be detected by an increase in the energy from a single auditory filter centered at the signal frequency. On the contrary, experimental manipulations (e.g., roving-level procedures) that degrade energy cues in tone-in-noise detection tasks show no effects on detection thresholds. Listeners must therefore rely on alternative cues instead of just spectral analysis of a stimulus to explain the data of level-invariant detection (where single-channel energy cues are severely disrupted). In "*profile analysis*" [5], this process is described as detecting changes in the overall shape of the spectrum. With across-channel cues, listeners are able to compare the shape or profile of the outputs of different auditory filters to enhance signal detection.

2.1.4. Temporal critical bands

Temporal discrimination tasks offer an alternative to spectral critical bands. In a temporal model, the detection cues are thought to be temporal in nature and based on changes in the cadence of neural discharge. These temporal models contrast with energy detection models that assume a rate-place neural code. Recently, auditory filter bandwidths were measured for a temporal process using an amplitude-modulation (AM) detection task [6]. The critical bandwidth for a temporal process (referred to as "*temporal critical band*") was observed to be consistently greater than that predicted by the critical band theory. Therefore, these findings decrease confidence in previous estimates of peripheral filtering.

2.1.5. Transition bandwidths

Discontinuous threshold functions also contradict spectral critical bandwidths by implying that the discrimination tasks evoke different and separate auditory processes. For instance, "*transition bandwidths*" [7] assume that envelope cues dominate at narrow bandwidths, while across-channel level comparisons dominate at wide bandwidths. This concept stresses that there are changes in the underlying process, unlike the constraining boundaries of a solitary process (as hypothesized in critical bandwidth or energy integration theories). For transition bandwidths, the changes to another dominant auditory process are thought to be due to a central mechanism (whereas critical bandwidths are only associated with the periphery). Therefore, transition bandwidths allow for multiple filtering processes to occur.

2.1.6. The volley theory

The divergence of positions between spectral bandwidths and temporal bandwidths shares similar controversies as the *place theory* and the *temporal theory* of pitch perception. The place theory states that the perception of sound depends on where each component of frequency produces vibrations. The temporal theory states that the perception of sound depends on the temporal patterns of neurons responding to sound in the cochlea. The "*volley theory*" [8] postulates that groups of neurons in the auditory system respond to firing action potentials that are slightly out-of-phase with one another so that they can be combined to encode and send a greater frequency of sound to the brain for analysis, as shown in **Figure 3**. In the next sections, we describe the importance of resolving these theories and assumptions to improve real-world solutions for data *compression* and speech processing. For instance, we will compare the efficiency of systems that use only one filterbank or multiple filterbanks.

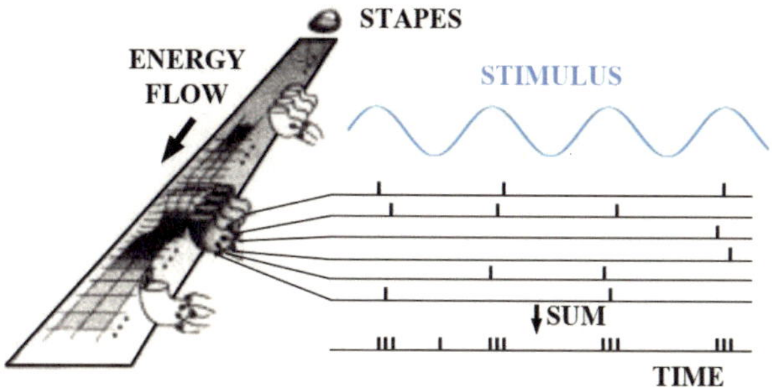

Figure 3. Temporal properties of nerve firing according to the "volley theory" of temporal coding.

2.2. Filterbanks

2.2.1. Audio coding and data compression

Audio coding formats that use lossy data compression take advantage of human auditory masking properties [9]. For instance, the MP3 format hides noises under the signal spectrum based on the masking property that sounds near the threshold of another sound will either be completely masked or reduced in loudness. These auditory masking properties also play critical roles in both speech coding applications and objective quality measures. In the next section, we will cover the impact of auditory masking on the coding of *cochlear implants* (devices that require data compression due to the electroneural bottleneck).

2.2.2. Cochlear implants

The cochlear implant is a surgically implanted electronic device that restores partial hearing to a person who is deaf or hearing impaired [10–12]. This neural prosthesis provides similar functions of the inner ear by electrically stimulating the auditory nerve. Cochlear implants consist of an external microphone, a speech processor, a transmitter, an internal receiver, and a multielectrode array stimulator. The microphone is placed on the ear and picks up incoming sounds from the environment. The speech processor filters these incoming sounds into different frequency channels and sets the appropriate electrical stimulation parameters. Next, a transmitter coil powers and transmits the processed sound signals through the skin to the internal receiver. Finally, the receiver converts the signals into electric impulses that stimulate an electrode array. Electrode arrays are surgically coiled within the scala tympani of the cochlea so that individual electrode plates can electrically stimulate different regions of the auditory nerve. A sparse electric representation is sufficient for the restoration of hearing.

Cochlear implant performance is satisfactory in quiet settings, but the abnormal perception of electric pitch limits the performance in noise. Typical users only detect over a 10% change in pitch compared to normal-hearing listeners who easily detect <1% change. Electric pitch is degraded because only a limited number of electrodes (~22 electrodes) can be inserted into the cochlea versus the >3000 inner hair cell transducers in a normal cochlea. In addition, the current spread from each electrode is uncontrollably broad and large areas of nerves can be unintentionally activated. Spectral mismatches can also occur from degraded nerve survival or inaccurate frequency-to-electrode allocation [11].

Speech recognition in noise becomes especially difficult without the ability to adequately separate components of sound from interfering sources. **Figure 4** shows the cochlear implant coding scheme [12] that was discovered to greatly improve speech recognition. This sparse representation at the auditory periphery is unique as it presents electric pulse stimulations that feature both (1) temporal envelope information and (2) place information. Section 3.2.3 will discuss how this coding is simulated as temporal envelope bank (TBANK) features in deep learning systems [13].

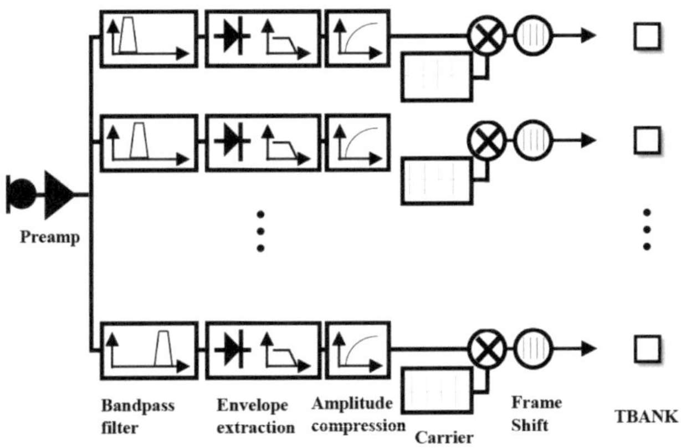

Figure 4. Temporal properties of a cochlear implant processor. In machine learning, temporal features can be derived from extracted temporal envelope bank (referred to as "TBANK").

2.3. Auditory masking in cochlear implants

To optimize current settings, psychoacoustic experiments were designed to investigate how the human auditory system processes complex sound interactions from electric stimulations. Specifically, auditory masking was investigated using electric stimulations as the probe or masker to understand how electric stimulations separate into individual sound sources. The diversified subject population with different types of hearing loss and electric configurations also provide alternative testing paradigms to reevaluate previous masking results obtained from normal hearing subjects. By measuring electric stimulations, the research field can gain new insight to study the interactions of peripheral and central auditory systems. In this section, we will review previous comparisons of ipsilateral *electric-on-electric* masking, *electric-on-acoustic* masking, and also contralateral *electric-on-electric* masking. We will then compare auditory masking curves in cochlear implants with the recently proposed concepts of profile analysis, temporal critical band, and transition bandwidths in normal hearing.

2.3.1. Comparison of electric-on-electric masking

Similar to the observations in normal hearing, electric masking studies [14] have shown that the amount of forward masking increases by decreasing the spatial separation between the

http://dx.doi.org/10.5772/66627

probe electrodes and the electric pulses from adjacent maskers. Both the amount of masking and the spread of neural excitation increase with electric masker levels. Cochlear implant excitation patterns were also shown to have a spatial bandpass characteristic with a peak in the region of the masked electrode [15].

2.3.2. *Comparison of electric-on-acoustic masking*

Electric-on-acoustic masking can also be measured for cochlear implant users who have preserved residual acoustic hearing following implantations (**Figure 5**). In a unilateral cochlear implant user with functional hearing preserved in the implanted ear, electric stimulations were observed to interact in the peripheral and central auditory system [16]. The masking growth function in **Figure 5** shows the detection thresholds of an electrode increased when the level of a 125-Hz acoustic masker increased from 90 to 110 dB. The 250-Hz acoustic masker also elevated electric detection in a similar manner. This data is consistent with the central theory of auditory masking and even provides new supporting evidence since the acoustic stimulations had to have been confined to the functional hair cells or nerves (as there is no known mechanism that acoustic stimulations could have directly activated a nerve fiber).

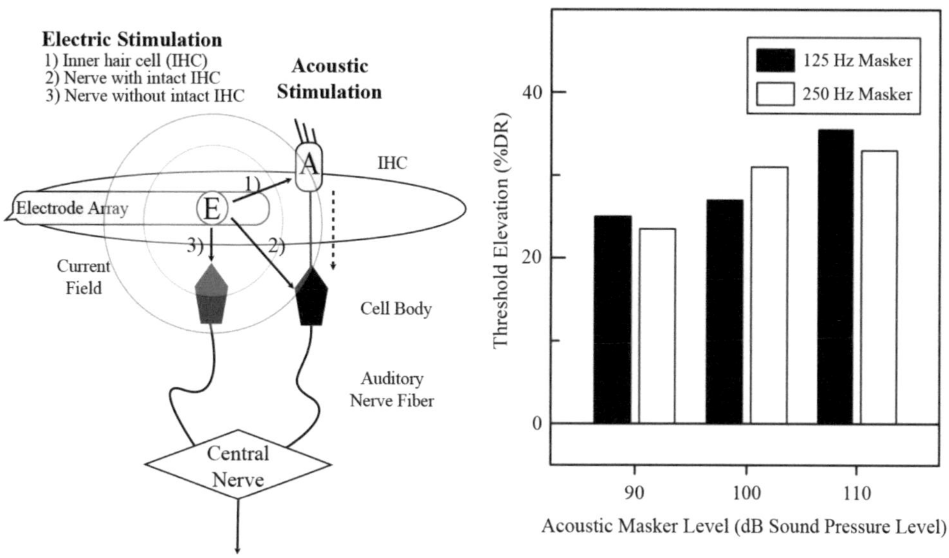

Figure 5. Ipsilateral masking data from [16]. The left panel shows a schematic representation of the acoustic (A) masking and the electric (E) masking mechanisms in hybrid hearing. The right panel shows the masking of an electrode probe by acoustic maskers at 125 or 250 Hz.

2.3.3. *Comparison of contralateral electric-on-electric masking*

Contralateral electric-on-electric masking can also be measured in bilateral cochlear implant users [17]. **Figure 6** shows the complete set of central masking data, with threshold elevation normalized so that each function peaks at 1. Each of the bilateral subjects was tested twice, alternating the ear used as the masker or probe (n = 14). As shown in **Figure 6**, the contralateral masking electrodes elevated the detection thresholds in both the left and the

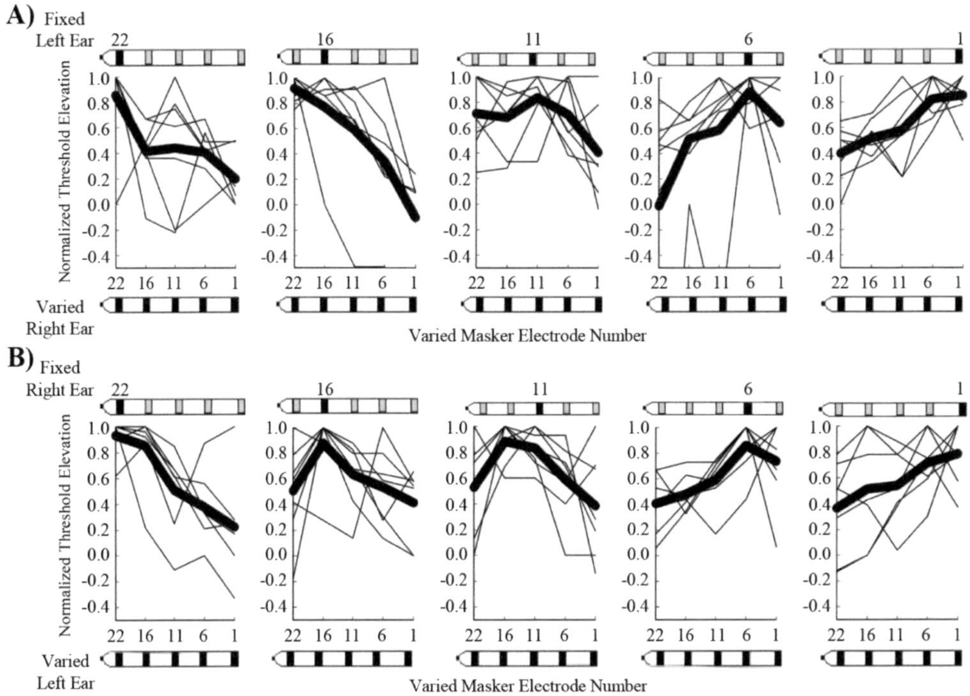

Figure 6. Central masking data measured and replotted for seven bilateral cochlear implant subjects from [17]. The curves are sorted into panels according to the location of the probe electrode number (black contacts) in either the (A) fixed left ear or (B) fixed right ear. Thin lines show the individual central masking curves and the thick lines show the mean data for each fixed probe electrode location. All curves are normalized so that the peak threshold is equal to 1.

right ears. The threshold elevation peaks generally occurred between interaural pairings sharing the same electrode number (which corresponds to electrodes with similar insertion depths across ears).

Figure 7 presents the same data to show the growth of masking as a function of the masker-probe electrode separation across ears. Masker-probe separation is calculated by subtracting the differences between the masker and probe electrode numbers. Place-matched masking conditions are categorized as "0" since both the masker and probe electrode numbers were identical across ears. When categorized in this manner, **Figure 7** shows the amount of central masking diminished with masker-probe electrode separation. In [17], this data was reorganized to analyze the growth of masking. A two-way repeated measure analysis of variance (ANOVA) showed a significant main effect of masker-probe electrode separation and threshold elevation [$F(2.122, 27.581) = 3.667$, $p = 0.036$]. There was also a significant main effect of masker-probe electrode separation, ear used as the probe electrode, and threshold elevation [$F(2.563, 33.323 = 9.472$, $p < 0.001$]. The masking growth pattern for each ear was also fitted with exponential equations and displayed similar spatial constants and significant R^2 values ($R^2 > 0.97$). The results demonstrate that the amount of central masking diminished with masker-probe electrode separation at similar rates on both sides.

http://dx.doi.org/10.5772/66627

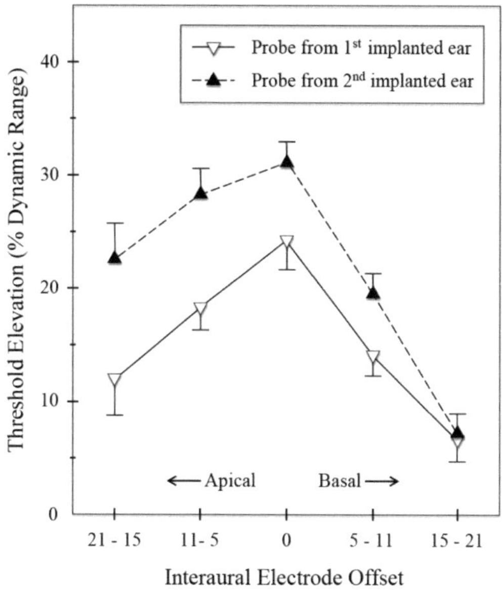

Figure 7. Threshold elevation as a function of the interaural electrode offset between the masker and the probe (n = 14). "Apical" refers to all masking conditions where the masker was apically positioned from the probe, whereas "basal" refers to all conditions where the masker was basally positioned from the probe. The 1st and 2nd implanted ears refer to the ears on each side of a participating subject that were sequentially implanted in two separate surgeries.

Figures 6 and **7** show bilateral cochlear implant stimulation contralaterally masked in a place-dependent manner. For electric-on-electric signals, the average thresholds peaked when the position of the masker and probe electrodes were place-matched across ears and diminished with electrode separation. These place-dependent findings have also been reconfirmed in a recent work [18] using different electrode arrays and testing apparatus. However, both studies [17–18] directly counter a previous conclusion in [19] that central masking with bilateral users gives rise to increased threshold, but not in a place-dependent manner (as is the case for contralateral masking in normal hearing). This previously accepted hypothesis in [19] was most likely concluded from data that was obscured by a limited test population (n = 2), electrical malfunctions (arrays with multiple electrical shorts), subjects reporting discomfort (uncomfortably high-pitched sensations), and electrodes that were inserted with primitive surgical techniques (offsets in electrode place accuracy of 6–9 electrodes).

2.3.4. *Comparison of masking in cochlear implants and normal hearing*

It will be important to optimize the configurations of cochlear implant stimulation as it has been reported that electrical pulse trains and acoustic sine waves do not fuse or merge well into a single percept [17, 20]. The presence of electric masking has indicated regions where electric and acoustic signals share similar frequencies as normal acoustic masking. However, the data in **Figure 6** show a large amount of individual variability as many of the bilateral participants displayed unmatched masking patterns across ears. This individual variability could be the result of several factors. First, cochlear implant users are likely to have irregular patterns of auditory nerve survival, which could cause the current to stimulate auditory fibers that are too apical or too basal from the intended location. "Dead regions" in auditory nerves may also prevent the adjacent masking electrodes from stimulating distinct place-frequencies. Second, different surgical procedures could result in variability between the insertion depths of a user's electrode array. This variability could be significant since neural activation patterns depend on the density of neurons in a particular region of the cochlea and on the radial distance between the electrode array and neural targets in the modiolus.

In general, cochlear implant subjects have exhibited electric-masking patterns that are much broader compared to what has been observed in normal hearing [14–20]. A reduction in the magnitude of contralateral versus ipsilateral masking functions was observed in [18], but this reduction was not as great as observed in normal hearing. Together, these findings of broader masking with cochlear implants both support and are supported by the concepts of:

1. Distorted *profile analysis*, where cochlear implant users are unable to adequately use across-channel cues to compare the shape of the output of different auditory filters.
2. Reliance on *temporal critical bands*, where cochlear implant users relied on filter bandwidths that were consistently broader than predicted by critical band theory.
3. Rapidly changing *transition bandwidths*, where cochlear implant users used separate and different auditory processes to handle either the narrow or wide bandwidths.
4. Distorted *volley theory* of encoding, where cochlear implant users were unable to combine the phases of action potentials to analyze a greater frequency of sound.

These findings all decrease confidence in previous estimates of peripheral filtering as well as the assumptions made in *critical band theory*, especially when combined with recent evidence in normal-hearing listeners that suggest a flexible selection of spectral regions upon which to base across-frequency comparisons [21]. Furthermore, the wide bandwidths observed in the initial filters of the cochlear implant subjects directly contradicts the theory that extraction of envelope information should be constrained to a single auditory filter, as theorized in [22]. For these reasons, *transition bandwidths* [7, 23] are the most plausible solution as they explain patterns that were observed in both normal hearing and electric hearing experiments (as this concept allows an interplay to occur between temporal or spectral processes). In the section on machine hearing research, a novel method based on "*deep learning*" is utilized to prove the computational efficiency of transition bandwidths in artificial neural network systems.

3. Machine hearing research

3.1. Motivation to compare human and machine hearing systems

There are several factors that have confounded cochlear implant research. Psychoacoustic experiments are often rendered inconclusive due to large individual variabilities in cochlear implant subjects. The physical limitations of uncontrollable test populations include variable nerve survival before implantation, inter-implant intervals and usage time, neuroplasticity after implantation, age at testing, and surgical insertion depths. These physical limitations have significant effects on the amount of masking [16, 17]. In addition, individual variability can arise due to cognitive factors or subjective testing protocols. For instance, the evaluation of cochlear implants can be unintentionally influenced by decision rules or dynamic ranges based on loudness judgment, visual feedback, sequential test order, unrealistic simulations, and even the content material used in subjective studies such as speech recognition [24, 25]. Therefore, alternative methods such as computational simulations and mathematical models should be used in order to account for these uncontrollable factors of individual variation.

We can only appreciate how sophisticated the human auditory system truly is when trying to simulate perceptual processing on a computer. By building a computational model, we gain new insight and develop quantitative ways to analyze each step of signal processing. Computational models are well suited to investigate how information from independent fibers are distributed and the extent to which distinct bandpass filterbanks are constructed within neural architectures [4]. In this chapter, we use artificial neural networks in order to measure response properties of auditory fibers using realistic representations of different integrative processes. Machine learning can provide algorithms for understanding learning in neural systems and can even benefit from these ongoing biological studies [26].

3.2. Deep neural networks (DNNs)

3.2.1. Automatic speech recognition: an auditory perspective

There have been many attempts to incorporate principles of human hearing into machine systems [27]. The motivation for these previous attempts was simply that human perception is much more stable than machines over a range of sources of variability. Therefore, it was reasonable to expect that the functional modeling of the human subsystems could provide plausible direction for machine research. One of the first auditory-inspired features (**Figure 2**) was based on the mel-scale warping of the spectral frequency axis (referred to as "FBANK"), which is then parameterized as mel-frequency cepstral coefficients (referred to as "MFCC") [28]. The usual objective for selecting an appropriate representation is to compress the input data by eliminating the information that is not pertinent for analysis and to enhance those aspects of the signal that contributes significantly to the detection of differences. In *automatic speech recognition* (ASR), these MFCC features were shown to allow better suppression of insignificant spectral variation in the higher-frequency bands. Concatenating other types of auditory-inspired spectro-temporal features with MFCCs can also boost performance [29]. In [30], cochlear implant speech synthesized from subband temporal envelope was shown to contain sufficient information to rival MFCC features in terms of accuracy. These acoustic simulations of cochlear implants [31] were subsequently proposed as general indicators to conduct useful subjective studies. In [32], the cross-disciplinary methods of cognitive science and machine learning were converged to promote the shared views of computational [33] foundations. Our study [32] expanded on [30] by comparing cochlear implant results using the Bayesian model of human concept learning [34] and proposed hidden Markov models (HMMs) for computationally predicting cochlear implant performance. In the next sections, we will further expand upon previous studies by introducing state-of-the-art tools based on *deep neural network* algorithms and presenting new results comparing the efficiency of profile analysis, temporal critical band, and transition bandwidths in cochlear implant simulations.

3.2.2. Spectral filterbank (FBANK) features as input to deep learning systems

Deep neural networks (DNNs) (**Figure 8**) make use of gradient-based optimization algorithms to adjust parameters throughout a multilayered network based on the errors at its input [35]. In DNNs, multiple processing layers learn representations of data with multiple levels of abstractions. In deep hierarchal structures, the internal layers of DNNs provide learned representations of the input data. The benefit of studying filterbank learning in DNNs is that the filterbank input can be viewed as an extra layer of the network, where these filterbank parameters are updated along with the parameters in subsequent layers [36, 37].

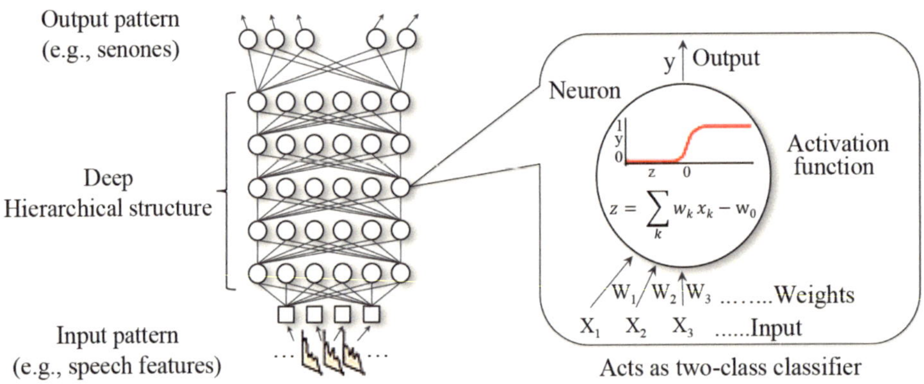

Figure 8. Structure of a deep neural network (DNN). Deep learning allows multiple layers of nonlinear processing.

In machine learning, speech is viewed as a two-dimensional signal where the spatial and temporal dimensions have vastly different characteristics. For instance, the time-dynamic information in the high-frequency regions is different compared to low-frequency regions. Although FBANK is popular, Sainath et al. [36, 37] argued that features designed based on the critical band theory might not guarantee appropriate frameworks for the end goal of reducing error rates. Since the power-spectra removes information from the signal by computing from a fixed window-length, FBANK features often lack the necessary temporal information. By starting with a raw signal representation to learn filterbanks jointly in a DNN framework, the results computed in [36] share many similarities as concepts from psychoacoustic studies:

1. Consistent with *critical band theory*, the computational results showed a similarity between learned and mel-filters in the low-frequency regions.

2. Consistent with *transition bandwidths*, the computational results showed the learned filters had multiple peaks in the mid-frequency regions (indicating that multiple important critical frequencies are being picked up, rather than just one like the mel).

http://dx.doi.org/10.5772/66627

3. Consistent with the *volley theory*, the computational results showed the learned filters are high-pass filters compared to mel-filters (which are bandpass at high-frequency regions).

3.2.3. Temporal envelope bank (TBANK) features

Our work in [13, 32] derived an alternative input feature (**Figure 4**) for ASR based on temporal envelope bank (referred to as "TBANK") which was inspired by *temporal critical bands* [6] and the broad temporal masking patterns of cochlear implants [16, 17]. The TBANK features have been evaluated as an input feature for DNNs [38] and as a temporal alignment feature for DNNs [39]. In the present study, we will combine both FBANK and TBANK features to improve the temporal dimension and its correlation with the frequency or spatial-domain properties in DNNs. **Figure 9** shows FBANK+TBANK (referred to as □□, "double-BANK") features, which were inspired by psychoacoustic results showing the flexible usage of across-channel cues [21], transition bandwidths [7, 23], and the volley theory [8].

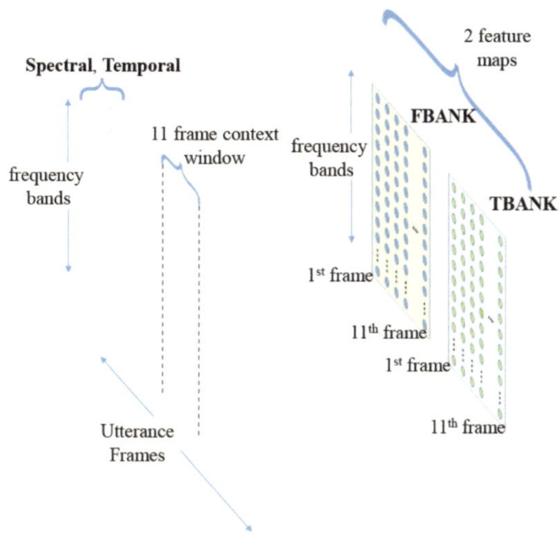

Figure 9. A simplified FBANK+TBANK (referred to as □□, "*double-BANK*") representation of speech.

In Section 3.3, we will use the same procedures in [38, 39] for the Aurora-4 robustness task (with a cochlear implant speech processor available at: www.tigerspeech.com/angelsim).

3.3. Computational results

3.3.1. Comparison of FBANK and TBANK on a computational ASR task

"Raw" TBANK features were derived from 32 channels of band envelope (**Figure 4**) via white-noise carriers [38]. These features were designed to preserve temporal and amplitude cues in each spectral band, but remove the spectral detail within each band as explained in [12]. Δ and $\Delta\Delta$ dynamic features were computed from derivative values with respect to time [40]. In **Table 1**, context-dependent DNN-HMMs were trained using 40-dimensional FBANK (described in [36]), 120-dimensional FBANK+Δ+ΔΔ (described in [41]), and our 80-dimensional □□ (FBANK+TBANK) input representation. It should be noted that the computational cost of changing the size of the input layer is negligible. **Table 1** shows inclusion of TBANK in the □□ (FBANK+TBANK) input features yielded a 14% improvement compared to FBANK and an 11% improvement over the FBANK+Δ+ΔΔ representation.

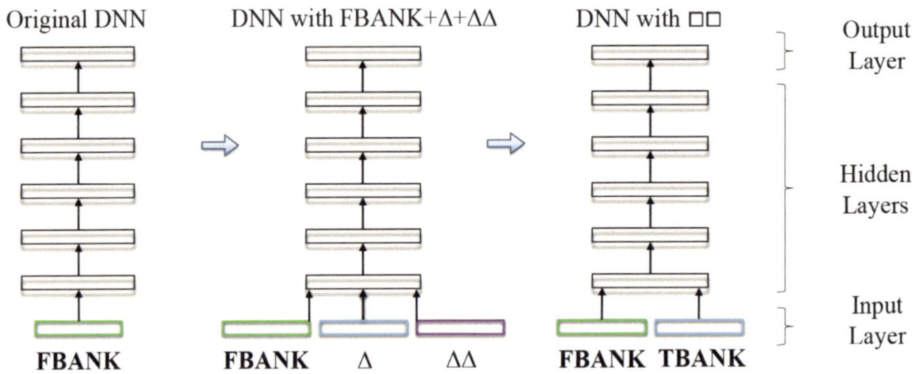

Parameterization	Test set A
FBANK	2.88
FBANK+Δ+ΔΔ	2.76
FBANK+TBANK	**2.47**

Note: **Bold** indicates better score.

Table 1. DNN performance (error rate %) on clean training set.

3.3.2. Comparison of FBANK and TBANK on temporal alignment task

Table 2 shows error rates for *Gaussian mixture model* (GMM)-HMMs when trained and tested on TBANK (**Figure 4**) alignment features (**Figure 10**) with white-noise carrier [13, 39]. TBANK models models aligned the training data to create senone labels for training the DNN. The results in **Table 2** show the temporally aligned DNN gives fewer errors when subsequently trained and tested on FBANK features.

Tree-building features	Error % (GMM)	Error % (DNN)
MFCC	5.08	2.88
16 band envelopes	5.44	**2.80**
24 band envelopes	**5.03**	**2.63**
32 band envelopes	5.90	**2.82**

Note: **Bold** indicates better score.

Table 2. Comparison of different tree-building features to generate a state-level alignment on the training set. TBANK features had 16, 24, or 32 band envelopes via white-noise carrier.

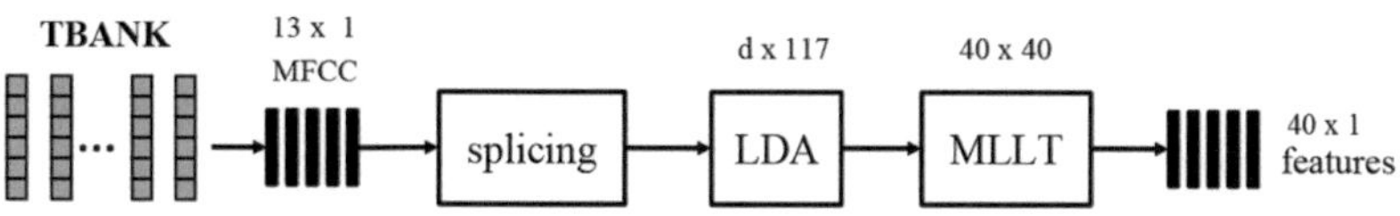

Figure 10. Generation of temporal alignment features using extracted TBANK, as in [39].

Designing a representation that both preserves relevant detail in the speech signal and also provides stability/invariance to distortions is a nontrivial task. Therefore, **Figure 11** derives slowly varying amplitude modulation (AM) and frequency modulation (FM) from speech to design novel features (referred to as frequency amplitude modulation encoding "FAME") with different modulations, as proposed in [42] and computed in ASR [31, 39]. In the FAME condition, the FM is smoothed in terms of both rate and depth and then modulated by the AM. The "slow" FM tracks gradual changes around a fixed frequency in the subband. The FAME stimuli are obtained by additionally frequency modulating each of the band's center frequency before amplitude modulation and subband summation. Finally, FAME stimuli were used to derive alternative features via extracted TBANK (**Figure 10**) for tree building and temporal alignment in GMM systems.

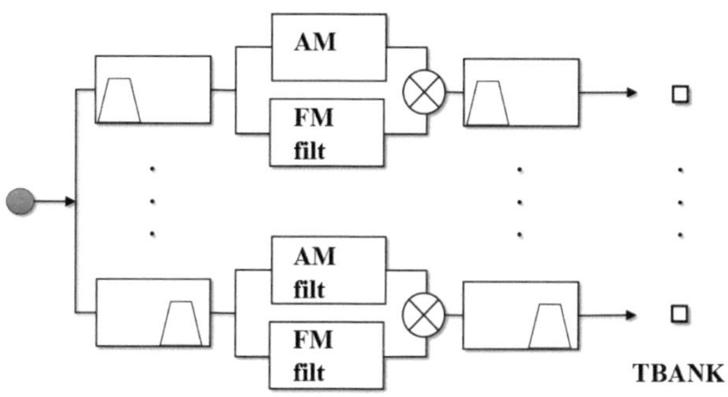

Figure 11. Signal processing diagram of *frequency amplitude modulation encoding* (FAME).

Compared to band envelope features (**Figure 4**), **Table 3** shows AM and FM lowered the error rate in GMM systems used during forced alignment to generate frame-level DNN training labels. These results expand upon [31] and provide additional evidence that FAME preserves more of the relevant detail compared to other carriers.

Tree-building TBANK features	Error rate % (GMM-Alignment)
16 band envelopes	5.44
16 bands of FAME	**5.21**

Note: **Bold** indicates better score.

Table 3. Comparison of alternative TBANK features for GMM alignment systems.

Table 4 shows error rates for GMM systems trained and tested on an additive configuration of □□ (MFCC + FAME) (**Figure 12**). This configuration was inspired by a frequency-dependent model that explains the loudness function in human auditory systems [43]. In this two-stage model, the first stage of processing is performed by a mechanical mechanism in the cochlear (for high-frequency stimuli) and by a neural mechanism in the cochlear nucleus (for low-frequency stimuli). **Table 4** shows the DNN gives fewer errors during time alignment with this additive configuration of □□ (MFCC + FAME) when subsequently trained and tested on FBANK. By digitally adding the different high-frequency FAME information (via TBANK) to the low-frequency MFCC information, **Table 4** shows this additive □□ (MFCC + FAME) feature representation allowed a better alignment in GMM systems during the generation of senone training labels for training the DNN.

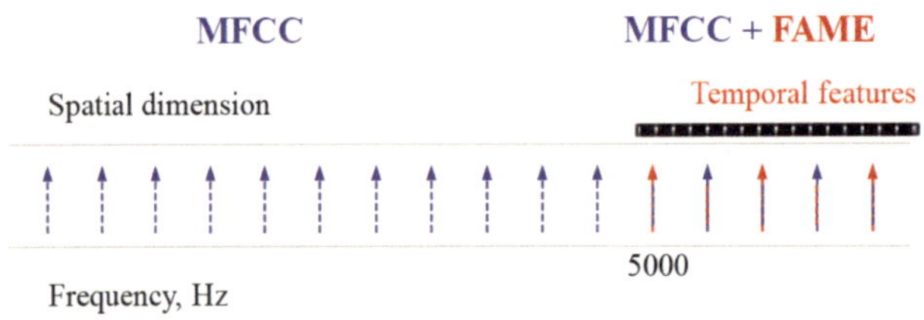

Figure 12. A digitally additive configuration of □□ alignment features (MFCC + FAME).

Table 5 provides further analysis [39] of deletion, substitution, or insertion errors to quantify the effects of the digitally additive □□ (MFCC + FAME) configuration. Misclassification leads to substitution errors. An imperfect segmentation leads to deletion errors (when some sounds are completely missed) or insertion errors (from extra boundaries). By reducing the extra segment boundaries, **Table 5** shows how front-end FAME processing using the FM extraction at high-frequency regions solves the segregating and binding problems [42] in ASR systems. The □□ results also demonstrate the computational efficiency of multiple filterbanks, which supports temporal critical bands [6] and transition bandwidths [7, 23].

Tree-building features	WER% (GMM)	WER% (DNN)
MFCC	5.08	2.88
MFCC + FAME	**4.82**	**2.75**

Note: **Bold** indicates better score.

Table 4. MFCC vs. □□ alignment feature (three additive FAME bands at high-frequency regions).

Tree-building features	(GMM) Deletion, substitution, insertion	(DNN) Deletion, substitution, insertion
MFCC	19, 189, 64	13, 114, 27
MFCC + FAME	20, **177**, **61**	18, **101**, 28

Note: **Bold** indicates less errors.

Table 5. Error type (deletion, substitution, insertion) analysis.

3.3.3. Discussion relating human hearing with machine hearing research

Many computational algorithms [9, 27, 28, 29, 30, 31, 35, 40, 41, 42] have been inspired by auditory processing pathways in the human nervous system. Traditionally, the critical band theory is commonly accepted for baseline DNN features [35] due to the ability of MFCC and FBANK to allow better suppression of insignificant spectral variation in the higher-frequency bands. However, recent progress in deep learning systems has allowed computational models that are composed of multiple layers of parallel processing to learn representations of filterbank features with multiple levels of abstraction. In fact, some DNN researchers have questioned the efficiency of spectral features derived from critical band theory. In [36], error rates were shown to improve by using a filterbank learning approach rather than just having a fixed set of filters. Therefore, [36] was the first computational study to contradict the energy detector or power spectrum models of critical band theory using purely quantitative and statistical results.

In the present study, we compared masking in cochlear implants and □□ (FBANK+TBANK) input representations in deep learning. The data provides statistical evidence supporting the efficiency of profile analysis, temporal critical bands, and transition bandwidths. Therefore, results in both human hearing and machine hearing oppose the historically accepted critical band theory. Furthermore, all of these findings decrease confidence in previous estimates of peripheral filtering as presumed [3, 19, 22] and adopted in [27, 28]. Moreover, the similarity and compatibility of the results in both human and machine hearing could provide new insight into the ability to process sound and may lead to advances in cochlear implant methods [44] or alternative neural network architectures [45]. For example, [36] indicated that using a nonlinear perceptually motivated log function was appropriate in deep learning, since their results showed that using log nonlinearity with positive weights was preferable.

4. Conclusions

In this chapter, we presented psychoacoustic results that support a recent theory in auditory processing [7, 23]: that the auditory system is actually composed of multiple filterbanks in the processing of sound (instead of just a solitary peripheral filterbank as previously assumed). Psychoacoustic results using electric stimulation in cochlear implant users suggest distorted *profile analysis* (where users are unable to adequately use across-channel cues to compare the shape of the output of different auditory filters), a reliance on *temporal critical bands* (where users relied on filter bandwidths that were consistently broader than predicted by critical band theory), rapidly changing *transition bandwidths* (where users employed separate and different auditory processes to handle either narrow or wide bandwidths), and a distorted *volley theory* of encoding (where users were unable to combine phases of action potentials to analyze a greater frequency of sound). In addition, the results from our deep learning system confirmed the computational effectiveness of combining both spectral filterbanks (FBANK) and temporal filterbanks (TBANK). The combined input representations (each with its own filtering properties) are formed into □□ (double-BANK) features to improve the processing of information in multiple parallel processes. These □□ features all outperformed FBANK features in deep neural network (DNN) systems.

Glossary

Human hearing research

Auditory masking: perceptual phenomenon that occurs when the threshold of audibility for one sound is raised in the presence of another sound.

Cochlear implant: a surgically implanted electronic device that restores a sense of hearing.

Critical band theory: estimates the bandwidth of spectral frequencies within which a second sound is predicted to interfere with the perception of the first sound by auditory masking.

Electric-on-acoustic masking: reproduction of masking by using cochlear implant electrodes.

Electric-on-electric masking: production of masking using only cochlear implant electrodes.

Energy detector model: the nonlinear power spectrum model approximation of auditory responses (which is the inspiration for acoustic features such as FBANK and MFCC).

Place theory: pitch perception depends on the location along the basilar membrane.

Profile analysis: a signal is detected by noting a change in the spectrum at some frequency.

Temporal critical bands: critical bandwidth for a temporal process (e.g., temporal envelope).

Temporal theory: pitch perception depends on the temporal firing patterns of neurons.

Transition bandwidths: occurrence of an interplay between spectral and temporal processes.

Volley theory: groups of neurons respond to a sound by firing action potentials slightly out-of-phase to encode a greater representation of sound that is sent to the brain.

Machine hearing research

Automatic speech recognition: a computational method that allows recognition of language.

Data compression: algorithm that reduces the audio transmission and storage requirements.

Deep learning: branch of machine learning that models high level abstractions in the data via multiple layers of processing and nonlinear transformations within hierarchal structures.

Deep neural networks: artificial neural network inspired by the hierarchal modeling of brains.

Double-BANK (□□) features: the combination of features (e.g.: FBANK+TBANK) as inspired by the observance of temporal critical bands and transition bandwidths in the auditory system.

Frequency amplitude modulation encoding (FAME): alternative features derived via TBANK.

Gaussian mixture model hidden Markov model (GMM-HMM): Bayesian method to align DNNs.

Spectral filterbanks: acoustic features (MFCC or FBANK) inspired by the nonlinear spacing of power spectrum or energy detector models, and critical band theory.

Temporal filterbanks: acoustic features (e.g.: TBANK) inspired by temporal critical bands.

http://dx.doi.org/10.5772/66627

Acknowledgements

In this chapter, some parts of this work was performed when the author was with the Hearing and Speech Laboratory, University of California, Irvine, USA, with Fan-Gang Zeng. The author is now working with the Center for Information Technology Innovation (CITI), Academia Sinica, Taipei, Taiwan, with Yu Tsao.

Author details

Payton Lin

Address all correspondence to: paytonlin20@gmail.com

Center for Information Technology Innovation, Academia Sinica, Taipei, Taiwan

References

[1] Wegel, R. L., & Lane, C. E. (1924). The auditory masking of one pure tone by another and its probable relation to the dynamics of the inner ear, *Phys. Rev.*, 23, 266–285.

[2] Zwislocki, J. J. (1972). A theory of central auditory masking and its partial validation, *J. Acoust. Soc. Am.*, 52 (2B), 644–659.

[3] Fletcher, H. (1940). Auditory patterns, *Rev. Mod. Phys.*, 12, 47–65.

[4] Berg, B. G. (2004). A temporal model of level-invariant, tone-in-noise detection, *Psychol. Rev.*, 111, 917

[5] Spiegel, M. F., & Green, D. M. (1982). Signal and masker uncertainty with noise maskers of varying duration, bandwidth, and center frequency, *J. Acoust. Soc. Am.*, 71(5), 1204–1210.

[6] Shim, A. I., & Berg, B. G. (2013). Estimating critical bandwidths of temporal sensitivity to low-frequency amplitude modulation, *J. Acoust. Soc. Am.*, 133(5), 2834–2838.

[7] Berg, B. G. (2007). Estimating the transition bandwidth between two auditory processes: Evidence for broadband auditory filters, *J. Acoust. Soc. Am.*, 121(6), 3639–3645.

[8] Wever, E. G., & Bray, C. W. (1937). The perception of low tones and the resonance-volley theory, *J. Psychol.*, 3(1), 101–114.

[9] Schroeder, M. R., Atal, B. S., & Hall, J. L. (1979). Optimizing digital speech coders by exploiting masking properties of the human ear, *J. Acoust. Soc. Am.*, 66, 1647–1652.

[10] Choi, C. T., & Lee, Y. H. (2012). A review of stimulating strategies for cochlear implants, in Cochlear Implant Research Updates, Dr. Cila Umat (Ed.), InTech Open Access Publisher.

[11] Noble, J. H., Hedley-Williams, A. J., Sunderhaus, L., Dawant, B. M., Labadie, R. F., Camarata, S. M., & Gifford, R. H. (2016). Initial results with image-guided cochlear implant programming in children, *Otol. Neurotol.*, 37(2), e63–e69.

[12] Wilson, B. S. (2013). Toward better representations of sound with cochlear implants, *Nat. Med.*, 19(10), 1245–1248.

[13] Lin, P., Wang, S.-S., & Tsao, Y. (2015). Temporal information in tone recognition, in *IEEE ICCE*.

[14] Lim, H. H., Tong, Y. C., & Clark, G. M. (1989). Forward masking patterns produced by intracochlear electrical stimulation of one and two electrode pairs in the human cochlea, *J. Acoust. Soc. Am.*, 86, 971–980.

[15] Chatterjee, M., & Shannon, R. V. (1998). Forward masked excitation patterns in multi-electrode electrical stimulation, *J. Acoust. Soc. Am.*, 105, 2565–2572.

[16] Lin, P., Turner, C. W., Gantz, B. J., Djalilian, H. R., & Zeng, F.-G. (2011). Ipsilateral masking between acoustic and electric stimulations, *J. Acoust. Soc. Am.*, 130(2), 858–865.

[17] Lin, P., Lu, T., & Zeng, F.-G. (2013). Central masking with bilateral cochlear implants, *J. Acoust. Soc. Am.*, 133(2), 962–969.

[18] Aronoff, J. M., Padilla, M., Fu, Q. J., & Landsberger, D. M. (2015). Contralateral masking in bilateral cochlear implant patients: a model of medial olivocochlear function loss, *PloS one*, 10(3), e0121591.

[19] van Hoesel, R., & Clark, G. (1997). Psychophysical studies with two binaural cochlear implant subjects, *J. Acoust. Soc. Am.*, 102, 495–507.

[20] James, C., Blamey, P., Shallop, J. K., Incerti, P. V., & Nicholas, A. M. (2001). Contralateral masking in cochlear implant users with residual hearing in the non-implanted ear, *Audiol. Neurootol.*, 6, 87–97.

[21] Buss, E., Hall, III, J. W., & Grose, J. H (2013). Monaural envelope correlation perception for bands narrower or wider than a critical band, *J. Acoust. Soc. Am.*, 133, 405–416.

[22] Patterson, R. D., & Moore, B. C. J. (1986). Auditory filters and excitation patterns as representations of frequency resolution, in *Frequency Selectivity in Hearing*, London: Academic Press, pp. 123–177.

[23] Berg, B. G. (2013). A decision weight analysis of transition bandwidths, *J. Acoust. Soc. Am.*, 121(6), 3639–3645.

[24] Dorman, M. F., Loizou, P. C., & Rainey, D. (1997). Speech intelligibility as a function of the number of channels of stimulation for signal processors using sine-wave and noise-band outputs, *J. Acoust. Soc. Am.*, 102(4), 2403–2411.

[25] Whitmal, N.A., Poissant, S.F., Freyman, R.L., & Helfer, K.S. (2007). Speech intelligibility in cochlear implant simulations: effects of carrier type, interfering noise, and subject experience, *J. Acoust. Soc. Am.*, 122(4), 2376–2388.

[26] Jordan, M.I., & Mitchell, T.M. (2015). Machine learning: trends, perspectives, and prospects, *Science*, 349(6245), 255–260.

[27] Morgan, N., Bourlard, H., & Hermansky, H. (2004). Automatic speech recognition: an auditory perspective, in *Speech Processing in the Auditory system*, S. Greenberg, W.A. Ainsworth, A.N. Popper, & R.R. Fay (Ed.), New York: Springer, 309–338.

[28] Davis, S. B., & Mermelstein, P. (1990). Comparison of parametric representations for monosyllabic word recognition in continuously spoken sentences, in *IEEE Trans. ASSP.*, 28(4), 357–366.

[29] Schädler, M. R., Meyer, B. T., & Kollmeier, B. (2012). Spectro-temporal modulation subspace-spanning filter bank features for robust automatic speech recognition, *J. Acoust. Soc. Am.*, 131(5), 4134–4151.

[30] Do, C.-T., Pastor, D., & Goalic, A. (2010). On the recognition of cochlear implant-like spectrally reduced speech with MFCC and HMM-based ASR, *IEEE Trans. Audio, Speech Language Process.*, 18(5), 1065–1068.

[31] Do, C.-T. (2012). Acoustic simulations of cochlear implants in human and machine hearing research, research, in *Cochlear Implant Research* Updates, Dr. Cila Umat (Ed.), InTech Open Access Publisher.

[32] Lin, P., Chen, F., Wang, S.-S., Lai, Y.-H., & Tsao, Y. (2014). Automatic speech recognition with primarily temporal envelope information, in *Proc. Interspeech.*

[33] Gershman, S.J., Horvitz, E.J., & Tenenbaum, J. B. (2015). Computational rationality: a converging paradigm for intelligence in brains, minds, and machines, *Science*, 349(6245), 273–278.

[34] Tenebaum, J. B., (1999). Bayesian modeling of human concept learning, in *Advances in Neural Information Processing Systems, 11 (NIPS-99)*, M.S. Kearns, S.A. Solla, & D.A. Cohn (Ed.), MIT Press, 59–65.

[35] Hinton, G., Deng, L., Yu, D., Dahl, G. E., Mohamed, A. R., Jaitly, N., Senoir, A., Vanhoucke, V., Nguyen, P., Sainath, T. N., & Kingsbury, B. (2012). Deep neural networks for acoustic modeling in speech recognition: the shared views of four research groups, *IEEE Signal Processing Magazine*, 29(6), 82–97.

[36] Sainath, T. N., Kingsbury, B., Mohamed, A., & Ramabhadran, B. (2013). Learning filter banks within a deep neural framework, in *IEEE ASRU*, 297–302.

[37] Sainath, T. N., Kingsbury, B., Mohamed, A., Saon, G., & Ramabhadran B. (2014). Improvements to filterbank and delta learning within a deep neural network framework, in *Proc. ICASSP*, 6839–6843.

[38] Lin, P., Lyu, D.-C., Chang, Y.-F., & Tsao, Y. (2015). Speech recognition with temporal neural networks, in *Proc. Interspeech*.

[39] Lin, P., Lyu, D.-C., Chang, Y.-F., & Tsao, Y. (2015). Temporal alignment for deep neural networks, in *Proc. IEEE GlobalSip*.

[40] Sagayama, S., & Itakura, F. (1978). On individuality in a dynamic measure of speech, in *Proc. Spring Meeting of Acoust. Soc. Japan* (in Japanese), 589–590.

[41] Furui, S. (1986). On the role of spectral transition for speech perception, *J. Acoust. Soc. Am.*, 80(4), 1016–1025.

[42] Zeng, F.-G., Nie, K., Stickney, G., Kong, Y.-Y., Vongphoe, M., Bhargave, A., Wei, C., & Cao, K. (2005). Speech recognition with amplitude and frequency modulations, in *Proc. Nat. Acad. Sci. USA (PNAS)*, 2293–2298.

[43] Zeng, F.-G., & Shannon, R.V. (1994). Loudness-coding mechanisms inferred from electric stimulation of the human auditory system, *Science*, 264, 564–566.

[44] Francart, T., & McDermott, H. J. (2013). Psychophysics, fitting, and signal processing for combined hearing aid and cochlear implant stimulation, *Ear Hearing*, 34(6), 685–700.

[45] Sainath, T. N., Kingsbury, B., Saon, G., Soltau, H., Mohamed, A. R., Dahl, G., & Ramabhadran, B. (2015). Deep convolutional neural networks for large-scale speech tasks, *Neural Networks*, 64, 39–48.

Chapter 9

Treatment of Partial Deafness: The Polish School in World Science

Henryk Skarżyński and Piotr Henryk Skarżyński

Additional information is available at the end of the chapter

http://dx.doi.org/10.5772/67234

Abstract

Introduction of the method of treatment of partial deafness with cochlear implants has given many patients the previously inaccessible chance to (re)enter the world of sounds. This method of treatment had been developed and introduced to the world's medicine by H. Skarżyński in 2002, after the extensive research since 1997. This task involved creation of a multispecialty team of experts, development of a special surgical method, and concept of the therapy reflecting on the world largest number of hearing improving surgeries being performed for 13 years averaging 15,000 otosurgical procedures yearly. This chapter introduces the treatment of partial deafness, considered as the Polish School in world science and medicine.

Keywords: partial deafness, partial deafness treatment, otosurgery, cochlear implant, hearing preservation, inner ear structure preservation

1. Introduction

Treatment of partial deafness, both congenital and acquired, with application of cochlear implants is for many patients regardless of their age practically the only chance of entering or returning to the world of sounds. Cochlear implants have been in use for more than 40 years and had been applied in more than 200 thousand people globally. Application of cochlear implants in treatment of classic partial deafness is, on the other hand, the matter of the last 15 or so years. This method of treatment, which is applied to an inner ear which is in a part fully functional and in another part completely deaf, had been introduced to the world medicine by

Skarżyński in 2002 [1]. This important breakthrough had been preceded by research studies which had been conducted in the Institute of Physiology and Pathology of Hearing since 1997, regarding preservation of even the smallest residual hearing which would then be supplemented with a "new hearing" achieved through a cochlear implant [2–4]. Development of a special surgical method and concept of the therapy had been a great challenge requiring involvement of many specialists: ear surgeons and other physicians, clinical engineers, and many other professionals working in the field of hearing rehabilitation [5, 6]. This treatment method had been applied at the beginning to patients whose preoperative hearing was at the level of residual hearing and since 2002 to those whose hearing in low-frequency ranges was good. In these patients their preoperative hearing levels would enable from 5 to 16% of speech understanding [1]. When this hearing is supplemented with electric stimulation obtained with a cochlear implant, patients can achieve complete speech understanding and free communication with their environment [7, 8]. This had been a groundbreaking approach in science and medicine as it had demonstrated the previously negated feasibility of electric stimulation within the partially functional inner ear [9].

Presentation of this program and a resultant Polish School are a reflection of the largest in the world number of hearing improving surgeries being performed for 13 years—on average 15 thousand otosurgical procedures yearly. Established criteria which an achievement or event should fulfill in order to be considered a school in modern science are commonly known and involve a significant achievement and confirmation of the results and importance of the school through the large clinical material supported by the longitudinal follow-up. A very important, although difficult to achieve, indicator confirming the existence and importance of school's output is the marks of appreciation, awards, citations, and opinions in relevant fields of science. The partial deafness treatment (PDT), considered as the Polish School in world science, meets all the abovementioned criteria and many more.

The step-by-step surgical procedure has been described by Skarżyński et al. in 2010 [7]. Cochlear implantation in the partial deafness treatment is in all patients undergoing this procedure performed in the worse hearing ear. The procedure is performed in all cases using the six-step Skarżyński round window approach for partial deafness treatment with different straight electrodes. It can be a 28 mm, 25 mm, or 24 mm slim straight electrode with different numbers of contacts and diameters 0.3 mm at the tip and 0.6 mm at the proximal end. The surgical steps are in order:

1. Antromastoidotomy
2. Posterior tympanostomy to allow visualization of the round window niche
3. Puncture and incision of the round window membrane
4. Insertion or partial insertion of the electrode array into the scala tympani
5. Electrode fixation in the round window niche
6. Fixation of the device in the bony well

Steroids are administered as a routine in every case: 0.1 mg/kg/day dexamethasone i.v. in two doses per day for 3–4 days.

http://dx.doi.org/10.5772/67234

2. Results

Program of treatment of deafness combining acoustic hearing with electric hearing obtained through cochlear implantation initiated by H. Skarżyński in 1997 had assembled in the Institute of Physiology and Pathology of Hearing a group of more than 50 specialists: physicians, clinical engineers, psychologists, educators, speech and language therapists, and technicians. They all have contributed to the scientific output of the school with their research, clinical, teaching, and organizational work. Leaders of the Institute's program have authored several hundreds of publications and presentations in collaboration with 52 scientists from all continents from 34 leading countries globally. In the years 2000–2016, the team of the Institute has presented, sometimes with international collaborators, 2135 presentations counting only international and continental series of congresses in otorhinolaryngology, audiology, and related fields in Europe, Asia, Australia, and both Americas and Africa. These presentations included many invited lectures, discussion panels, and expert round tables. Simultaneously the same group has published 1465 papers reporting all aspects related to diagnostics, treatment, and rehabilitation of the partial deafness. Subsequent studies, analyses, and reports of longitudinal follow-up studies are related to the largest in the global medicine group of 317 patients with partial deafness.

Establishment and development of the Polish School in Otosurgery had several landmark dates and events. In 2000, on congresses in Antwerp [2] and Berlin [3], H. Skarżyński and A. Lorens have presented first reports about the quality of preserved nonfunctional residual hearing. Preservation of even such small level of hearing after cochlear implantation is a significant assistance in the process of hearing and speech rehabilitation. It means also that the structures of the inner ear have been preserved in the unchanged condition, thus that ear could be useable later, when new, innovative, better technologies for improving hearing will be developed and implemented. At the same time, implementation of the partial deafness treatment with a cochlear implant at the present stage of development of technology and medicine still enables sustained development of hearing, speech, and one or even more languages.

The second milestone, related to the typical partial deafness, has been the first surgery in an adult performed by H. Skarżyński in 2002 [1]. That patient had been able preoperatively to perceive sounds well in the low-frequency range up to 500 Hz, with total deafness in all other frequencies. Successful preservation of the low-frequency hearing complemented with electric stimulation for reception of the rest of frequency range provided an incentive for the dynamic development of research and clinical practice in that direction. After 2 years of follow-up of all implanted adult patients, in 2004 H. Skarżyński had performed the first in the world implantation in a child with this type of hearing [10]. Another landmark has been the first in the world presentation in 2009 [11] and publication in 2010 [12] introducing and explaining Skarżyński's concept of treatment in relation to various groups of patients with partial deafness. It involved inclusion of three principal criteria:

a. Application of Skarżyński's surgical method of six steps [13].

b. Selection and implementation of the surgical approach to the inner ear through the round window membrane as the most physiological way of entry to the cochlea.

c. Availability of different types of elastic electrode arrays, including Cochlear CI422 slim straight electrode designed by Skarżyński [14].

Further works on developing the program of treatment of partial deafness had been continued in the Institute of Physiology and Pathology of Hearing simultaneously with different forms of activities aimed at popularizing this method on different continents. Promotion of this treatment method included, of course, presentations on all major global and continental scientific congresses, supplemented by "live" demonstration surgeries performed by H. Skarżyński in Asia, Europe, and America. Simultaneously, for the needs of spreading clinical knowledge and providing an optimal training program, the Institute has started a series of international surgical training workshops called the window approach workshops (WAW). Since the beginning of the WAW program till 2016, there had already been 24 editions, with more than 3500 ear surgeons from all over the world participating. The WAW program includes hands-on training, patient assessment, and demonstration surgeries. Since 2010, the Institute actively participates also in the Live International Otolaryngology Network (LION) yearly global broadcast, with H. Skarżyński presenting surgeries of partial deafness treatment with various types of electrodes and implant systems. These regularly organized live surgical training broadcasts involve demonstrations of surgeries transmitted from several centers from the whole world simultaneously—from Australia, Asia, Europe, and Americas. These broadcasts enjoy always a very wide audience of surgeons and other medical specialists.

Presentation of the Polish School of treatment of partial deafness had been preceded by a huge work and contribution of an international group of leading specialists involved in implementation of the program of treatment of total deafness. The program had been spearheaded by such eminent researchers and surgeons as W. House and T. Balkany in the USA, Ch. Chouard in France, K. Burian in Austria, E. Lehnhardt in Germany, and G. Clark and W. Gibson in Australia. The leader and many members of the team of the Institute of Physiology and Pathology of Hearing had been visiting these leading members of the international community of specialists involved in treatment of total deafness programs. Many of these leaders had participated in conferences organized by the Institute in Poland. Practical preparations for initiation of the program of treatment of deafness in Poland had been initiated by H. Skarżyński with the support of the Foundation of Medical Development "Homo-Homini" in 1991. Following these preparations, first surgeries of treatment of total deafness in Poland had been performed by H. Skarżyński on 16 and 17 July 1992. They had reverberated widely in Polish society and mass media as well as in science and medicine [15, 16]. Further progress of the Polish program of treatment of total deafness has brought about further groundbreaking events and overcoming further barriers and limitation, including the gradual widening of indications for treatment of deafness with cochlear implants. It had been a foundation for the program of treatment of partial deafness. In its initial stage, in the years 2002–2008, the program had involved combining the electric hearing with the preserved natural hearing up to the level of 500 Hz. In following years electrical complementation had been extended to the level of 750 Hz and 1000 Hz. The top achievement had been first in the world publications, in 2014 and 2015, in which Skarżyński et al. had presented the possibility of treatment of partial deafness with preservation of natural hearing up to 1500

Hz [17, 18]. In clinical practice this approach is an opportunity created by modern science and medicine for patients with this type of hearing impairment at any age, but the most important is the opportunity for people in advanced age. In the group of people over 70 years, as many as ¾ have different kinds of hearing impairment negatively impacting their ability to communicate with their environment. In a global scale, there are tens of millions of people suffering from the typical partial deafness above 1500 Hz. They are not deaf. In diagnostic studies conducted in conditions of silence, their speech understanding may reach the level of 40–60%. In the standardized conditions of hearing testing in noise, which better mirrors the situations of everyday functioning, their levels of speech understanding drop to 11–22%. It is a cause of their gradual isolation from the society, withdrawal from active participation in social life. In a growing proportion these patients develop deep depression. If we consider that this senior group of citizens grows steadily in line with increasing life expectancy in the developed countries, it is not difficult to arrive at the conclusion that partial deafness today is an important social problem.

3. Summary

At the turn of the twenty first century, the problem of preservation of the nonfunctional residual hearing and thus preservation of the intact inner ear structure had been addressed by several research teams in the world. The trend started by the team of the Institute of Physiology and Pathology of Hearing, especially first results from children and adults published since 2000, had brought about the realization that an intact inner ear might in future be useful when novel, yet unknown techniques for preservation/restoration of good hearing at any age become available. Particularly noteworthy are in this context studies of the research groups from Frankfurt, von Ilberg et al. [19]; Iowa City, Gantz [20]; Kansas City, Staecker [21]; Vienna, Baumgartner et al. [22]; Melbourne, Briggs [23]; Antwerp, Van de Heyning et al. [22, 24]; and Matsumoto, Usami et al. [25]. Until present day these centers have developed various programs of partial deafness treatment with residual hearing up to 250 and 500 Hz in adults and make preparations for conducting similar surgeries in children. Present indications for acoustic and electric stimulation of the damaged inner ear have been included in the newest concept published by Skarżyński et al. in 2014 [17], presented in **Figure 1**.

A crucial issue in development of the Polish School in modern science had been the search for standardized method of assessment of the results of therapy achieved by different research groups in various groups of patients different with regard to their size and qualities. On the initiative of Skarżyński and the team of the Institute of Physiology and Pathology of Hearing, a global HearRing group had initiated the works that resulted in developing the first scientific scale which was published in 2012 by Skarżyński et al. [26]. This scale enables archiving and comparing the results of growing groups of patients provided with cochlear implants. Participation of several tens of prominent researchers from the whole world in development of this scale was not only helpful in its elaboration; it facilitates its steady popularization in modern science and medicine [27].

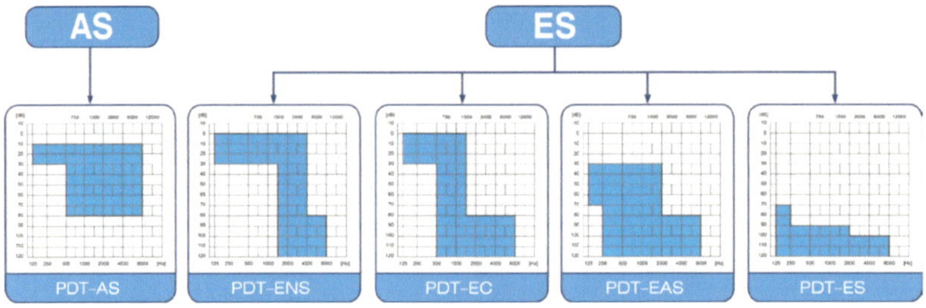

Figure 1. The newest concept of complementation of damaged hearing in indicated ranges: (a) acoustic complementation with hearing aids and middle ear implants (acoustic stimulation, AS), (b) electric support for the effective electric-natural hearing (partial deafness treatment-electronatural stimulation, PDT-ENS), (c) electric complementation of the preserved hearing only in the low-frequency range up to 500 Hz (partial deafness treatment-electric complement, PDT-EC), (d) combined electric and acoustic stimulation with a hearing aid and cochlear implant (partial deafness treatment-electro-acoustic stimulation, PDT-EAS), and (e) only electric stimulation with preservation of the inner ear structure and nonfunctional residual hearing (partial deafness treatment-electric stimulation, PDT-ES).

A final argument summarizing the position of the international scientific community toward strengthening of the Polish School is personal citations and awards and distinctions bestowed for these achievements by the various international scientific and expert groups. Erixon et al. in the Ear and Hearing, which has one of the highest Impact Factor journals in this field, have written in 2015: "Skarzynski et al. (2012) called the first group electrical complement patients and the second group electro-acoustic stimulation patients" [28]. Von Ilberg with an international group of collaborators in a multicenter study published in the Audiology and Neurotology in 2011 [19] has mentioned: "The most expanded indication for electro-acoustic stimulation (EAS) has been reported by the Warsaw group, who implanted candidates with markedly better acoustic hearing in the frequencies between 125 and 500 Hz. Some of the recipients showed extremely sloping audiograms, using the natural preserved acoustic LFH, without the need of any additional acoustic amplification." The same paper mentions further "a small number of studies reporting on children fitted with EAS have recently been published by Skarzynski et al." In its summary it says "Skarzynski and his group have demonstrated convincing results in their first studies on children" and further "however, Skarzynski stressed that this kind of surgery on children should not be attempted without significant successful experience with adults" and still further "by introducing this method, it became possible to improve hearing preservation, with rates going up to 95–100% in most EAS candidates." Guimares et al. in the Brazilian Journal of Otorhinolaryngology in 2015 have said: "Some classifications for hearing preservation have been proposed to assess the degree of preservation of residual hearing, and the most commonly employed is that proposed by Skarzynski (…)" [29].

It should be underlined that the real effects of the Polish School are shown by the increasing abilities of Polish patients in their sustained development of hearing, speech, learning of languages, and development of artistic potential—vocal and musical. The best example of this success is their achievements demonstrated during the first International Music Festival "Beats of Cochlea" [30].

From among nearly two hundred distinctions and awards won by H. Skarżyński and his team in Poland and internationally in relation to the implementation and promotion of the Polish School, three awards are particularly noteworthy. The first is the '21st Century Award—chief award in the global competition "21st Century Achievement Award Winners" in the category "Healthcare" for the System of Remote Fitting and Rehabilitation in Washington in 2010, in relation to the development and implementation of the telemedical care for patients with partial deafness. The second is the golden medal in the global Prix Galien competition—the first award considered as "Oscar" or "Nobel" of the medical world, awarded for creation of the first "National Network of Teleaudiology" for patients after cochlear implantation, in Monte Carlo in 2014. The third personal distinction of the international community has been the highest citation for H. Skarżyński, as one of the four scientists from the whole world, for his contribution to the development of science and medicine and providing the optimal possibilities of communication of the modern societies. This award has been given to H. Skarżyński in recognition of his leadership and inspirational example for the international society through establishment of the internationally known medical center dedicated to the surgical treatment of hearing disorders and tireless advocacy for people with hearing disorders all over the world.

4. Conclusions

1. The principal idea of the Polish School in the international medical science is a demonstration of the full advantages of patients with partial deafness, preservation of the unchanged structures of the inner ear allowing unlimited development of hearing, speech, and language and chances for application of new future technologies.
2. The perspectives of popularizing of the Polish School in global medical science create a real chance of help for tens of millions of people, particularly in the advanced age.

Glossary

Six-step Skarżyński procedure—surgical procedure of cochlear implantation developed by Skarżyński H. [7] for hearing preservation combining the atraumatic round window electrode insertion with different straight electrodes.

HearRing preservation classification—the first scientific scale which enables comparing the rate of hearing preservation after cochlear implantation developed by the HearRing group published in 2012 by H. Skarżyński et al. [26].

Partial deafness (PD)—a condition where patient has in one ear normal low-frequency hearing but no hearing in the high-frequency range; hearing loss occurs in at least one frequency critical to speech understanding.

Partial deafness treatment—management of partial deafness (PD) consisting in preservation of preoperative hearing through minimally traumatic surgical implantation procedure along with the use of different means of acoustic and electric stimulation.

Author details

Henryk Skarżyński[1,2]* and Piotr Henryk Skarżyński[2,3,4]

*Address all correspondence to: skarzynski.henryk@ifps.org.pl

1 Oto-Rhino-Laryngology Surgery Clinic, Institute of Physiology and Pathology of Hearing, Warsaw, Kajetany, Poland

2 World Hearing Center of the Institute of Physiology and Pathology of Hearing, Kajetany Poland

3 Institute of Sensory Organs, Kajetany, Poland

4 Heart Failure and Cardiac Rehabilitation Department, Medical University of Warsaw, Warsaw, Poland

References

[1] Skarżyński H., Lorens A., Piotrowska A., A new method of partial deafness treatment, Medical Science Monitor, 2003, 9(4), 20–24.

[2] Skarżyński H., Results of non-functional residual hearing and inner ear structures preservation, 5th European Symposium on Paediatric Cochlear Implantation, 2000, Antwerp, Belgium

[3] Lorens A., Results of non-functional residual hearing and inner ear structures preservation, European Federation of Oto-Rhino-Laryngological Societies, 2000, Berlin, Germany

[4] Lorens A., Geremek A., Walkowiak A., Skarżyński H., Residual Acoustic Hearing in the Ear Before and After Cochlear Implantation, in: 4th European Congress of Oto-Rhino-Laryngology Head and Neck Surgery ``Past-Present-Future", Monduzzi Editore, Berlin, 2000, 135–138.

[5] Obrycka A., Lorens A., Piotrowska A., Skarżyński H., Middle ear implant. A chance to eliminate some restrictions in sound perception inherent in hearing aids, Audiofonologia, 2004, 26, 91–94. (article in Polish)

[6] Pankowska A., Geremek-Samsonowicz A., Skarżyński H., Cochlear implants in partial deafness. Tasks and forms of rehabilitation of children, in: Speech-language therapy for

the deaf, theory and praxis, Ewa Muzyka-Furtak ed., Harmonia Universalis Gdańsk, 2015, 329–342, (article in Polish)

[7] Skarżyński H., Lorens A., Piotrowska A., Skarżyński P.H., Hearing preservation in partial deafness treatment, Medical Science Monitor, 2010, 16(11), CR 555–CR 562

[8] Skarżyński H., Ten years' experience with a new strategy of partial deafness treatment, Journal of Hearing Science®, 2012, 2(2), RA11–RA18.

[9] von Bekesy G., Simplified model to demonstrate the energy flow and formation of traveling waves similar to those found in the cochlea, Proceedings of National Academy of Sciences United States of America, 1956, 42(12), 930–944.

[10] Skarżyński H., Lorens A., Piotrowska A., Anderson I., Partial deafness cochlear implantation in children, International Journal of Pediatric Otorhinolaryngology, 2007, 71(9), 1407–1413.

[11] Skarżyński H., Treatment of Partial Deafness, 9th European Symposium on Pediatric Cochlear Implantation (ESPCI2009), 14–17 V, 2009, Warsaw, Poland

[12] Skarżyński H., Lorens A., Partial deafness treatment, Cochlear Implants International, 2010, 11(Supplement 1), 29–41.

[13] Skarzynski H., Lorens A., Piotrowska A., Anderson I., Preservation of low frequency hearing in partial deafness cochlear implantation (PDCI) using the round window surgical approach, Acta Oto-Laryngologica, 2007, 127, 41–48.

[14] Skarżyński H., Podskarbi-Fayette R., A new cochlear implant electrode design for preservation of residual hearing: a temporal bone study, Acta Oto-Laryngologica, 2010, 130(8), 888–896.

[15] Skarżyński H., Application of cochlear implants in treatment of partial deafness, Gazeta Lekarska, 1992, 8, 16–17. (article in Polish)

[16] Successful surgery – hope for thousands of deaf people (Izabella Wit-Kossowska), Życie Warszawy, Warsaw, 17.07.1992, (article in Polish)

[17] Skarżyński H., Lorens A., Skarżyński P.H., Electro-natural stimulation (ENS) in partial deafness treatment: a case study, Journal of Hearing Science, 2014, 4(4): CS67–CS71.

[18] Skarżyński H., Lorens A., Dziendziel B., Skarżyński P.H., Expanding pediatric cochlear implant candidacy: A case study of electro-natural stimulation (ENS) in partial deafness treatment, International Journal of Pediatric Otorhinolaryngology, 2015, 79(11), 1896–1900.

[19] von Ilberg C.A., Baumann U., Kiefer J., Tillein J., Adunka O.F., Electric-acoustic stimulation of the auditory system: a review of the first decade, Audiology and Neurootology, 2011, 16(Suppl 2), 1–30.

[20] Gantz B., Eppsteiner R., Shearer A., Hildebrand M., Deluca A., Ji H., Dunn C., Black-Ziegelbein E., Casavant T., Braun T., Scheetz T., Scherer S., Hansen M., Smith R.,

Prediction of cochlear implant performance by genetic mutation: the spiral ganglion hypothesis, Hearing Research, 2012, 292(1–2), 51–58.

[21] Prentiss S., Sykes K., Staecker H., Partial deafness cochlear implantation at the University of Kansas: techniques and outcomes, Journal of American Academy of Audiology, 2010, 21(3), 197–203.

[22] Van de Heyning P., Adunka O., Arauz S.L., Atlas M., Baumgartner W.D., Brill S., Bruce I., Buchman C., Caversaccio M., Dillon M., Eikelboom R., Eskilsson G., Gavilan J., Godey B., Green K., Gstoettner W., Hagen R., Han D., Iwasaki S., Kameswaran M., Karltorp E., Kleine Punte A., Kompis M., Kuthubutheen J., Kuzovkov V., Lassaletta L., Li Y., Lorens A., Manikoth M., Martin J., Mlynski R., Mueller J., O'Driscoll M., Parnes L., Pillsbury H., Prentiss S., Pulibalathingal S., Raine C.H., Rajan G., Rajeswaran R., Riechelmann H., Rivas A., Rivas J.A., Senn P., Skarzynski P.H., Sprinzl G., Staecker H., Stephan K., Sugarova S., Usami S.I., Wolf-Magele A., Yanov Y., Zernotti M.E., Zimmerman K., Zorowka P., Skarzynski H., Standards of practice in the field of hearing implants, Cochlear Implants International, 2013, 14(Suppl 2), S1–S5.

[23] Briggs R.J., Future technology in cochlear implants: assessing the benefit, Cochlear Implants International, 2011, 12(Suppl 1), S22–S25.

[24] Mertens G., De Bodt M., Van de Heyning P., Cochlear implantation as a long-term treatment for ipsilateral incapacitating tinnitus in subjects with unilateral hearing loss up to 10 years, Hearing Research, 2016, 331, 1–6.

[25] Nakagawa T., Yamamoto M., Kumakawa K., Usami S.I., Hato N., Tabuchi K., Takahashi M., Fujiwara K., Sasaki A., Komune S., Yamamoto N., Hiraumi H., Sakamoto T., Shimizu A., Ito J., Prognostic impact of salvage treatment on hearing recovery in patients with sudden sensorineural hearing loss refractory to systemic corticosteroids: a retrospective observational study, Auris Nasus Larynx, 2016, 43(5), 489–494.

[26] Skarżyński H., van de Heyning P., DeMin H., Li Y., Bo L., Caversaccio M., Rivas J.A., Raine Ch., Arauz S., Zernotti M., Manoj M., Kameswaran M., Sprinzl G., Zorowka P., Staecker H., Parnes L., Gavilan J., Lassaletta L., Green K., Usami S., Muelle J., Atlas M., Rajan G., Godey B.,Karltorp E., Yanov Y., Kuzovkov V., Adunka O., Buchman C., Baumgartner W.D., Gstoettner W., Hagen R., Skarżyński P.H., Lorens A., Hearing preservation classification, Journal of Hearing Science®, 2012, 2(2), SR95–SR96

[27] Skarżyński H., van de Heyning P., Agrawal S., Arauz S.L., Atlas M., Baumgartner W., Caversaccio M., de Bodt M., Gavilan J., Godey B., Green K., Gstoettner W., Hagen R., Han DM., Kameswaran M., Karltorp E., Kompis M., Kuzovkov V., Lassaletta L., Levevre F., Li Y., Manikoth M., Martin J., Mlynski R., Mueller J., O'Driscoll M., Parnes L., Prentiss S., Pulibalathingal S., Raine C.H., Rajan G., Rajeswaran R.J. Rivas A., Rivas A., Skarżyński P. H., Sprinzl G., Staecker H., Stephan K., Usami S., Yanov Y., Zernotti M.E., Zimmermann K., Lorens A., Mertens G., Towards a consensus on a hearing preservation classification system, Acta Oto-Laryngologica, 2013, 133(Suppl 564), 3–13

[28] Erixon E., Rask-Andersen H., Hearing and patient satisfaction among 19 patients who received implants intended for hybrid hearing: a two-year follow-up, Ear and Hearing, 2015, 36(5), e271–e278.

[29] Guimares et al., Hearing preservation and cochlear implants according to inner ear approach, Brazilian Journal of Otorhinolaryngology 2015, 81(2), 190–196.

[30] Beats of Cochlea, 1st International Music Festival for Children, Youths and Adults with Hearing Disorders, Festival Book, 2015

Section 6

New aspects of Auditory periphery

Chapter 10

Various Aspects of Auditory Fatigue Caused by Listening to Loud Music

Andrzej Dobrucki, Maurycy J. Kin and
Bartłomiej Kruk

Additional information is available at the end of the chapter

http://dx.doi.org/10.5772/64611

Abstract

This chapter presents results of research on influence of auditory fatigue on some aspects of listening condition measured among various groups of listeners. Three experiments have been carried out. The aim of the first one was to find the influence of the kind of headphones used by young people on their hearing loss. The second experiment was concerning the temporary threshold shift (TTS) caused by the listening of loud musical signals after several time of sound exposure. The main interest of the third experiment was the detection ability of changes in spectrum of musical samples obtained after several time of listening to the loud music. It turned out that except for frequency of 4 kHz there is no relation between the types of preferred headphones and the shift of hearing threshold while for the frequency of 4 kHz, a statistically important influence of the headphone types on the threshold values was observed. The second and third experiments were carried out under conditions which normally exist in a studio or on the stage when the sound material is recorded and/or mixed. It turned out that after several loud music listening sessions the average value of temporary threshold shift reached more than 3 dB for 1 kHz and increased up to 6–7 dB with an exposure time of 120 min. On the basis of results obtained from the third experiment, it was found that the decrease in ability to detect the spectrum changes for longer noise exposure exists particularly for lower changes (of ±1.5 dB) and at all frequency regions under investigation. It may suggest that the hearing system gets tired for the region of higher frequencies faster than for other bands after listening to loud music. The results may also be influenced by the mental fatigue which occurred after several time duration of permanently played loud sounds, together with demanding tasks. Such conditions involving the mental engagement in a noisy environment, which is referred to the natural scenery of the studio work can significantly reduce the time of exhaustion which causes the decrease of accuracy in solving several tasks. It should be also noted that the tendencies observed within young people culture in listening loud music in order to be isolated from the environment is actually causing not the TTS phenomenon but permanent threshold shift (PTS).

Keywords: listening fatigue, perception of spectral changes, temporary threshold shift

1. Introduction

The act of listening to musical sounds is usually considered as a kind of recreation, or an impulse to take a rest. But the music can also be considered as a noise not only from the musical structure and composers' point of view—in some cases, listening to the music may not be only a kind of recreation—for particular professionals it is their work. Reinforcement and recording engineers as well as sound producers are the examples of a trade in which the listening process and its conditions may reflect in the final quality of the work. The people working in these professions are subjected to hearing problem, in the same manner as the noise-exposed workers in an industry. Of course, listening to the musical sounds is different from a simply industrial noise from the psychological point of view: musical sounds are usually nice and desired while the noise means that a particular signal is assessed as awful and unpleasant. Also, the time-frequency structure of musical signals differs from the consistency of noise which makes listening to music a pleasant act. In the modern entertainment industry, there is one fact which may be considered while talking about the reinforcement of sound, it is the sound focusing techniques which enable to focus energy within a selected region using the special transducers, the line arrays in this case [1]. The energy dose of sound is a basic acoustic variable that determines the magnitude of sound, and the other function of sound focusing technique is to increase the clarity of sound by increasing the magnitude of the direct wave and decreasing the reflections from unwanted directions which result finally in higher sound levels. From the measurement point of view, it is not so simple to determine the actual sound level in all areas occupied by the audience. Moreover, it can be found that the sound level measured by the microphone in a sound field may be different than the level in the ear canal, so the maximum impulsive noise levels were high in the ear canal but the implications for the causes of hearing loss are indistinct because of ear amplification of 3–4 dB in the region of 1–3 kHz [2]. It should be also added that the sound sources (as a loudspeaker set, or PA systems) situated very close to the ear might increase the risk of hearing loss.

It may be fairer to say that working with louder music as well as listening to it over a long period of time may systematically lead to a permanent hearing damage or to a listening fatigue, which makes proper attention being impossible. In the past few years, the trend in sound production industry has been to increase loudness of musical recordings, particularly. Many radio stations as well as record companies have applied large amounts of dynamic range compression and other means of recording process in order to be perceived in today's noisy world. The trend called as "loudness wars" has been reflected in the higher subjective impressions in psychological domain, and the slogan "louder sounds are sold better" has come true [3]. Many young people want to single their minds out of different backgrounds by the use of special kinds of headphones and they listen to the sound material louder, beside the fact that the listened material is louder in comparison to the recordings made in the previous century. Also, the contemporary designed and produced equipment allows the listeners to consume the music in accordance with their way of life [4, 5] and with higher concentrated energy of sound in order to make the proper sensations for the audience [1].

The way of stimuli presentation (via headphones or loudspeaker, or naturally listening of the event) seems to be an important thing causing the hearing loss. Young people do not take into account that the popular or rock music causes the same effects like the higher and longtime exposure to the noise when the earphones are used for listening, due to the average sound level and duration of exposure which simply leads to a listening fatigue. Young people say, we listen to the music that sounds nicely for us and it is not like noise, so why may it be dangerous for our hearing? Sometimes, one can find many pieces of classical music from the twentieth century which are very loud while performed. As an example, the fourth Symphony of Dmitri Shostakovich if given in some fragments, the sound level exceeds 100 dB in the audience area of the concert hall. The main differences between classical and pop-music are in the time duration of continuous exposure to the sound, a character of musical structure and spectral consistence of stimuli. In popular music, the method used for musical production is very often based on the sound compression, and this compression itself may increase the potential risk of hearing damage [6–8] or a listening fatigue which makes proper attention being impossible.

The typical effect of listening to loud sounds is the temporary threshold shift (TTS) or permanent threshold shift (PTS) which play a huge role in the proper assessment of sound while working in a recording studio. The negative effects of TTS may occur when someone is under the noise, or another loud acoustical signal, exposure for a particular time interval, and then having a rest only after the whole work, without breaks for recreation process. The higher sound levels usually influence human concentration in a negative way, like the chaotic visual structures [9] which are based on psychology of perception. The results of a permanent hearing threshold shift of the people working in the entertainment industry as well as the influence of the kinds of equipment used have been presented [10, 11]. The recommendations of a daily dose of noise for sound makers as well as for musicians are not stated because of the nature of work apart from the fact that it may cause permanent or temporary hearing damages.

Physiological and psychological processes connected to a reaction to sound consist of sensational and emotional reactions. The sensational reaction is the effect of a physiological process, which occurs during listening. It arises when stimuli overdraw sensitivity levels, while the emotional reaction is more complex and difficult to analysis because it is not a direct result of received signal features but depends on the habits and conditions of the listener [12]. Noise related to some activities, for example teaching in classrooms, is correlated with performer's fatigue, increases tension and discomfort, and an interference of teaching and speech recognition [13]. Several studies have been conducted to investigate the effects of noise exposure patterns, including noises of different spectra, interrupted noise exposure patterns, and short-duration noise exposures on TTS in order to find and determine the maximum time duration of acting noise at a particular level, and the resting time, after that the ear can recover to the before-noise-state [14–16]. From these studies, a temporary decrease in auditory sensitivity in normal ear was found after exposure to continuous noise levels weighted by A-curve above 80 dB for long periods. The set of audiograms characteristic for particular hearing loss caused by various types of noise are also presented in the literature and those results can give the directions to the protections in order to avoid the permanent hearing damage. Laboratory studies regarding the human response from noise exposure provide a better control over noise exposure variables, because the TTS—which can be studied under controlled conditions in the laboratory—behaves almost consistently. It is a relatively simple matter to determine combinations of levels, duration, and temporal pattern that produce the same TTS as the standard daily noise dose.

It is known from literature [14, 15, 17, 18] that the greatest effect of TTS occurs first for the range of 2–6 kHz, and this upward shift disappears after a time, usually in 24 hours, but may last as long as a week. If exposure to noise occurs repeatedly without sufficient time between exposures to allow recovery of normal hearing, threshold shift may become chronic, and eventually permanent. This is a specific danger when people who work in noisy environments are exposed to further noise afterward while driving, at home or at places of entertainment.

The facts mentioned above may reflect in an increase of hearing thresholds of the young people consuming today's music in the way that "louder means better". Of course, the higher hearing thresholds induce difficulty in collecting, understanding, and interpreting many information from the human environment which influences the sense of safety and causes the changes in the way of thinking and living together in society. It also may be interesting if the European Standard EN ISO 7029 still remains true in the light of youngsters' way of life and this aspect is the aim of presented research. According to this standard, the hearing thresholds increase with the age of a subject, starting from 0 dB, as recommended for 20-year-old people. The authors' research [10] showed that for young people who use to listen to the loud music via headphones the hearing thresholds have been shifted up to 6 dB. Although such hearing is still qualified as "normal" [19] (see also Section 3.1), according to the EN ISO 7029 this value of hearing threshold shift is typical for 40–50 years-old people. The population of young people with shifted threshold of hearing is growing up year-by-year.

2. Description of research

2.1. Audiometric tests

The research was aimed at young people (16–25 years old) because they are the most vulnerable to hearing loss caused by frequent loud noise exposure in their own choices. Some of the people are working for the entertainment industry in professional way so they were divided into three groups reflecting their activities:

- young classical musicians or music academy students,
- sound engineers of Front of House/Public Address (FOH/PA) systems and
- sound engineers working in recording studios.

The ordinary young users of portable audio equipment were representative as the reference group for this range of age, so the total number of subjects was more than 80 people. After the interviews and giving instructions, the audibility of people was measured by the means of Maico M 53 audiometers. Audiometric tests were conducted in an anechoic chamber and in the recording studio of the Wrocław University of Science and Technology. These places meet the requirements of maximum allowable amount of background-sound pressure level [20]. Therefore, during the test, any masking phenomenon from outer signals does not occur [20, 21]. Before the measurements all audiometers had been basically calibrated and checked aurally, also they had been calibrated subjectively in accordance with the ISO recommendations.

Threshold of hearing levels were determined by the air conduction audiometry. The measurements were carried out according to the applicable standards [20], by ascending methods and with the use of continuous sinusoidal signals. All measurement points were repeated twice in order to eliminate random errors for some of the inexperienced subjects.

2.2. Detection of spectral changes of musical signals vs. TTS

The detection of spectrum changes of musical signals was the subject of investigation in the first part of research. Sixteen subjects in the age ranging from 22 to 25 years, participated in the experiment and all of them are professional recording or reinforcement engineers. Moreover, they have experience in psychoacoustic experiments. They featured the normal hearing, that is, the absolute threshold was not more than 10 dB HL in the entire frequency range (125 Hz–16 kHz) which has been confirmed by the air conduction measurements with the Maico M53 audiometers. The threshold measurements were carried out according to the applicable standards [20, 22] by ascending stimuli methods and with the use of continuous sinusoidal signals with steps of 2 dB. All measurement points were repeated twice in order to eliminate random errors. Because the described experiment was addressed to the people working with or listening to higher sound levels of the music, the loud music as a disturbing noise typical for musical material in the studio or at the concerts, was presented without any break which reflects a typical way of sound exposure at entertainment event or studio works.

Ten musical pieces had been equalized at octave bands of 125 Hz, 1 kHz, and 8 kHz as center frequencies, with ±1.5 dB, ±3 dB and finally ±6 dB boosts of a sound material. It should be added that these frequencies as well as introduced spectral changes were chosen as typical values of correction parameters in low, medium, and high regions of frequency in mixing consoles often used in live-reinforcement applications. The 10-second samples have been prepared with a digital audio workstation and then recorded digitally by a TASCAM DA-30 DAT recorder. As a trial, test stimuli samples have been presented in pairs, where the first one contained the original (nonequalized signal) and the second one, the processed signal. The time interval between samples was set at 1 s, and between pairs as 2 s. The test samples have been presented via active TLC loudspeakers and played back from DAT recorder. The subjects' task was to answer if these samples sounded the same, or not. Every combination of signal-equalization occurred at least three times because of the statistical significance. The length of the test sequences did not exceed 5 min. The test signals contained pieces of various musical styles (pop rock, jazz, symphony, chamber music, heavy metal, etc.). The musical material used as a disturbing noise contained mostly pop and rock pieces frequently broadcasted in radio stations. The sound pressure levels in octave bands in the range of 63 Hz–4 kHz were practically constant at 87–93 dB and decreased to about 80 dB at 31 Hz and 8 kHz octave bands. These conditions of levels were maintained for both test and disturbing signals. Similar stimuli have been used in other experiments [11] as a reflection of typical distributions of sound pressure levels in musical selections performed by American rock and roll groups. This method of an experimental performance was chosen in order to limit the effect of fatigue of the subjects during the test sequence as well as the fact that listeners' attention should not be devoted on the new audio material. Also, the fixed sample sequence was used with an intention to minimize some artifacts which can appear in subjective assessment and simply refers to an accuracy increase because the attention of listeners was focused only on the noticeable changes between presented samples, without additional tasks about scaling and identifying the reason of the differences [23, 24].

In this experiment, the TTS phenomenon for the listeners was also the subject of research. The hearing thresholds were measured after every session of music exposure which enabled observation of the TTS caused by listening of loud musical signals in several periods of exposure. In this case, the thresholds of hearing were measured in the same way that at the beginning of experiment, i.e., by ascending stimuli methods and with the use of continuous sinusoidal signals with steps of 2 dB. These measurements were repeated twice.

3. Analysis of the results

3.1. Average hearing threshold

Figure 1 shows the values for threshold of hearing for the left and right ear of the population tested before the experiment. These values have been averaged over results obtained for 276 listeners. It can be easily seen that the threshold of hearing is uniformly shifted by about 7–8 dB. In order to confirm the results, various types of statistical testing have been applied. When a calculated value of particular statistics for a tested factor is less than the critical value, depending mainly on the number of repetitions and the level of significance α (usually stated as 0.05), the influence of this factor is not important from statistical point of view, so it can be fairer to say that this factor does not influence the obtained results. In this case, the Bartlett test has been used. This test features the distribution asymptotic to χ^2 thus it can be applied even to a small population. This kind of test enables to confirm homogene-

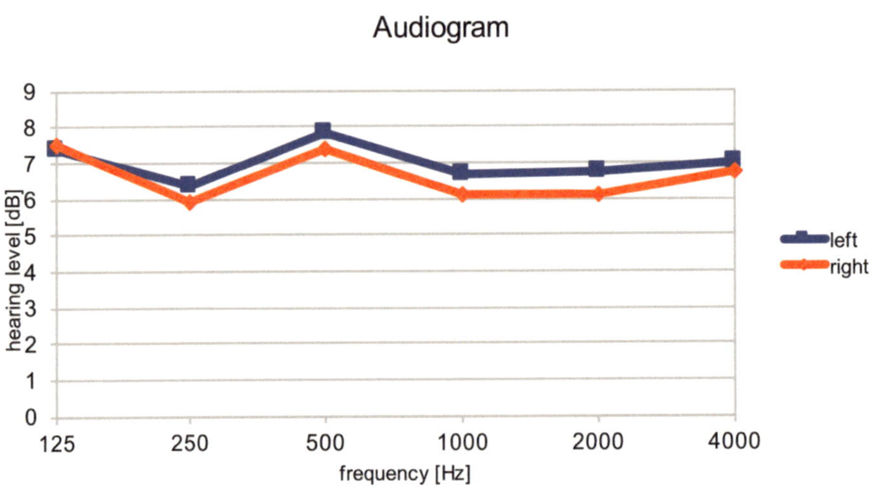

Figure 1. The average values of the threshold of hearing shift for the tested population.

http://dx.doi.org/10.5772/64611

F (Hz)	250	500	1000	2000	4000	8000
$\bar{x}_L$	7.40	6.34	7.83	6.65	6.73	7.01
σ_L	6.07	6.06	6.19	6.21	8.65	10.36
$\bar{x}_R$	7.52	5.93	7.36	6.12	6.09	6.74
σ_R	5.70	5.44	6.00	6.82	9.86	9.81

Table 1. The average values and standard deviations for hearing thresholds for left and right ears measured for all the 276 subjects.

ity of variances of obtained results, with the assumption that they featured a normal distribution. The results of statistical treatment showed that the variances of obtained results were homogenous ($\chi^2 = 24.893 < \chi_\alpha^{\ 2} = 39.977$, at $\alpha = 0.05$) for all frequencies. According to the classification of the Bureau International Audiophonology [19], five types of hearing loss can be distinguished:

- hearing loss up to 20 dB: normal hearing
- hearing loss in the range 21–40 dB: a mild degree of hearing loss
- hearing loss in the range 41–70 dB: a moderate degree of hearing loss
- hearing loss in the range 71–90 dB: a severe degree of hearing loss
- hearing loss greater than 91–120 dB: very severe hearing loss.

According to this classification, the tested young people belong to the group of normal hearing, but the shift in the threshold of hearing points with the slow tendency to begin a permanent damage of hearing which is caused by a long-term work with loud music (see Section 3.3). These values, however, are the average ones and the greatest hearing losses can be balanced by the results for the people with otological normal values that is shown in the **Table 1** as the values of standard deviations, especially for higher frequencies. Thus, it was decided to divide the whole group into the categories which could influence the obtained results and reflect the hearing loss for some specific conditions of working activity as well as kinds of equipment used by the people.

3.2. The influence of different kind of headphones on the threshold of hearing

In this section, results of pure tone audiometry for users of different types of headphones are presented. These results present "the worse" ear (left or right) for each subject, and these values have been averaged over the people who declare to use particular types of headphones. They are shown in **Figure 2**.

It can be seen that the type of headphones used has a major impact on the threshold of hearing values. On the basis of analysis of variance, it was found that for all tested groups of people using different types of headphones and particular frequencies there was a good convergence between all the subjects' notes and thresholds did not depend on the listener in all cases at

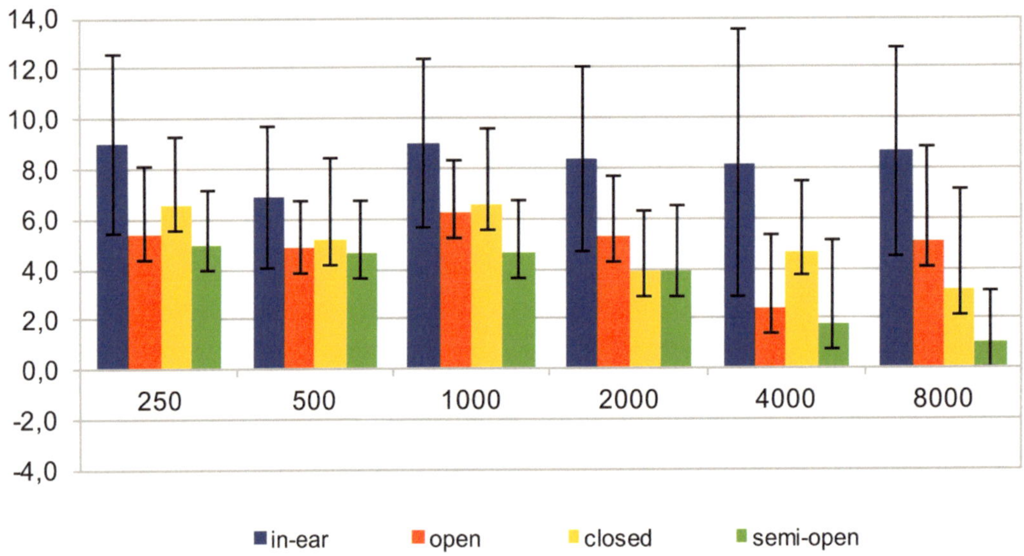

Figure 2. The influence of different kind of headphones on the threshold of hearing. Standard deviation values are presented as vertical lines on the tops of the bars.

the 95% of confidence ($p < 0.02$). It was decided to use the *F*-Snedecor statistics because of nonequal numbers of particular groups of users declaring the specific kinds of earphones. It turned out that except for frequency of 4 kHz there is no relation between the types of preferred headphones and the shift of hearing threshold ($F < F_{\alpha} = 2.75$, where, F and F_{α} are calculated and critical values of *F*-Snedecor test, respectively, at $\alpha = 0.05$). For the frequency equal to 4 kHz, the influence of the headphone types on the threshold values was observed ($F = 3.35 > F_{\alpha}$). It means that the most unfavorable for the hearing are the in-earphones, especially at high frequencies to which our hearing system is the most sensitive. The air in the ear canal is a natural protection from high-sound pressure. Using inside earphones the length of the channel is reduced, through which natural protection becomes less effective. A good alternative are semi-open headphones that in a small way can isolate us from the outside noise. They additionally ensure good hygiene of the ear and by their design, they protect from very high-sound pressure acting directly on the ear membrane. The results of upward threshold shifts obtained for the 4 kHz frequency are presented in **Table 2**.

In order to determine how the particular kinds of headphones are injurious for hearing conditions, the structure index test as a statistical treatment was applied. This test allows to classify the groups of results as influenced by a particular factor, the kind of headphones and its influence on the hearing threshold values in this case. The results of such testing for these series reflect the degree of hearing damage caused by the type of used headphones, with $u_{\alpha} = 1.96$ at $\alpha = 0.05$. It turned out that for the frequency of 4 kHz the most dangerous type of headphone for the hearing threshold is the in-ear one ($|u| = 4.73$), while an influence of the semi-open is inessential statistically ($|u| = 1.05 < u_{\alpha}$). The degree of injury for hearing damage obtained for the open and the closed headphones are lower than for the in-ear headphones ($|u| = 2.52$ and $|u| = 2.12$, respectively).

In-ear	Open	Closed	Semiopen
8.2	2.4	4.7	1.8

Table 2. The average values for upward shift of hearing thresholds at 4 kHz for various types of headphones used by investigated subjects (in dB).

3.3. Threshold of hearing in terms of professional work

Some of tested people have been working in the profession for 7 years. By analyzing these data, it can be concluded that even 3–4 years of working in the entertainment industry, especially as the front-of-house engineers may cause a slight loss in hearing ability. By comparing other professional groups, it can be assumed that the results coincide in a large extent and the type of work (noise level) has no longer such effect on the threshold of hearing. In **Figure 3**, hearing thresholds are presented depending on the profession. In **Figure 3**, there are also results for the ordinary user of portable equipment – there are the subjects nonpracticing in any kind of sound-engineering profession as well as musicians. These results present "the worse" ear (left or right) for each subject, and these values have been averaged over the people within the particular group of profession as well as "amateur" listeners.

On the basis of analysis of variance, it turned out that for frequency values of 500 Hz, 1 kHz as well as 4 kHz the influence of working activity on the threshold of hearing has been observed ($F > F_\alpha = 3.29$, where F and F_α are calculated and critical values of F-Snedecor test, respectively, at $\alpha = 0.05$). For the other frequencies, there is no relation between the profession of work and the shift of hearing threshold values. As it was mentioned in previous chapter, the hearing loss at 4 kHz can be interpreted as the beginning of permanent hearing damage resulting from the exposure to the sound at high levels while the upward threshold shifts that appeared

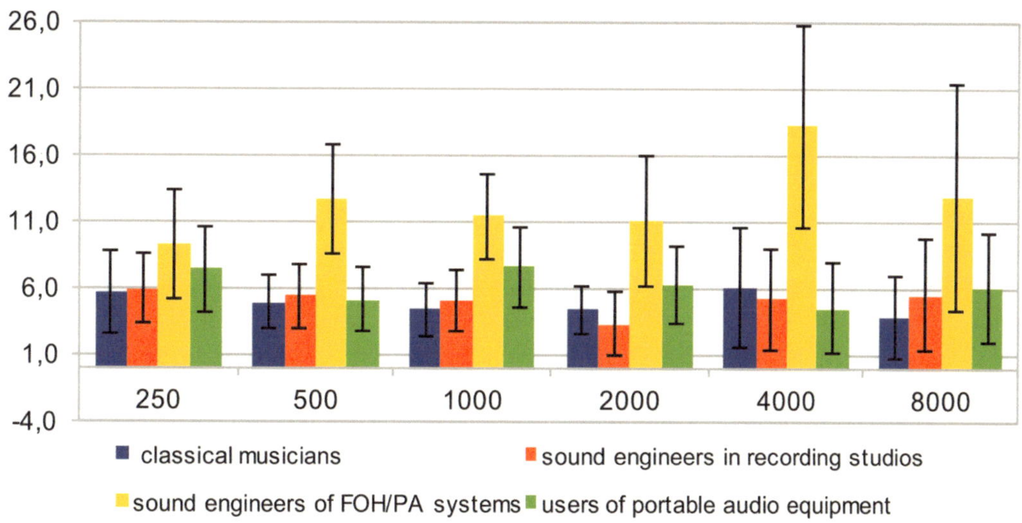

Figure 3. Thresholds of hearing depending on the profession. Standard deviation values are presented as vertical lines on the tops of the bars.

for lower frequencies (500 and 1000 Hz) are the results of the exposure to hyper-compressed musical sounds in these frequency bands, especially occurring on stage in order to increase the total loudness impression.

3.4. Detection of spectral changes vs. auditory fatigue

In **Figure 4**, results of this part of the research are presented. They are expressed as the percentage of correct answer number obtained before and after the loud music exposure. Subjects listened to the test trials containing the introduced several spectral modifications and have to denote if they perceived them. Thus, results may be expressed as a percentage of correct answers in a dependence of degree of introduced corrections for several noise-like exposures. For statistical treatment, the Bartlett's test was applied allowing the confirmation of homogeneity of variances of obtained results. On the basis of this test, for every exposure, the results were homogeneous ($\chi^2 = 4.922 < \chi_\alpha^2 = 28.869$, at $\alpha = 0.05$). Thus, the obtained results may be averaged over the total number of subjects and over the all styles of musical material. It is clearly noticeable that the differences before and after exposure for particular frequency are significant ($\chi^2 = 9.103 > \chi_\alpha^2 = 5.986$, at $\alpha = 0.05$).

It can be noted that the decrease in ability to detect the spectral changes for longer noise exposure has been observed particularly for lower changes and all frequency regions. Moreover, the number of false alarms (i.e., the case when the subjects signalized that some correction had been introduced, but no spectral changes have been really done) is less than 5% of the number of total answers at a specific condition which means that listeners mostly have not perceived the small changes in spectra. The changes of ±1.5 dB are perceived with detection ability higher than 70% only at the beginning of the test for middle and higher frequency regions. When subjects are exposed to noise for a longer period, their ability to detect changes in the spectrum of musical signals is less effective. For the noise exposure longer than 1 h the ability gets worse, especially for 8 kHz octave band where the only larger (±6 dB) equalization of the musical sounds may be perceived properly. This fact can be explained by the nature of frequency analysis made by the hearing system: this range of frequency is responsible for the proper reproduction of temporal structure of transient sounds [25], and the influence of rise time, especially, for the loudness impression has been reported [26]. The loudness changes may be perceived effectively when the "carrier" sound levels are higher than the hearing threshold of 10–20 dB [27]. When the changes of spectra in this frequency region do not exceed ±3 dB the difference of spectrum could be detected less effectively than in other investigated frequency bands because of the lower loudness impression in this region after several times of sound exposure. For octave bands of 125 Hz as well as for 1 kHz, the perceived spectral changes at the level of 70% have been noted for ±3 dB, or greater. It may suggest that the hearing system gets tired for the region of higher frequencies faster than for other bands after listening to a loud music. It can be shown that the trend is almost the same for every frequency of notched/boosted bands: when the attenuation, or amplification in a particular octave band increases, the percentage of correct answer reflecting the ability of detection of changes in the spectrum of musical signals also increases. It can also be observed that the differences between obtained values for increasing time of loud music exposure gets lower when the changes in spectra increase: the difference of ability of perception of spectrum

http://dx.doi.org/10.5772/64611

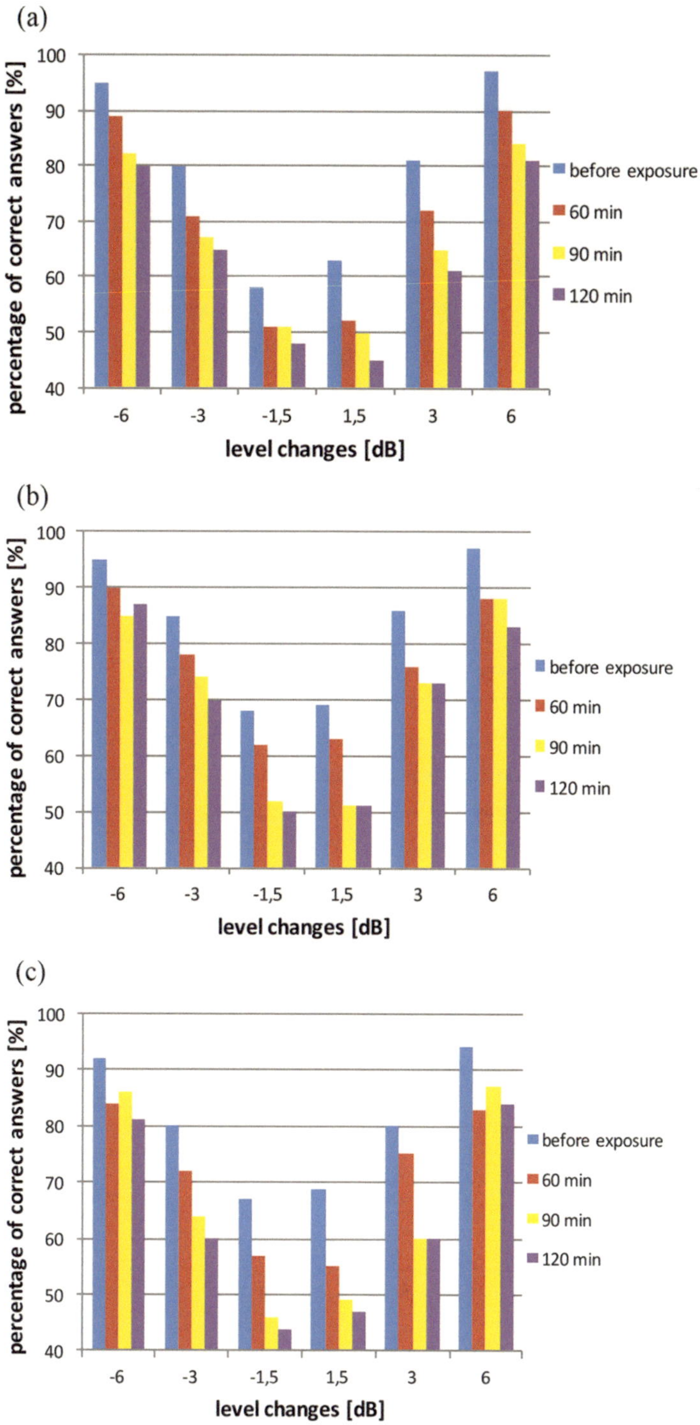

Figure 4. Detection of spectrum changes for frequencies of 125 Hz (a), 1 kHz (b) and 8 kHz (c) for different values of level changes in particular octave band.

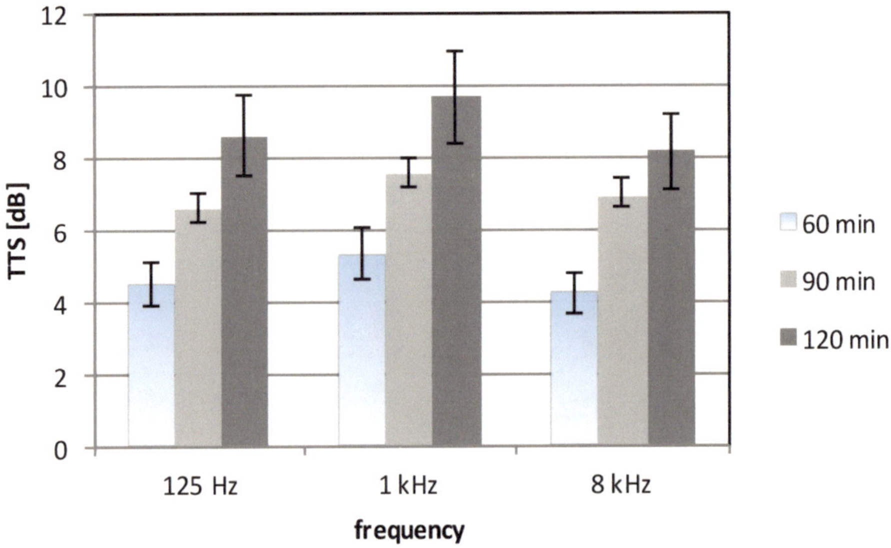

Figure 5. Average values of TTS after noise exposure of 1 h, 1.5 h and 2 h.

changes between fresh-ear listening and perception after 2 h-exposure takes 20% for ±1.5 dB spectrum modification, and then decreases to about 10% for ±6 dB attenuation/amplification. These results are convergent to the ones obtained in experiments on the profile analysis [28–30]: the values reported in a literature are equal to 2–3 dB for similar frequency regions, which can be compared to the values obtained for detection ability at 70% of correct answer number measured before the exposure to the music treated as a disturbing noise.

The obtained results can also be discussed in the light of TTS values presented in **Figure 5**. They have been averaged over all listeners. As it can be seen, the greatest values of TTS have been obtained for 1 kHz (about 9.5 dB, after 120 min of exposure) but the way of change is monotonic for all investigated frequencies. Moreover, the differences between the TTSs after the loud music exposure of 1 and 2 h are about 4 dB, for all frequencies. These values are

Spectral change/ standard deviation	-1.5 dB	+1.5 dB	-3 dB	+3 dB	-6 dB	+6 dB
σ_0	18.2	14.0	8.4	6.6	4.8	3.9
σ_{60}	27.3	22.8	20.3	18.6	15.0	11.5
σ_{90}	31.1	33.2	24.7	24.3	13.2	12.7
σ_{120}	36.0	34.3	25.3	24.2	16.5	15.8

Table 3. Standard deviation values of percentage of correct answer for spectra changes of musical samples equalized at 125 Hz, measured at different times of loud music exposure (in %).

http://dx.doi.org/10.5772/64611

Spectral change/ standard deviation	-1.5 dB	+1.5 dB	-3 dB	+3 dB	-6 dB	+6 dB
σ_0	10.8	9.9	6.5	6.1	4.3	3.9
σ_{60}	22.1	20.3	16.3	15.2	10.8	10.2
σ_{90}	23.6	22.8	16.8	16.2	11.3	10.9
σ_{120}	28.2	30.8	16.5	16.6	11.0	11.2

Table 4. Standard deviation values of percentage of correct answer for spectra changes of musical samples equalized at 1000 Hz, measured at different time of loud music exposure (in %).

greater than those resulting from the detection ability presented in **Figure 4** because of the different stimuli used in both tests, although the character of changes is similar.

For a quality of the work activity in this particular profession it is important to detect these changes as accurate as possible, especially at a work as a studio recording engineer. However, the long exposure to the noise causes the worsening of attention, or listening fatigue. This phenomenon may be expressed as the standard deviations values of obtained results which is presented in **Tables 3–5**. These values may show that after every sound exposure, the attention of listeners gets lower causing an increase of uncertainty during evaluation of musical samples.

It can be seen that precision in spectral changes detection increases when these changes are greater (±6 dB, in this case). Another interesting fact is that after every acting noise (ranging from 60 to 120 min) the standard deviation values increase, but this change is not monotonic: sometimes exposure time does not influence the value of standard deviation of the obtained results which was confirmed by Bartlett test ($\chi^2 = 3.427 < \chi_\alpha^{\ 2} = 5.986$, at $\alpha = 0.05$), and sometimes this influence is significant (as for 125 Hz band, where $\chi^2 = 11.886 > \chi_\alpha^{\ 2} = 7.802$, at $\alpha = 0.05$). This means that the uncertainty for sound color evaluation for small differences of spectra is relatively high when some masking sounds appear simultaneously which increases the hearing system fatigue. For the lowest investigated equalization (±1.5 dB) the standard deviation for results after listening to loud music takes values greater than those presented for ±3 dB correction. Without the noise-like signal exposure, the standard deviation is almost the same as for ±3 dB (before listening to loud music) and this is in good agreement with previously reported

Spectral change/ standard deviation	-1.5 dB	+1.5 dB	-3 dB	+3 dB	-6 dB	+6 dB
σ_0	9.8	9.5	7.5	6.8	4.2	3.9
σ_{60}	20.7	21.2	12.3	13.5	11.0	10.7
σ_{90}	25.7	25.8	17.9	15.9	13.3	14.9
σ_{120}	26.3	24.5	17.8	16.3	16.8	15.5

Table 5. Standard deviation values of percentage of correct answer for spectra changes of musical samples equalized at 8 kHz, measured at different time of loud music exposure (in %).

research [31, 32] for amateurs as well as for professional sound engineers. Taking into account the obtained values for all kinds of spectral modification at given octave bands it can be clearly seen that longer exposure to loud signals causes greater uncertainty of sound color assessment but the relation is not proportional: the great increase has been noted when time exposure is 90 min and further prolongation of noise exposition up to 2 h does not influence the standard deviation values for lower and higher frequency regions, so it might be said that the concentration is kept at the same level. It should be also noted that the values of standard deviation are higher for 125 Hz for a modified frequency band than for higher frequencies which clearly means that uncertainty of spectrum change detection is worse for lower frequencies.

4. Conclusions

The audibility of timbral modifications depends on the frequency of modified region, the amplitude of peak (or notch) as well as the bandwidth. As it is reported in the literature, changes in sound quality, for example, made by introducing resonances or notches depend on musical material used in audition, the listening environment and reverberation used at a recording process [30]. The most important result of present experiment is that the audibility of spectral changes depends on the level of this modification as well as on the time of disturbing loud music exposure. Moreover, with discontinuous, irregular impulsive, or transient sounds characteristic for speech and musical signals, the test material is less resistible in comparison to the steady sounds. Obtained results are in good agreement with the ones reported in the literature as results of profile analysis [29] as well as the "classical" view on the timbre change perception [28]. It should be noted here that so called traditional view on the timbre perception is based on the intensity discriminations in particular frequency bands while the basic assumption of the profile analysis is that discrimination of the spectral changes is based on the evaluation of the overall spectrum shape involving the memory and interstimuli intervals. The results of experiments provided by both methods are similar in a case of such signals as used in our research. According to this, the ability of the distinguished changes in spectrum are 2–3 dB for listeners with normal hearing. It may be assumed that this fact takes place at the beginning of experiment (before exposure to the loud musical material). For the people with relatively small hearing loss (up to 20 dB) the predicted results of the peak or notch of spectrum modification may be shifted up to 5–6 dB which coincides with our results: the attenuation/amplification must be at 6 dB to be perceived with the greatest accuracy after longer (more than 1 h) presentation of loud music.

On the basis of the obtained results, it may be stated that the temporary threshold shift phenomenon is the important factor that determines perceptibility of changes in spectral and amplitude domains of musical signals. This conclusion results from the way of changes in obtained values for different time of loud music exposure. This is a usual phenomenon especially for 1 kHz because this range of frequency is the most sensitive for human hearing [33] and this fact can help the listeners to take a good decision during sound evaluation. Results of spectral changes detection are convergent with results reported in the literature. According to these results, the TTS measured immediately after loud music exposure ranges from 10 to 30 dB, depends on the level, time, and the temporal and spectral structure of noise or loud music [15, 18]. Moreover, if one can assume that TTS phenomenon causes similar effects that may be characteristic for the hearing loss, the decrease of sensitivity of the hearing system affects the perception of auditory signals in all their dimensions, that is, temporal and frequency resolution as well as loudness perception may be distorted or deteriorated. This effect may be observed in the discotheque attendants or in the people who are exposed to the noise level greater than 90 dB [17].

The results may also be influenced by the mental fatigue which occurred after permanently playing loud sounds for several time durations, together with demanding tasks. Such conditions involving the mental engagement in a noisy environment which is natural in the studio can significantly reduce the time of exhaustion which causes the decrease of accuracy in solving several tasks [9].

Nowadays portable players are getting cheaper, smaller, and offer more and better sound quality. Everything would be fine, if not the fact that listening to the loud music does not hurt. These devices induce young people to listen louder and louder, applying that noise directly on themselves. It is very easy to meet someone on the tram, the bus, or on the street with headphones in their ears and the music is reproduced so loud that it is possible to recognize songs that are played being in a distance from the listening person. The body does not give us a sign that the process of destroying the hearing has just began, and once damaged, hair cells would never regenerate. The results of the research conclude that if a person listens to loud music on MP3 player for 5 years for an hour a day it is enough to ruin a hearing system permanently. Thus, it should be noted that the tendency observed in young people to listen loud music in order to be isolated from the environment is still actual which will cause not the TTS but PTS. The most dangerous factor influencing the human hearing system reported in the literature [8, 10, 18] is the type of headphones used for every day listening. Most of young people listen to the music through inside earphones which causes that the reduction in the length of outer ear channel, and as a consequence, a natural protection becomes less effective. From sociological point of view, the young people like this kind of earphones because they take up little space and can be always carried in a pocket, but on the other hand, they are the worst for our hearing. Research has shown that 2–3 years of using this type of headphones leads to a slight hearing damage resulting with incomprehensibility of a whisper or a quiet voice. Listening to music is becoming an addiction primarily among young people, but unfortunately this fact is ignored in the mainstream media.

Glossary of used terms

A-weighting is the correction of the sound pressure level (SPL) as a function of frequency in such a manner that it reflects human feeling of loudness level of different frequencies. The A-weighting curve is defined in the International Standard IEC 61672:2003

Clarity of sound is the property of reproduced sound that allows the listener to distinguish the basic components of information. It depends on the degree to which the sound is free from any kind of distortion.

Closed headphones are the headphones which have the back of the earcups closed. Closed headphones isolate the ear from external ambient noise and minimize the music leakage out of the earpieces.

Dynamic compression is a signal processing operation that reduces the volume of loud sounds or amplifies quiet sounds by narrowing an audio signal's dynamic range. The device which realizes dynamic compression is called a compressor.

Earphones are electroacoustic transducers which converts an electrical signal into acoustical one and deliver it directly to the ear.

Energy dose is the integral of the square of acoustic pressure over time. The units of energy dose are Pa^2s and Pa^2h. It is also known as sound exposure.

Front of House (FOH) is the part of a performance venue which is open to the public, for example, an auditorium and foyer. Front of house sound engineer is normally positioned in a small sectioned-off area front of house, surrounded by the audience or at the edge of the audience area. From this position, he has unobstructed hearing and a clear view of the performance, enabling the operation of the speaker system, show control consoles and other equipment. In this case, Front of House can refer to both the general audience/public area or to the specific small section from where the show is operated.

Headphones are a pair of earphones connected with a bail which is put on the head. The bail provides the necessary downforce of earpieces to the ears.

Hearing level (HL) is defined in a similar way as the SPL (see below), except the reference level which is equal to normal threshold of hearing for a given frequency. Hearing level is applied in audiometry for determination of hearing loss.

Inside or inner earphones are very small earphones which are inserted directly into ear canal.

Loudspeakers are electroacoustic transducers, which convert an electrical signal into acoustical one and radiate it into space. The loudspeakers occur most often as loudspeaker sets, which consist of a few single loudspeakers, enclosure, filters, amplifiers etc.

Open headphones have the back of the earcups open. The sound in the ear canal does not depend on the downforce of the earphones to the ears. Open headphones do not block out ambient noise and allow audio leakage out of the earpieces.

Permanent threshold shift (PTS)is a permanent shift in the auditory threshold. It may occur suddenly or develop gradually over time. A permanent threshold shift results in permanent hearing loss.

Public address (PA) is an electronic sound amplification and distribution system, used to delivery sound with sufficiently high SPL to the public in large spaces: railway stations, airports, stadiums, department stores etc.

Semi-open headphones are a compromise between open and closed headphones. They combine all the positive properties of both designs.

http://dx.doi.org/10.5772/64611

Sound pressure level (SPL) is defined as twenty logarithms of the ratio the RMS (root mean square) value of an actual acoustic pressure and the reference level equal to 20 μPa. Unit of the SPL is decibel (dB).

Temporary threshold shift (TTS)is a temporary shift in the auditory hearing threshold. It may occur suddenly after exposure to a high level of noise, a situation in which most people experience reduced hearing. A temporary threshold shift results in temporary hearing loss.

Author details

Andrzej Dobrucki*, Maurycy J. Kin and Bartłomiej Kruk

*Address all correspondence to: andrzej.dobrucki@pwr.edu.pl

Department of Acoustics and Multimedia, Faculty of Electronics, Wroclaw University of Science and Technology, Wrocław, Poland

References

[1] Kim Y-H, Choi J-W. Sound Visualization and Manipulation. Singapore: Wiley; 2013.

[2] Jokitulppo J., Ikäheimo M., Pääkkönen R. Noise exposure measurements in real ears: an evaluation of MIRE-Technique use in the field and in the laboratory. Acta Acustica United with Acustica. 2008;**94**(5):734–739.

[3] Vickers E. The loudness war—do louder, hypercompressed recordings sell better? Journal of the Audio Engineering Society. 2011;**59**(5):346–352.

[4] Katz B. Mastering Audio: The Art and the Science. Oxford: Focal Press; 2007.

[5] Rumsey F. Mastering-art, perception, technologies. Journal of the Audio Engineering Society. 2011;**59**(6):436–440.

[6] Moore B.C.J. Effect of sound-induced hearing loss and hearing aids on the perception of music. Journal of the Audio Engineering Society. 2016;**64**(3):112–123.

[7] Pawlaczyk-Łuszczyńska M., Dudarewicz A., Zamojska A., Śliwińska-Kowalska A. Evaluation of sound exposure and risk of hearing impairment in orchestral musicians. International Journal of Occupational Safety and Ergonomics. 2011;**17**(3):255–269.

[8] Royster J.D., Royster L.H., Killion M.C. Sound exposures and hearing thresholds of symphony orchestra musicians. Journal of the Acoustical Society of America. 1991;**89**:2793–2803.

[9] Marcora S.M., Staiano W., Manning V. Mental fatigue impairs physical performance in humans. Journal of Applied Physiology. 2009;**106**(3):857–864.

[10] Dobrucki A.B., Kin M.J., Kruk B. Preliminary study on the influence of headphones for listening music on hearing loss of young people. Archives of Acoustics. 2013;**38**(3):383–387.

[11] Rintelmann W.F., Lindberg R.F., Simiteley E.K. Temporary threshold shift and recovery patterns from two types of rock-and-roll music presentations. Journal of the Acoustical Society of America. 1972;**51**:1249–1255.

[12] Brachmański S. Automatic classification of subjective measurements of logatom intelligibility in classrooms. In: Kongoli F., editor. Automation. Rijeka, Croatia: InTech; 2012.

[13] Smaldino J.J., Crandell C.C., Kreisman B.M., John A., Kreisman N. Room acoustics for listeners with normal hearing and hearing impairment. In: Valente M., Hosford-Dunn H., Roeser R.J., editors. Audiology Treatment. New York – Stuttgart: Thieme; 2008.

[14] Chiou-Jong C., Yu-Tung D., Yih-Min S., Yi-Chang L., Yow-Jer J. Evaluation of auditory fatigue in combined noise, heat and workload exposure. Industrial Health. 2007;**45**(4):527–534.

[15] Jaroszewski A., Rakowski A. Loud music induced threshold shifts and damage risk prediction. Archives of Acoustics. 1994;**19**:311–321.

[16] Kozłowski E., Młyński R. Effects of acoustic treatment on music teachers' exposure to sound. Archives of Acoustics. 2014;**39**:159–163.

[17] Jaroszewski A., Fidecki T., Rogowski P. Hearing damage from exposure to music. Archives of Acoustics. 1998;**23**:3–31.

[18] Jaroszewski A., Fidecki T., Rogowski P. Exposures and hearing thresholds in music students due to training sessions. Archives of Acoustics. 1999;**24**:111–118.

[19] BIAP. Recommendation 02/1: Automatic classification of hearing impairment [Internet]. October 26, 1996.

[20] ISO 8253-1:2010. Acoustics: Audiometric test methods–Part 1: Pure-tone air and bone conduction audiometry [Internet].

[21] ISO 7029:2000. Acoustics: Statistical distribution of hearing threshold as a function of age [Internet].

[22] PN-EN 26189. The measurements of hearing threshold by audiometric air conditions for hearing protection (in Polish) [Internet].

[23] Moore B.C.J. An Introduction to the Psychology of Hearing. London: Academic Press; 1997.

[24] Pawłowski T. Informational aesthetics. In: Selection of Aesthetic Papers. Kraków: Universitas; 2010.

[25] Gustafsson B. The loudness of transient sounds as a function of some physical parameters. Journal of Sound and Vibration. 1974;**37**:389–398.

[26] Kumagai M., Ebata M., Sone T. Effect of some physical parameters of impact sound on its loudness. Journal of the Acoustical Society of Japan. vol. 2 (1981), No. 1;15–26.

[27] Fastl H., Zwicker E. Psychoacoustics–Facts and Models. Berlin, Heidelberg, New York: Springer; 2007.

[28] de Bruijn A. Timbre classification of complex tones. Acustica. 1978;**40**(2):108–114.

[29] Green D.M. Profile analysis: A different view of audiology intensity discrimination. American Psychologist. 1983;**38**(2):133–142.

[30] Toole F.E., Olive S.E. The modification of timbre by resonances: Perception and measurement. Journal of the Audio Engineering Society. 1988;**36**(3):122–142.

[31] Kin M., Dobrucki A. Perception of changes in spectrum and envelope of musical signals vs. auditory fatigue. Archives of Acoustics. 2016;**41**:323–330.

[32] Kruk B., Kin M. Perception of timbre changes vs. temporary threshold shift. In: 138th AES Convention; May 2015; Warsaw. New York: Audio Engineeing Society; 2015. Preprint 9228.

[33] Scharf B. Recent measurements of loudness adaptation and the definition of loudness. In: Proceedings of the 14th International Congress on Acoustics; International Commision on Acoustics; 1992.

Chapter 11

Psychophysiological Evidence of an Autocorrelation Mechanism in the Human Auditory System

Yoshiharu Soeta

Additional information is available at the end of the chapter

http://dx.doi.org/10.5772/66198

Abstract

This article details a model for evaluations of sound quality in the human auditory system. The model includes an autocorrelation function (ACF) mechanism. Thus, we conducted physiological and psychological experiments to search for evidence of the ACF mechanism in the human auditory system. To evaluate physiological responses related to the peak amplitude of the ACF of an auditory signal, which represents the degree of temporal regularity of the sound, we used magnetoencephalography (MEG) to record auditory evoked fields (AEFs). To evaluate psychological responses related to the envelope of the ACF of an auditory signal, which is a measure of the repetitive features of an auditory signal, we examined perceptions of loudness and annoyance. The results of the MEG experiments showed that the amplitude of the N1m, which is found above the left and right temporal lobes around 100 ms after stimulus onset, was a function of the peak amplitude and its delay time or the degree of envelope decay of the ACF. The results of the psychological experiments indicated that loudness and annoyance increased for sounds with envelope decay of the ACF in a certain range. These results suggest that an autocorrelation mechanism exists in the human auditory system.

Keywords: auditory evoked field, pitch strength, loudness, annoyance

1. Introduction

Correlation is one of the most common and useful statistical concepts. It measures the strength and direction of a linear relationship between two variables. **Figure 1** shows some examples of correlations between pairs of variables, including white noise signals with different phases, pure tones with the same frequency and phase, pure tones with different frequencies, human voice signals and time-delayed versions of the same signal, environmental noise signals and time-delayed versions of the same signal, and environmental noise signals obtained at the left and right ears. The correlation coefficient ranges between −1 and 1, and characterizes the strength of the relationships between the two variables.

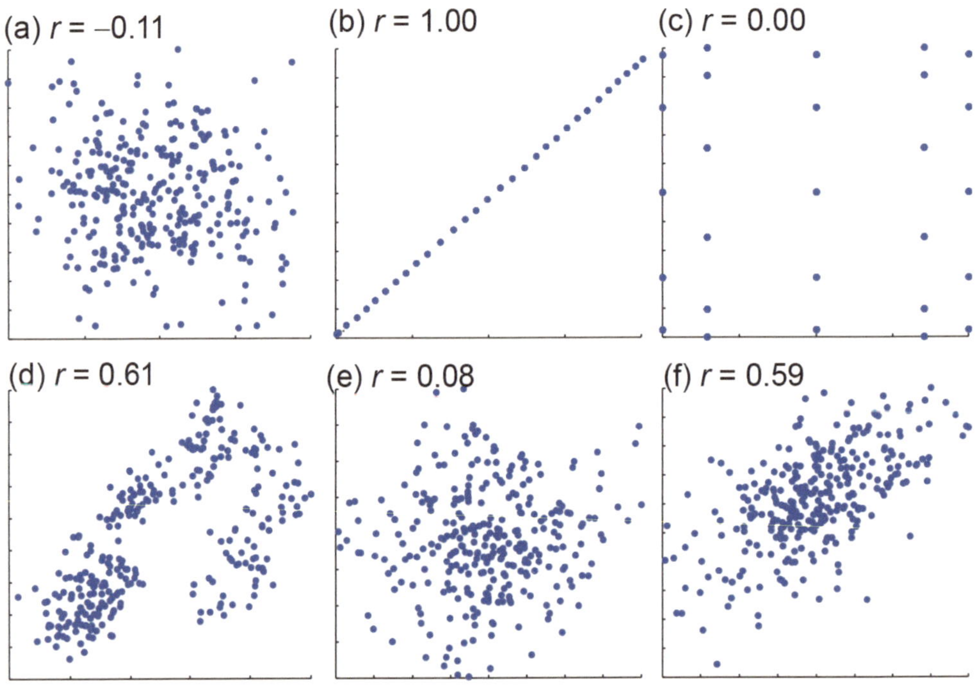

Figure 1. Relationship between two variables. (a) White noise signals with different phases, (b) pure tones with the same frequency, (c) pure tones with different frequencies, (d) human voice signals and time-delayed versions of the same signal, (e) environmental noise and time-delayed versions of the same signal, and (f) environmental noise signals obtained at the left and right ears.

When a signal is represented as a time series, it is characterized by periodicity or randomness as a function of time. **Figure 2** shows some examples of relationships between a signal and the time-delayed version of that signal. The signals included in the figure are white noise, pure tones, a human voice, and train noise. The way in which correlation coefficients change as a function of time can be evaluated using an autocorrelation function (ACF). An ACF is a set of correlation coefficients that characterize the relations between the points in a series and time-delayed version of the same set. In other words, the ACF is a time-domain function that measures how much a waveform resembles the delayed version of itself. While the values of an ACF can extend beyond −1 and 1, the normalized ACF (NACF) for a signal, $\phi(\tau)$, is defined by

http://dx.doi.org/10.5772/66198

$$\phi(\tau) = \frac{\Phi(\tau)}{\Phi(0)} \tag{1}$$

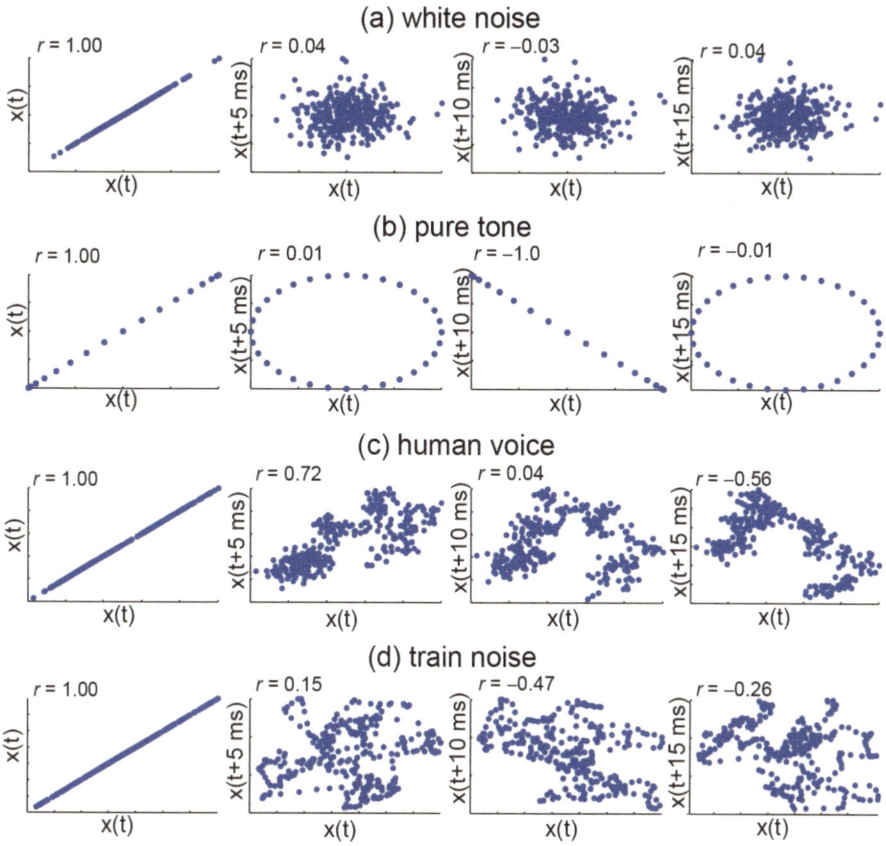

Figure 2. Relationships between a signal and a time-delayed version of the same signal. (a) White noise, (b) pure tones, (c) a human voice, and (d) train noise.

where

$$\Phi(\tau) = \frac{1}{2T}\int_{-T}^{+T} p(t)p(t+\tau)dt \tag{2}$$

That is, the ACF is normalized by the maximum value of the ACF at the point with zero delay, Φ(0), thus restricting the values to fit the range between −1 and 1. **Figure 3** shows some examples of the NACF. As white noise is random, the ACF is close to zero. As pure tones are completely periodic, the ACF is also periodic and the maximum and minimum values are 1 and −1, respectively. The human voice and environmental noise have periodic components, so the ACF values for these stimuli are high at the dominant frequency.

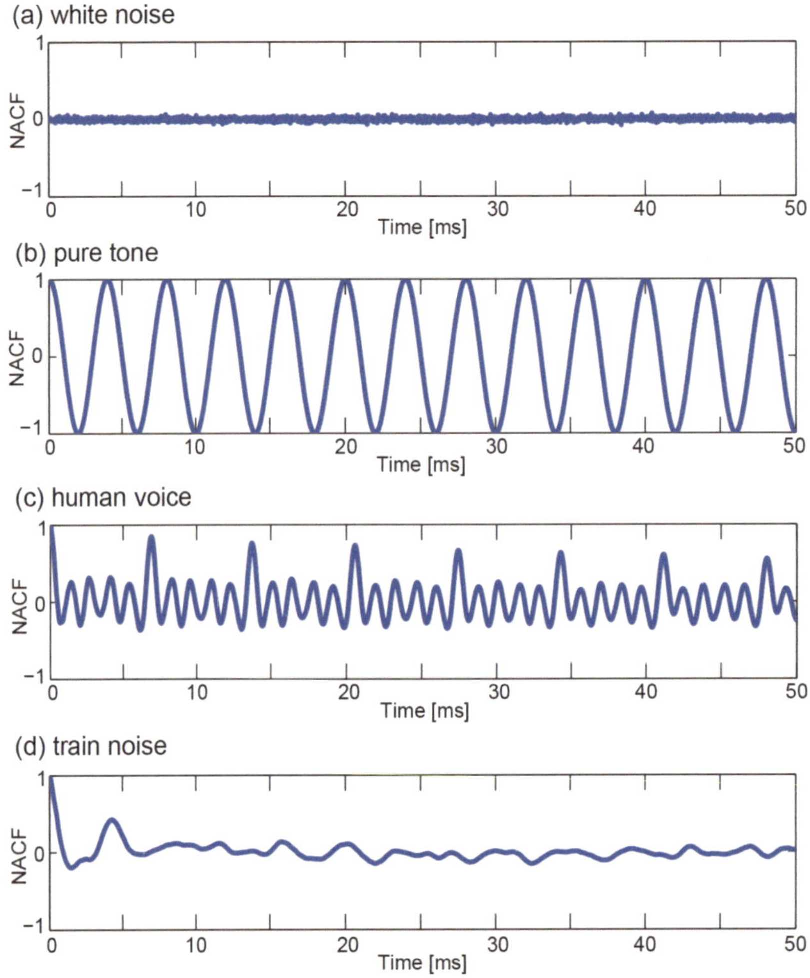

Figure 3. Examples of the NACF for (a) white noise, (b) pure tones, (c) the human voice, and (d) train noise.

Mathematically, the ACF contains the same information as the power spectrum of a given signal. For characterization of auditory signals, five factors are extracted from the ACF [1]. The first factor is the energy at the point with zero delay, given by $\Phi(0)$, which corresponds to the equivalent continuous sound pressure level (SPL). The second and third factors are the amplitude and delay time of the first maximum peak of the NACF, ϕ_1 and τ_1, which are related to the perceived pitch strength and pitch [2, 3]. The fourth factor is the effective duration of the envelope of the NACF, τ_e, which is defined by the 10th percentile delay. It represents a repetitive feature containing the auditory signal itself and is related to the preferred condition for the temporal factors of a sound field, such as reverberation time and the delay time of the first reflection [3, 4]. The fifth factor is the width of the amplitude of the NACF around the origin of the delay time, $W_{\phi(0)}$, which is defined as having a value of 0.5. It corresponds to the spectral centroid [1]. The definitions of the ACF factors are depicted in **Figure 4**.

http://dx.doi.org/10.5772/66198

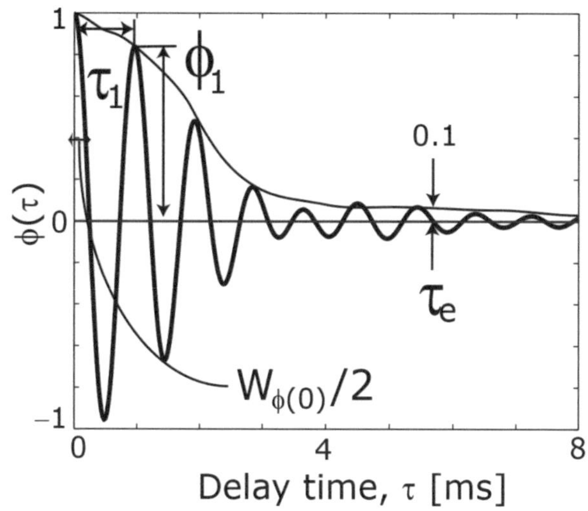

Figure 4. Definitions of the ACF factors, ϕ_1, τ_1, τ_e, and $W_{\phi(0)}$.

The ACF is one of the most famous models for describing the perception of pitch and pitch strength. Pitch is thought to be extracted by the ACF in the temporal model of pitch perception [e.g., 5–7] and pitch strength corresponds to ϕ_1, which represents the degree of temporal regularity of a sound [e.g., 1–3, 6]. It is possible to systematically manipulate the values of ϕ_1 using iterated rippled noise (IRN). IRN is produced by adding a delayed version of a noise signal to the original signal, and then repeating this delay and addition process [2]. Increasing the number of iterations increases the periodicity and ϕ_1 value.

Physiologically, IRN elicits signals in auditory nerve fibers [8, 9] and cochlear nucleus neurons [10–12], indicating that the pitch of IRN is represented in the firing patterns of action potentials locked to either the temporal fine structure or the envelope periodicity. That is, autocorrelation-like behavior in the fine structure of the neural firing patterns suggests that the pitch of IRN is based on an ACF mechanism. Indeed, the pooled interspike interval distributions of auditory nerve discharge patterns in response to complex sounds are similar to the ACF of the stimulus waveform, and ϕ_1 of the ACF corresponds to pitch strength [13, 14].

Therefore, to find the physiological counterparts of an ACF mechanism in the human auditory cortex, we used magnetoencephalography (MEG) to investigate the auditory evoked magnetic field (AEF) elicited by IRN and bandpass filtered noise (BPN). The ϕ_1 value can be manipulated systematically by changing the bandwidth of the BPN. A narrower bandwidth produces a higher ϕ_1. In MEG, the measured signals are generated by synchronized neuronal activity in the human brain. The time resolution is in the range of milliseconds. Thus, this technique can be used to examine rapid changes in cortical activity that reflects ongoing signal processing in the brain; electrical events in single neurons typically last from one to several tens of milliseconds [15]. With respect to the psychological aspect of sound perception, we evaluated the effects of the other ACF factor, i.e., τ_e, on loudness and annoyance because it can explain changes in loudness even when SPL conditions are unchanged.

2. AEFs in relation to the peak amplitude of the ACF, ϕ_1

2.1. AEFs in relation to IRN

MEG has been used to investigate how features of sound stimuli related to pitch are represented in the human auditory cortex. For instance, tonotopic organization of the human auditory cortex has been investigated as a spatial representation of pure tone in the auditory system according to frequency [16–18]. The frequency of pure tones has been found to influence the source location of AEF response components, such as the N1m, in the human auditory cortex. The periodicity of pitch-related cortical responses has been investigated as part of the temporal structure of sound [19, 20]. However, it is currently unclear whether periodic pitch is reflected in the location of the source of the AEF response in the human auditory cortex.

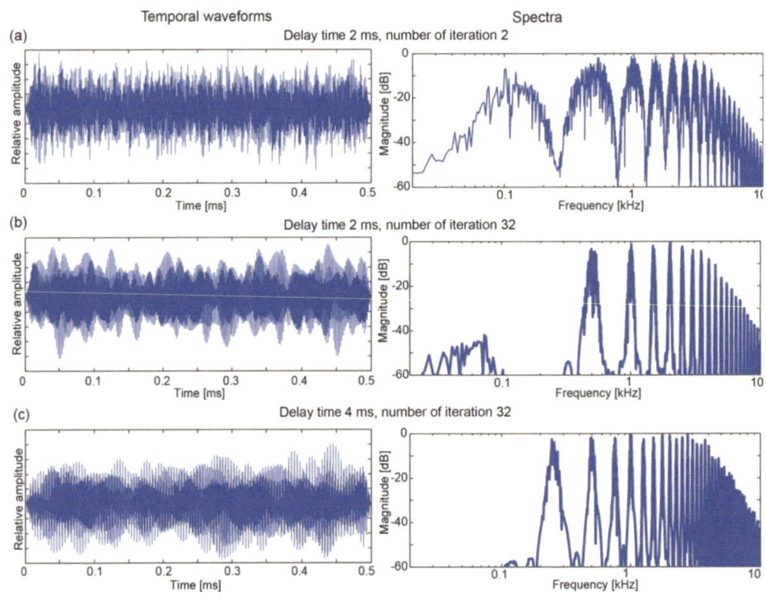

Figure 5. Temporal waveforms (left panels) and power spectra (right panels) of the IRN with different delay times (d) and number of iterations (n). (a) $d = 2$ ms, $n = 2$; (b) $d = 2$ ms, $n = 32$; (c) $d = 4$ ms, $n = 32$.

To evaluate responses related to the first maximum peak of the ACF, ϕ_1, which corresponds to pitch strength, in the auditory cortex, we recorded the AEFs elicited by IRNs with different iteration numbers. We anticipated that the N1m amplitude would increase with ϕ_1. The N1m is a typical component of the AEFs, which is generated in the auditory cortex approximately 100 ms after stimulus onset, offset, or a change in sound [21]. A large number of physical and psychological parameters have been reported to influence N1m responses, including intensity, frequency, interaural level or time difference, threshold, states of arousal, and selective attention. For example, the N1m is correlated with basic sensations such as loudness and pitch [1].

Ten normal-hearing listeners (22–36 years; all right-handed) took part in the experiment. We produced an IRN using a delay-and-add algorithm applied to BPN that was filtered using fourth-order Butterworth filters between 100 and 3500 Hz. The number of iterations of the delay-and-add process was set at 2, 4, 8, 16, and 32, and the delay was set to 2 and 4 ms, corresponding to pitch values of 500 and 250 Hz, respectively. The stimulus duration was 0.5 s, including rise and fall ramps of 10 ms. The sounds were digital-to-analog (D/A) converted with a 16-bit sound card and a sampling rate of 48 kHz. Sounds were presented at a SPL of 60 dB through insert earphones inserted into both the left and right ear canals. **Figure 5** shows the temporal waveforms and the power spectra of some of the IRN used in this experiment. **Figure 6** shows the ACF waveform of some of the IRN used in this experiment. The τ_1 value of IRN is the same value with the delay of the IRN. The ϕ_1 value increases as the number of iterations increases.

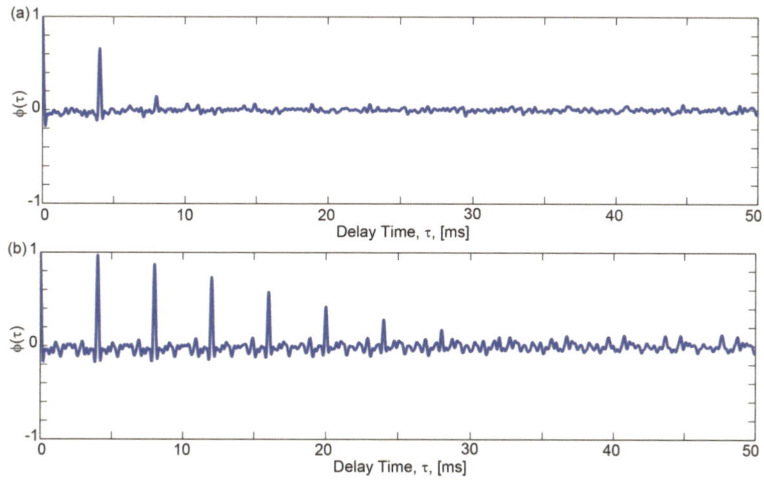

Figure 6. ACFs of the IRN with the delay time of 4 ms and number of the iterations: (a) 2 and (b) 32.

The AEFs were recorded using a 122 channel whole-head DC superconducting quantum interference device (DC-SQUID) magnetometer (Neuromag-122™; Neuromag Ltd., Helsinki, Finland) in a magnetically shielded room [15]. The IRNs were presented in a randomized order with a constant interstimulus interval of 1.5 s. To maintain listeners' attention level, listeners were instructed to watch a self-selected silent movie and ignore the stimuli during the experiment. The magnetic data were sampled at 0.4 kHz after being bandpass filtered between 0.03 and 100 Hz, then averaged approximately 100 times. The averaged responses were digitally filtered between 1.0 and 30.0 Hz. We analyzed a 0.7 s period starting 0.2 s prior to the stimulus onset, and an averaged 0.2 s prestimulus period served as the baseline.

We conducted source analysis for the measured field distribution based on the model of a single moving equivalent current dipole (ECD) [15]. Source estimates were based on a subset of 40–44 channels over each hemisphere. The dipole with the maximal goodness-of-fit over the analysis time window was chosen for further analysis. Only dipoles with a goodness-of-fit of more than 80% were included in the further analyses. The source waveforms for all stimuli were calculated using the best-fitting dipole in each hemisphere. The peak amplitudes and latencies of the N1m reported in the following sections are based on the source waveforms.

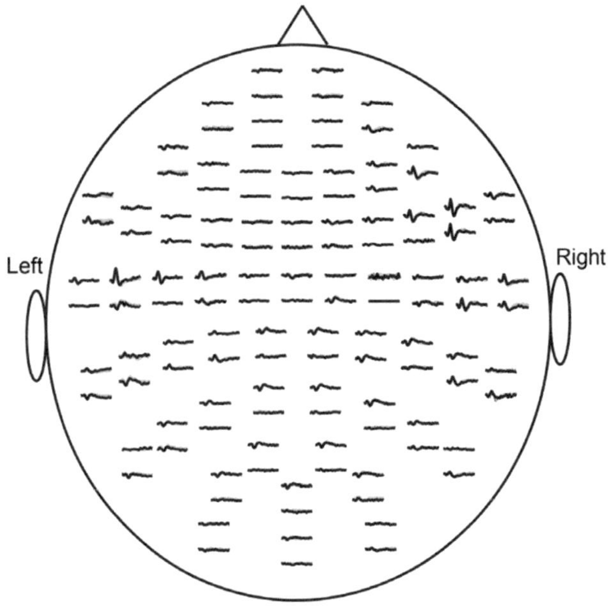

Figure 7. Typical waveforms of AEFs from 122 channels in a listener.

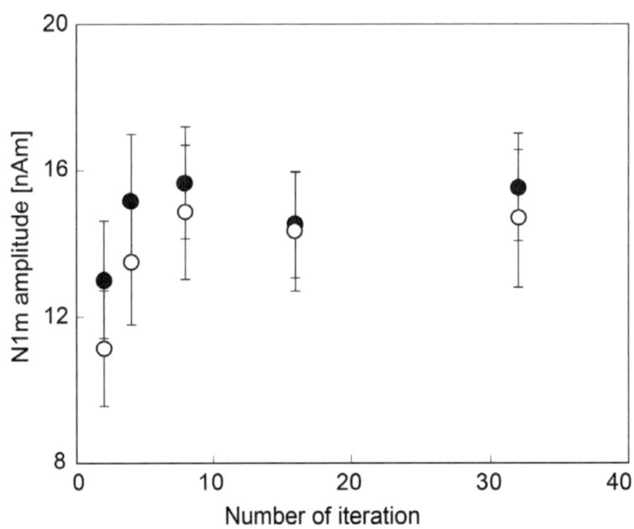

Figure 8. Mean amplitude of the N1m (± standard error) across 10 listeners and hemispheres as a function of the number of iterations with a delay time of 2 ms (○) or 4 ms (●).

Clear N1m responses were observed in both the left and right temporal areas in all listeners as shown in **Figure 7**. The N1m latencies were not systematically affected by the number of iterations of the IRN. **Figure 8** depicts the mean N1m amplitude across 10 listeners as a function of the number of iterations. A greater number of iterations of the IRN, i.e., a larger ϕ_1 value, produced a larger N1m amplitude. This suggests that a stronger pitch produces a larger N1m response. This result is consistent with previous studies [22, 23]. Previously, the amplitude of the AEF component elicited by periodic stimuli was compared with simulated peripheral activity patterns of the auditory nerve [24]. The researchers reported that the amplitude of the N1m was correlated with the pitch strength, estimated on the basis of auditory nerve activity. This finding is consistent with the present results.

Figure 9 shows the relationship between ϕ_1 of the IRN and the N1m amplitude. A larger ϕ_1 value produced a larger N1m response, with a correlation coefficient of 0.76 ($p < 0.05$). However, we found another factor that appears to influence N1m amplitude. To calculate the effects of each ACF factor on AEF responses, we conducted multiple regression analyses with the N1m amplitude as the outcome variable. We used a linear combination of ϕ_1, τ_1 and τ_e as predictive variables in a stepwise fashion. The final version indicated that ϕ_1 and τ_1 were significant factors:

$$\text{N1m amplitude} \approx a_1 * \phi_1 + a_2 * \tau_1 + b_1 \tag{3}$$

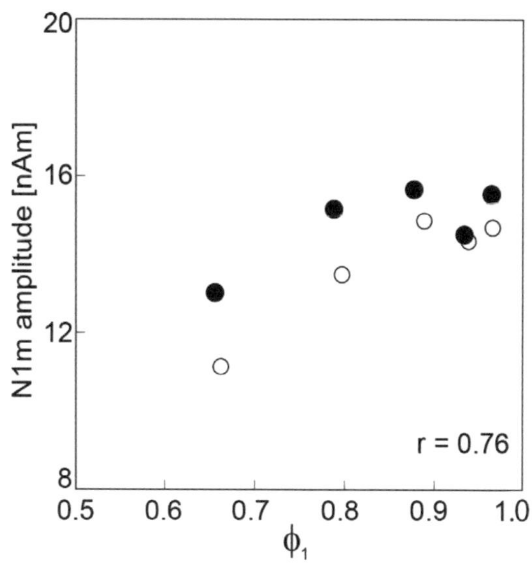

Figure 9. Relationship between ϕ_1 and mean N1m amplitude. The delay time of the IRN of 2 ms (○) or 4 ms (●).

The model was statistically significant ($p < 0.01$), and the correlation coefficient between the measured and predicted values was 0.88. The standardized partial regression coefficients of the variables a_1 and a_2 in Eq. (3) were 0.77 and 0.44, respectively. These results indicate that both the ACF factors ϕ_1 and τ_1 had significant effects on N1m responses, although ϕ_1 had a stronger effect.

2.2. AEFs in relation to BPN

To evaluate responses related to ϕ_1 in the auditory cortex, we also recorded the AEFs elicited by BPN with different bandwidths. Eight normal-hearing listeners (22–28 years; all right-handed) took part in the experiment. We produced BPN by repeated digital filtering of 10 s white noise signals. We set the magnitude of the Fourier coefficients to a cut-off slope of 200 dB/octave outside the desired bandwidth. For stimuli with a center frequency of 500 or 1000 Hz, the stimulus bandwidth was set at 1, 40, 80, 160 or 320 Hz. For stimuli with a center frequency of 2000 Hz, the stimulus bandwidth was set at 1, 40, 80, 160, 320 or 640 Hz. The maximum bandwidth was wider than the critical bandwidth for each center frequency [25]. The stimulus duration was 0.5 s, which we took from the 10 s BPN signal and set rise and fall ramps of 10 ms. The sounds were D/A converted with a 16-bit sound card and a sampling rate of 48 kHz. They were presented at a SPL of 74 dB through insert earphones inserted into both the left and right ear canals. **Figure 10** shows the temporal waveforms of the stimuli with a center frequency of 1000 Hz. As the bandwidth of the BPN increases, fluctuations in the envelope of the BPN waveform decrease. The ACF can characterize the BPN, that is, τ_1 corresponds to the center frequency of the BPN and the ϕ_1 value increases as the filter bandwidth decreases.

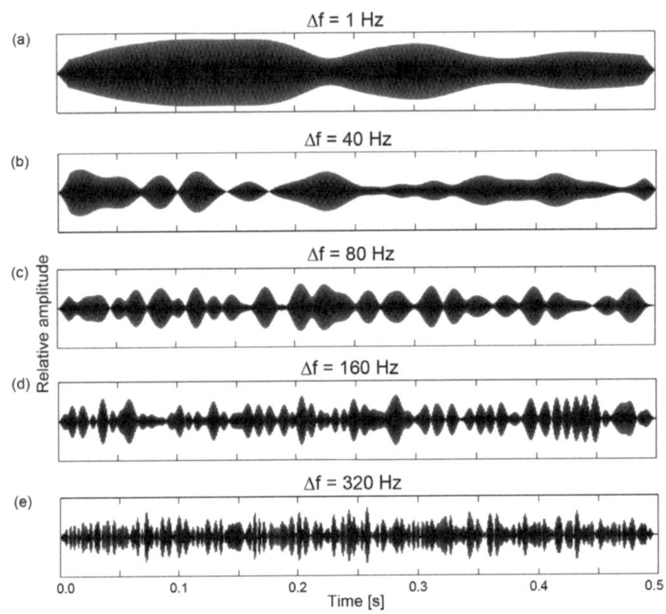

Figure 10. Temporal waveforms of BPNs with a center frequency of 1000 Hz and different bandwidths, Δf, (a) 1 Hz; (b) 40 Hz; (c) 80 Hz; (d) 160 Hz; (e) 320 Hz.

http://dx.doi.org/10.5772/66198

We recorded and analyzed the AEFs using methods similar to previous MEG experiments using IRN. The temporal waveforms of AEFs from 122 channels showed clear N1m responses in both the left and right temporal areas in all listeners. **Figure 11** depicts the mean N1m amplitude across eight listeners as a function of the BPN bandwidths. A narrower BPN bandwidths produced a larger N1m amplitude, that is, the larger the ϕ_1 value, the larger the N1m response. This result is consistent with previous IRN experiments.

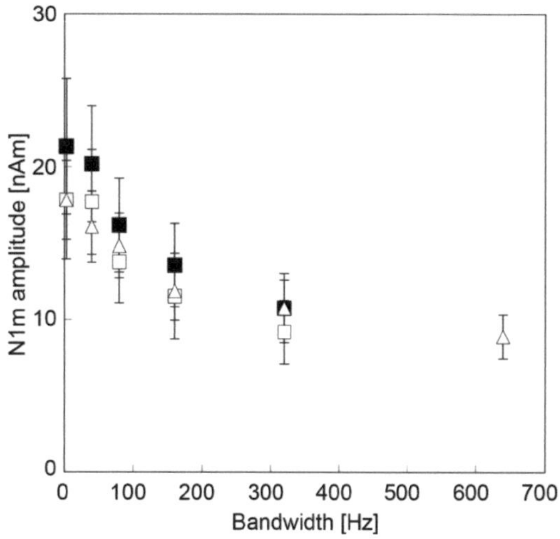

Figure 11. Mean amplitude of the N1m (± standard error) across eight listeners and hemispheres as a function of bandwidth with a center frequency of 500 Hz (□), 1000 Hz (■), and 2000 Hz (△).

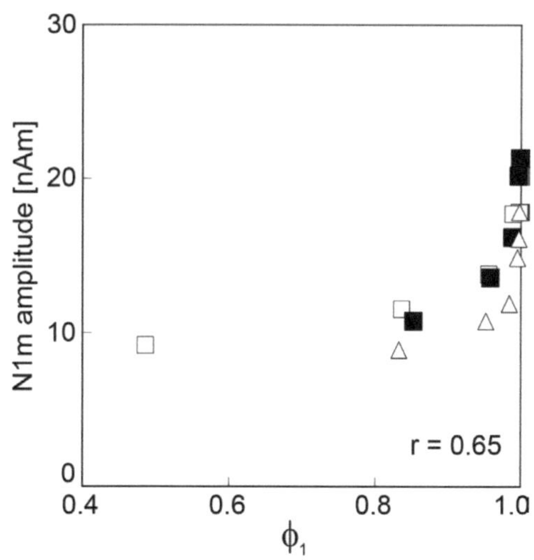

Figure 12. Relationship between ϕ_1 and mean N1m amplitude. Symbols denote the center frequency of the BPN as 500 Hz (□), 1000 Hz (■), or 2000 Hz (△).

Figure 12 shows the relationship between ϕ_1 of the BPN and the N1m amplitude. A larger ϕ_1 produced a larger N1m response. The correlation coefficient was 0.65 ($p < 0.05$). However, we identified another factor that influences N1m amplitude. To calculate the effects of each ACF factor on AEF response, we conducted multiple regression analyses with the N1m amplitude as the outcome variable. We used a linear combination of ϕ_1, τ_1, and τ_e as predictive variables in a stepwise fashion. The final version indicated that ϕ_1 and τ_e were significant factors:

$$\text{N1m amplitude} \approx a_3 * \phi_1 + a_4 * \tau_e + b_2 \tag{4}$$

The model was statistically significant ($p < 0.01$), and the correlation coefficient between the measured and predicted values was 0.78. The standardized partial regression coefficients of the variables a_3 and a_4 in Eq. (4) were 0.52 and 0.45, respectively. The results indicated that the ACF factors ϕ_1 and τ_e had significant effects on N1m responses.

3. Loudness and annoyance in relation to the effective duration of the ACF, τ_e

3.1. Loudness in relation to IRN

Previous investigations of the relationship between loudness and the BPN bandwidth have concluded that for sounds with the same SPL, loudness remains constant as bandwidth increases, up until the point at which the bandwidth reaches a critical band. For bandwidths larger than the critical band, loudness increases with bandwidth [25]. However, the loudness of a sharply filtered BPN increases with the effective duration of the ACF, i.e., τ_e, even when the bandwidth of the BPN is within the critical band [26]. The τ_e value represents the repetitive components within the signal itself and increases as the BPN bandwidth decreases. However, the envelope and SPL also vary with the BPN bandwidth. This variation of the envelope and SPL might therefore affect the loudness of a BPN signal [27, 28]. To eliminate the effects of these factors, we investigated the effects of τ_e on loudness using IRN. The envelope and SPL variation of the IRN are much smaller than those of the BPN [29].

We produced IRN by applying a delay-and-add algorithm to the BPN that was filtered from white noise using the fourth-order Butterworth filters ranging between 100 and 3500 Hz. The number of iterations of the delay-and-add process was set at 2, 4, 8, 16, and 32. The delay values were set at 0.5, 1, 2, 4, 8, and 16 ms, corresponding to pitches of 2000, 1000, 500, 250, 125, and 62.5 Hz, respectively. The duration of the stimuli was 0.5 s and the rise and fall ramps were 10 ms. The sounds were D/A converted with a 16-bit sound card and sampling rate of 48 kHz. The sounds were presented at a SPL of 60 dB through insert earphones inserted into the left and right ear canals. **Figure 13** shows the τ_e and ϕ_1 values of the IRN used in the experiment.

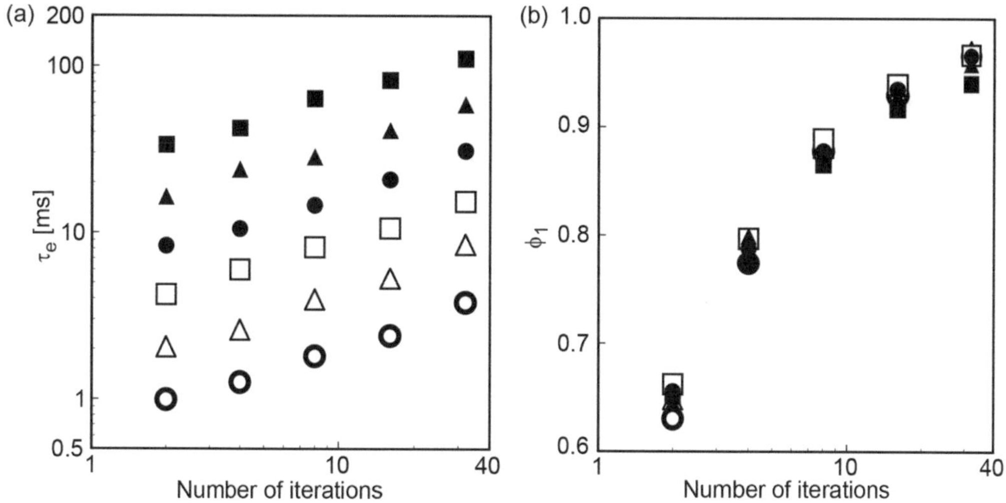

Figure 13. (a) τ_e and (b) ϕ_1 of the IRN used in the experiment as a function of the number of iterations with delays of (○) 0.5, (△) 1, (□) 2, (●) 4, (▲) 8 and (■) 16 ms.

Ten listeners (aged 21–37 years) with normal hearing took part in the experiment. We obtained loudness matches using a two-interval, adaptive forced-choice procedure converging on the point of subjective equality (PSE) following a simple 1-up, 1-down rule [30]. The experiment took place in a soundproof room. In each trial, the fixed (test) and variable (reference) sounds were presented in randomized order with equal probability at an interval of 500 ms. The test sound was an IRN and the reference sound was a 1-kHz pure tone. The listener was asked to indicate which sound they perceived as louder by pressing a key on a keyboard. For each

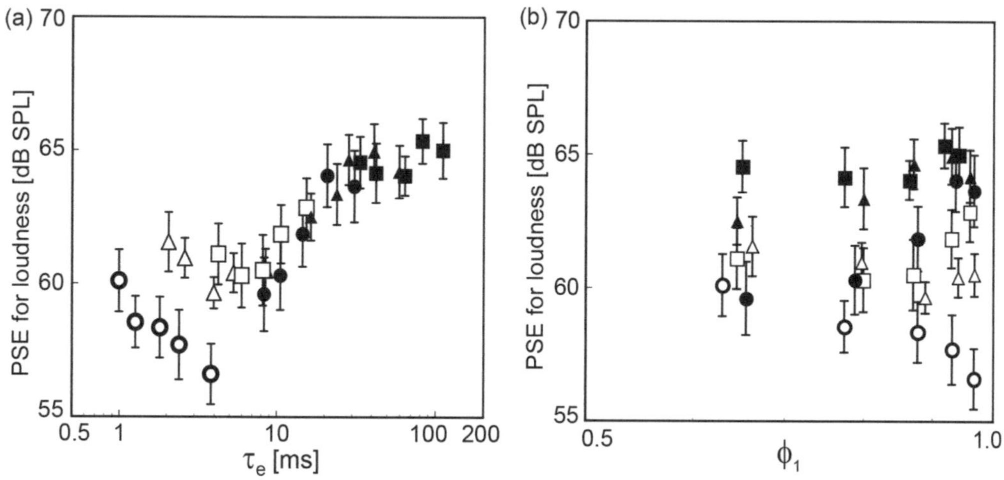

Figure 14. Mean PSE for loudness (± standard error) across 10 listeners as a function of (a) τ_e and (b) ϕ_1 for IRN with a delay of (△) 0.5, (□) 1, (○) 2, (●) 4, (▲) 8 and (■) 16 ms.

adaptive track, the overall level of the test sound was fixed at 60 dB SPL, and the starting level of the reference sound was 50 dB SPL. The level of the reference sound was controlled with an adaptive procedure: when the listener judged the reference sound to be louder than the test sound, the SPL of the test sound was lowered by a given amount, and when the listener judged the test sound to be louder than the reference sound, the SPL of the reference sound was increased by that same amount.

Figure 14 shows the PSE for loudness as a function of τ_e and ϕ_1 of the IRN. ϕ_1 was not correlated with the perceived loudness. When τ_e was between 10 and 100 ms, the perceived loudness increased with τ_e, clearly confirming that loudness is influenced by the repetitive components of sounds [26] in the τ_e range between 10 and 100 ms. The increase in loudness for the τ_e values between 10 and 100 ms was approximately 5 dB.

When τ_e was less than 5 ms, the loudness of the IRN increased with decreasing τ_e and the bandwidth of the IRN was larger than the critical bandwidth. These tendencies may explain the basis of the critical band effect, such that loudness remains constant as the bandwidth of the noise is narrower than the critical band, then increases with increasing bandwidth beyond the critical band [25]. Loudness models are able to predict these tendencies [31, 32].

The loudness model introduced previously [31, 32] was unable to predict loudness when the delays were 2 and 4 ms for stimuli with a pitch of 500 and 250 Hz, respectively. Loudness increases caused by a tonal component are predictable according to τ_e in a certain range. Previous studies have indicated that the τ_e values of various noise sources, such as airplanes [33], trains [34], motor bikes [35] and flushing toilets [36], are within the range of 1–200 ms. This suggests that τ_e is a useful criteria for measuring the loudness of various sounds. Thus, this value is likely helpful for the identification of sound sources.

3.2. Annoyance in relation to BPN

Annoyance is one of the most commonly studied features of environmental noise [37]. Basically, psychoacoustic annoyance depends on loudness and other factors such as timbre and the temporal structure of sounds. Loudness and annoyance have been distinguished previously: Annoyance is the reaction of an individual to noise within the context of a given situation, while loudness is directly related to SPL [38]. To evaluate whether annoyance is related to the effective duration of the ACF, i.e., τ_e, we examined the annoyance elicited by a pure tone and BPN stimuli with different bandwidths.

We used pure tone and BPN signals with center frequencies of 1000 and 2000 Hz as auditory signals. We used a maximum length bandpass filtered sequence signal (order 21; sampling frequency, 44,100 Hz) as the basic stimulus. To control the ACF of the BPN, we varied the filter bandwidth at 0, 40, 80, 160, and 320 Hz using a cut-off slope of 2068 dB/octave. The sounds were D/A converted with a 16-bit sound card and sampling rate of 48 kHz. The sounds were presented to both the left and right ears at an SPL of 74 dBA using headphones (Sennheiser HD-340). **Figure 15** shows τ_e of the stimuli used in the experiment.

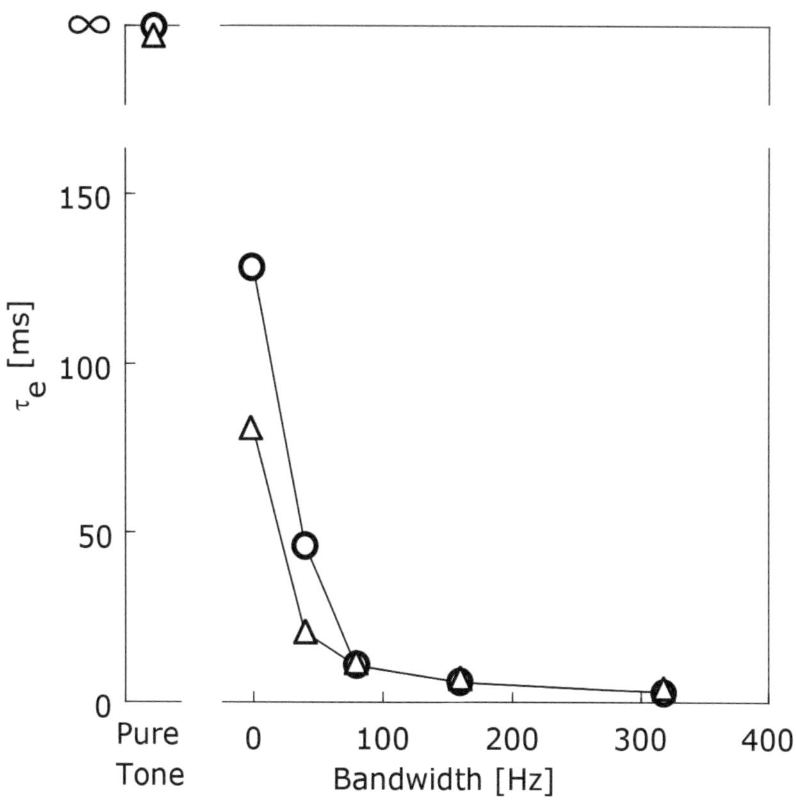

Figure 15. The measured effective duration of NACF, i.e., τ_e, of the signal as a function of the bandwidth. Different symbols indicate different frequencies: (○): 1000 Hz; (△): 2000 Hz.

Eight listeners aged 21–23 years with normal hearing took part in the experiment. We performed paired-comparison tests for all combinations of the pairs of the pure tone and BPN stimuli. The duration of the stimuli was 2.0 s, the rise and fall times were 50 ms, the silent interval between the stimuli was 1.0 s, and the interval between the pairs was 3.0 s, which was the time during which the listeners were expected to make a response. They were asked to judge which of the two sound signals was more annoying. We calculated the scale values of the annoyance rated by each listener according to Case V of Thurstone's theory [39].

The relationship between the scale values of annoyance and τ_e is shown in **Figure 16**. The averaged scale values of annoyance increased as τ_e increased within the critical band for both center frequencies of 1000 and 2000 Hz. The τ_e value represents the repetitive feature or tonal component of the auditory signals. Previous research suggests that tonal components increase the perceived annoyance and noisiness of broadband noise [35, 40, 41]. This is consistent with the present results. Two of the eight listeners reported the least annoyance for pure tone stimuli, with BPN stimuli with the widest bandwidth and a center frequency of 2000 Hz rated as the most annoying. In other words, annoyance increased as τ_e decreased. This could indicate that the effects of τ_e on annoyance are subject to individual variation.

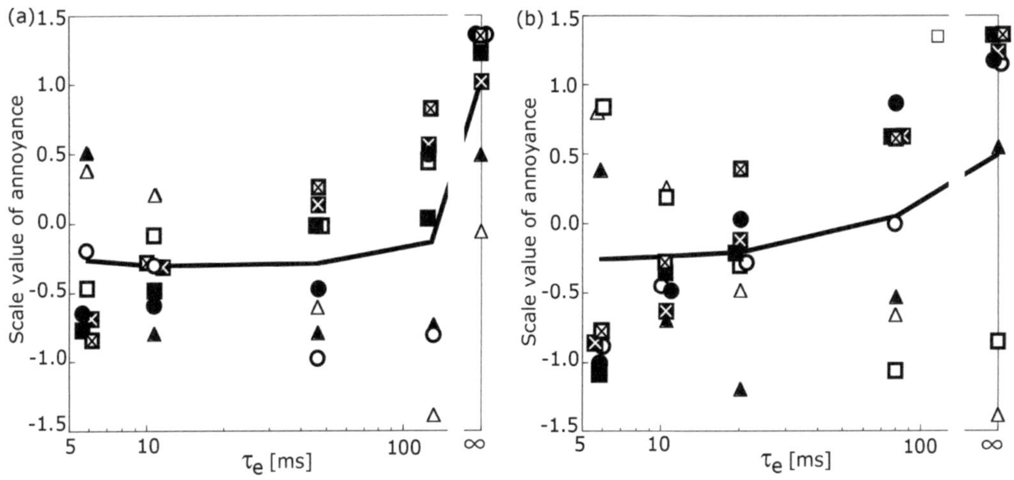

Figure 16. Scale value of annoyance as a function of τ_e for BPN with a center frequency of (a) 1000 Hz and (b) 2000 Hz. Each symbol represents one listener. The line represents the mean scale value of the eight listeners.

4. Concluding remarks

In this study, we investigate the effects of ACF factors on physiological and psychological responses. As a result, we found that the ACF factors ϕ_1, τ_1, and τ_e had significant effects on N1m response, suggesting that ACF factors are used as cues in the auditory cortex. We also found that the ACF factors ϕ_1 and τ_e influence loudness and annoyance, suggesting that ACF factors are used as a cue for perception. These results indicate that the human auditory system has an autocorrelation-like mechanism.

Acknowledgements

This work was supported by Grants-in-Aid for Scientific Research (B) (Grant No. 15H02771) from the Japan Society for the Promotion of Science.

Appendix

Auditory evoked fields (AEFs): Magnetic fields evoked by any abrupt sound or change in a continuous sound in the auditory cortex.

Butterworth filters: A kind of signal processing filter widely used for bandpass filtering.

Bandpass filtered noise (BPN): A noise in which frequency components are limited by bandpass filtering.

http://dx.doi.org/10.5772/66198

Envelope: Approximate shape of a sound wave form calculated by joining the peak amplitude.

Equivalent current dipole: A dipole estimated from the measured magnetic fields in the human brain, widely used in MEG analysis.

Interspike interval: Observed time between spikes from a single neuron.

Magnetoencephalography (MEG): A noninvasive technique for investigating human brain activity by measuring the magnetic fields produced by electric currents flowing in neurons.

Multiple regression analysis: A statistical technique for predicting a dependent variable from independent variables.

Paired-comparison tests: A psychophysical method that measures a linear distance among paired stimuli.

Point of subjective equality (PSE): Any of the points along a stimulus dimension at which a variable stimulus is judged by a listener to be equal to a standard stimulus.

Pure tone: A tone with a frequency component and a sinusoidal wave.

Tonotopic organization: Spatial arrangements in which sounds of different frequencies are processed in the auditory system.

Two-interval, adaptive forced-choice procedure: A psychophysical experimental design in which listeners are instructed to make a response between two alternatives within a timed interval, and the next alternative is determined by the previous response.

White noise: A random signal with equal intensity at all frequencies.

Author details

Yoshiharu Soeta

Address all correspondence to: y.soeta@aist.go.jp

National Institute of Advanced Industrial Science and Technology (AIST), Osaka, Japan

References

[1] Soeta Y, Ando Y. Neurally based measurement and evaluation of environmental noise. Tokyo: Springer Japan; 2015. DOI: 10.1007/978-4-431-55432-5.

[2] Yost WA. Pitch strength of iterated ripple noise. Journal of the Acoustical Society of America 1996;100:3329–3335. DOI: 10.1121/1.416973.

[3] Ando Y. Auditory and visual sensations. New York: Springer; 2010. DOI: 10.1007/b13253.

[4] Ando Y. Architectural acoustics: blending sound sources, sound fields, and listeners. New York: Springer-Verlag; 1998.

[5] Licklider JCR. A duplex theory of pitch perception. Experimenta. 1951;7:128–134. DOI: 10.1007/BF02156143.

[6] Wightman FL. The pattern-transformation model of pitch. Journal of the Acoustical Society of America 1973;54:407–416. DOI: 10.1121/1.1913592.

[7] Meddis R, Hewitt M. Virtual pitch and phase sensitivity of a computer model of the auditory periphery. I: Pitch identification. Journal of the Acoustical Society of America. 1991;89:2866–2882. DOI: 10.1121/1.400725.

[8] Fay RR, Yost WA, Coombs S. Psychophysics and neurophysiology of repetition noise processing in a vertebrate auditory system. Hearing Research 1983;12:31–55. DOI: 10.1016/0378-5955(83)90117-X.

[9] ten Kate JH, van Bekkum MF. Synchrony-dependent autocorrelation in eighth-nerve-fiber response to rippled noise. Journal of the Acoustical Society of America 1988;84:2092–2102. DOI: 10.1121/1.397054.

[10] Shofner WP. Temporal representation of rippled noise in the anteroventral cochlear nucleus of the chinchilla. Journal of the Acoustical Society of America 1991;90:2450–2466. DOI: 10.1121/1.402049.

[11] Shofner WP. Responses of cochlear nucleus units in the chinchilla to iterated rippled noises: analysis of neural autocorrelograms. Journal of Neurophysiology 1999;81:2662–2674.

[12] Winter IM, Wiegrebe L, Patterson RD. The temporal representation of the delay of iterated rippled noise in the ventral cochlear nucleus of the guinea-pig. Journal of Physiology 2001;537:553–566. DOI: 10.1111/j.1469-7793.2001.00553.x.

[13] Cariani PA, Delgutte B. Neural correlates of the pitch of complex tones. I. Pitch and pitch salience. Journal of Neurophysiology. 1996;76:1698–1716.

[14] Cariani PA, Delgutte B. Neural correlates of the pitch of complex tones. II. Pitch shift, pitch ambiguity, phase invariance, pitch circularity, rate pitch, and the dominance region for pitch. Journal of Neurophysiology. 1996;76:1717–1734.

[15] Hämäläinen MS, Hari R, Ilmoniemi RJ, Knuutila J, Lounasmaa OV. Magnetoencephalography theory, instrumentation, and applications to noninvasive studies of the working human brain. Reviews of Modern Physics 1993;65:413–497. DOI: 10.1103/RevModPhys.65.413.

[16] Elberling C, Bak C, Kofoed B, Lebech J, Sarmark G. Auditory magnetic fields from the human cerebral cortex: location and strength of an equivalent current dipole. Acta Neurologica Scandinavica 1982;65:553–569. DOI: 10.1111/j.1600-0404.1982. tb03110.x.

[17] Romani GL, Williamson SJ, Kaufman L. Tonotopic organization of the human auditory cortex. Science 1982;216:1339–1340. DOI: 10.1126/science.7079770.

[18] Pantev C, Hoke M, Lehnertz K, Lütkenhöner B, Anogianakis G, Wittkowski W. Tonotopic organization of the human auditory cortex revealed by transient auditory evoked magnetic fields. Electroencephalography and Clinical Neurophysiology 1988;69:160–170. DOI: 10.1016/0013-4694(88)90211-8.

[19] Langner G, Sams M, Heli P, Schulze H. Frequency and periodicity are represented in orthogonal maps in the human auditory cortex: evidence from magnetoencephalography. Journal of Comparative Physiology A 1997;181:665–676. DOI: 10.1007/s003590050148.

[20] Cansino S, Ducorps A, Ragot R. Tonotopic cortical representation of periodic complex sounds. Human Brain Mapping 2003;20:71–81. DOI: 10.1002/hbm.10132.

[21] Näätänen R, Picton T. The N1 wave of the human electric and magnetic response to sound: a review and an analysis of the component structure. Psychophysiology 1987;24:375–425. DOI: 10.1111/j.1469-8986.1987.tb00311.x.

[22] Soeta Y, Nakagawa S, Tonoike M. Auditory evoked magnetic fields in relation to the iterated rippled noise. Hearing Research 2005;205:256–261. DOI: 10.1016/j.heares.2005.03.026.

[23] Krumbholz K, Patterson RD, Seither-Preisler A, Lammertmann C, Lütkenhöner B. Neuromagnetic evidence for a pitch processing center in Heschl's gyrus. Cerebral Cortex 2003;13:765–772. DOI: 10.1093/cercor/13.7.765.

[24] Seither-Preisler A, Krumbholz K, Lutkenhoner B. Sensitivity of the neuromagnetic N100m deflection to spectral bandwidth: a function of the auditory periphery? Audiology Neurootology. 2003;8:322–337. DOI: 10.1159/000073517.

[25] Zwicker E, Flottorp G, Stevens SS. Critical bandwidth in loudness summation. Journal of the Acoustical Society of America 1957;29:548–557. DOI: 10.1121/1.1908963.

[26] Sato S, Kitamura T, Ando Y. Loudness of sharply (2068 dB/Octave) filtered noises in relation to the factors extracted from the autocorrelation function. Journal of Sound and Vibration 2002;250:47–52. DOI: 10.1006/jsvi.2001.3888.

[27] Zhang C, Zeng FG. Loudness of dynamic stimuli in acoustic and electric hearing. Journal of the Acoustical Society of America 1997;102:2925–2934. DOI: 10.1121/1.420347.

[28] Moore BCJ, Vickers D, Baer T, Launer S. Factors affecting the loudness of modulated sounds. Journal of the Acoustical Society of America 1999;105:2757–2772. DOI: 10.1121/1.426893.

[29] Soeta Y, Nakagawa S. Effect of the repetitive components of a noise on loudness. Journal of Temporal Design in Architecture and the Environment. 2008;8:1–7.

[30] Levitt H. Transformed up–down procedures in psychophysics. Journal of the Acoustical Society of America 1971;49:467–477. DOI: 10.1121/1.1912375.

[31] Moore BCJ, Glasberg BR, Baer T. A model for the prediction of thresholds, loudness, and partial loudness. Journal of the Audio Engineering Society 1997;45:224–240.

[32] Zwicker E, Fastl H. Psychoacoustics. Facts and models. New York: Springer; 2010. 1999. DOI: 10.1007/978-3-662-09562-1.

[33] Fujii K, Soeta Y, Ando Y. Acoustical properties of aircraft noise measured by temporal and spatial factors. Journal of Sound and Vibration 2001;241:69–78. DOI: 10.1006/jsvi.2000.3278.

[34] Sakai H, Hotehama T, Prodi N, Pompoli R, Ando Y. Diagnostic system based on the human auditory-brain model for measuring environmental noise – an application to the railway noise. Journal of Sound and Vibration 2002;250:9–21. DOI: 10.1006/jsvi.2001.3884.

[35] Fujii K, Atagi J, Ando Y. Temporal and spatial factors of traffic noise and its annoyance. Journal of Temporal Design in Architecture and the Environment. 2002;2:33–41.

[36] Kitamura T, Shimokura R, Sato S, Ando Y. Measurement of temporal and spatial factors of a flushing toilet noise in a downstairs bedroom. Journal of Temporal Design in Architecture and the Environment. 2002;2:13–19.

[37] Berglund B, Berglund U, Lindvall T. Scaling loudness, noisiness, and annoyance of aircraft noise. Journal of the Acoustical Society of America 1975;57:930–934. DOI: 10.1121/1.380535.

[38] Hellman RP. Loudness, annoyance, and noisiness produced by single-tone-noise complexes. Journal of the Acoustical Society of America 1982;72:62–73. DOI: 10.1121/1.388025.

[39] Thurstone LL. A law of comparative judgment. Psychological Review 1927;34:273–289.

[40] Kryter KD, Pearsons KS. Judged noisiness of a band of random noise containing an audible pure tone. Journal of the Acoustical Society of America 1965;38:106–112. DOI: 10.1121/1.1909578.

[41] Hargest TJ, Pinker RA. The influence of added narrow band noises and tones on the subjective response to shaped white noise. Journal of the Royal Aeronautical Society. 1967;71:428–430. DOI: 10.1017/S0001924000055512.

Chapter 12

Cochlea – A Physiological Description of a Finely Structured Sense Organ

Raphael R. Ciuman

Additional information is available at the end of the chapter

http://dx.doi.org/10.5772/66316

Abstract

The whole inner ear or the cochlea, responsible for hearing perception, represents a unique sense organ, including the organ of Corti and the inner ear endo- and perilymph. The fluid homeostasis of the lymph spaces with its parameters volume, concentration, osmolarity and pressure, as well as the finely aligned hair cell receptors, their supporting cells and structures embedded in these unique fluid spaces, corresponds to the specific necessities for adequate response to continuous stimulation and the outstanding discrimination capacity of the hearing system. The manuscript gives an overview and describes the structural characteristics and distinct physiological hearing qualities of the cochlea in comparison with the other human receptor cells and sense organs.

Keywords: cochlea, organ of Corti, endolymph, stria vascularis, inner hair cells, outer hair cells, stereocilia, supporting cells, efferent innervation

1. Introduction

The whole inner ear or the cochlea, responsible for hearing perception, can be described as unique sense organ, including the organ of Corti and the inner ear endo- and perilymph. The fluid homeostasis of the lymph spaces with its parameters volume, concentration, osmolarity and pressure corresponds to the specific necessities for adequate response to continuous stimulation and the outstanding discrimination capacity of the hearing system. Discrimination of loudness is regulated mainly by discharge intensity of stimulus transmission, rhythm by discharge duration and discrimination of frequency and tone colour timbre by harmonized fine regulation of the geometrically and functionally aligned hearing structures along the cochlear duct. Surrounded by endolymph, the inner and outer hair cells with their distinct geometrically arranged finger-like processes, the stereocilia, are the mechanoelectrical transducers of the mechanoreceptor organ ear. The complex afferent and efferent innervation of the hair cells respond to further fine processing of the hearing stimulus. In this context, the efferent innervation supplies further qualities, in particular noise protection, mediation of selective attention and improvement of signal-to-noise ratio. It also supports adaptation and frequency selectivity by modification of the micromechanical properties of the outer hair cells. The past five decades of molecular biological research involved immense achievements in understanding of the physiological and biochemical mechanisms leading to current genetic-based, nanotechnology-based and stem cell research [1, 2].

2. Hearing system qualities

The human cochlea consists of about two and a half turns and is about 9 cm in length from the oval window to the helicotrema, corresponding to a frequency gradient starting with high frequencies at the base and proceeding to low frequencies at the apex.

The middle ear main function is to achieve mechanical gain by the ossicles as a lever and the tympanic membrane and oval window as a plane focuser. Besides, the middle ear makes the stimulus processable by harmonizing the sound wave resistance (impedance) of air and perilymph and the hair cells, respectively (**Figure 1**).

Adaptation mechanisms are characteristical for a sense organ, and as the cochlea has to process travelling waves continuously, it involves all molecular structures and biochemical processes of the inner ear. Adaptation lowers the system requirements, protects from overstimulation and reflects the environmental necessities of stimulus perception. In addition, it characterizes tone and music perception. Contrastingly, to the chemical receptors of the olfactory and gustatory system and the dermal mechano-, and thermoreceptors, sound adaptation does not lead to no stimulus perception at all. Generally speaking, the adaptation time constant is faster in hair cells at the high-frequency end than at the low-frequency end, what probably contributes to frequency selectivity [3].

Different adaptation mechanisms contribute to inner ear function, namely voltage-dependent hair-cell properties, structural hair-bundle characteristics and afferent transmitter release. Fast adaptation operates around the most sensitive portion of the hair cell activation, whereas larger displacements of the hair bundle induce slow adaptation [4]. Fast adaptation has been identified in both cochlear and vestibular hair cells, but is the main form of adaptation in cochlear hair cells. Slow adaptation has been identified in all but mammalian auditory hair cells, and is the predominant adaptation mechanism found in vestibular hair cells [5–7]. (Comparison of the adaptation mechanisms of the human sense organs and receptor cells is described at the end of the article in **Table 1**. Comparison of the perception qualities of the human sense organs and further comparison are listed in **Table 2**. Comparison of the structural characteristics of the human sense organs.)

http://dx.doi.org/10.5772/66316

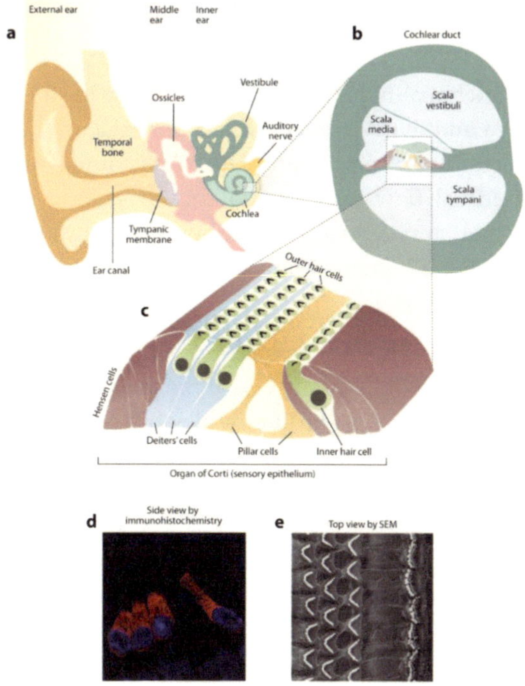

Figure 1. Schematic illustration of the human ear. (**a**) The ear consists of the outer, middle and inner ear. (**b**) A section through the cochlear duct illustrates the fluid-filled compartments of the inner ear. (**c**) The organ of Corti resides in the scala media, with sensory hair cells surrounded by supporting cells that include Deiters, Hensen and pillar cells. (**d**) Immunohistochemistry with the inner ear hair cell marker myosin VI, marking the cytoplasm of inner and outer hair cells, and 4,6-diamidino-2-phenylindole (DAPI), marking the nuclei. (**e**) Scanning electron microscopy image of the top view of the sensory epithelium reveals the precise arrangement of one row of inner hair cells and three rows of outer hair cells, separated by the pillar cells (with permission from Ref. [75]. Copyright © 2009, Annual Reviews. All rights reserved).

3. Supporting structures

3.1. Communication routes of the inner ear filled with endo- or perilymph

The cochlea consists of three scalae that contain endo- and perilymph. The scala media contain endolymph, where osmotic and ionic characteristics are close to the intracellular hair cell milieu (high potassium content, K^+ = 144 mval/l), and the scala tympani and vestibuli contain perilymph, which can be compared to cerebrospinal fluid (high sodium content, Na^+ = 140 mval/l). There exist three communication routes between the intracranial spaces and the inner ear, the vestibular aqueduct, the cochlear aqueduct and the internal auditory canal [8]. The vestibular aqueduct contains the endolymphatic duct that begins with the union of the utricular and saccular ducts and ends in a blind pouch, the endolymphatic sac, which is embedded between two dural blades, located in the epidural space and shows immunological competence. The cochlear aqueduct contains the perilymphatic or periotic duct and possesses communication with the subarachnoidal space (**Figure 2**).

The aqueducts provide functionality for continuous response to stimulation to both inner ear sense systems, the cochlea and the vestibular organs, maculae of the utricle and saccule and cupulae of the three semicircular canals, by pressure equilibrium, participate in inner ear fluid regulation, make longitudinal flow feasible and thus possess a key role in guaranteeing adequate response to stimulation. Pressure equilibrium is primarily the function of the cochlear aqueduct, whereas fluid circulation is dependent on an intact vestibular aqueduct, but various interactions exist.

The main drainage of the inner ear is maintained by two to four veins of the cochlear aqueduct, and to a lesser extent by one or more, usually two at the proximal termination-located vessels of the vestibular aqueduct [9–11]. The protein and ionic composition, the endolymphatic potential and resting potential of the hair cells show differences in the distinct parts of the endolymphatic fluid spaces. These gradients and the fluid circulation are essential for adequate response to stimulation. Procedures which expand the endolymphatic space induce endolymph flow towards the base of the cochlea, contributing to the removal of electrolytes and volume. Procedures which reduce cochlear endolymph volume lead to apically directed flow in the cochlea, contributing to the addition of electrolytes and volume [12].

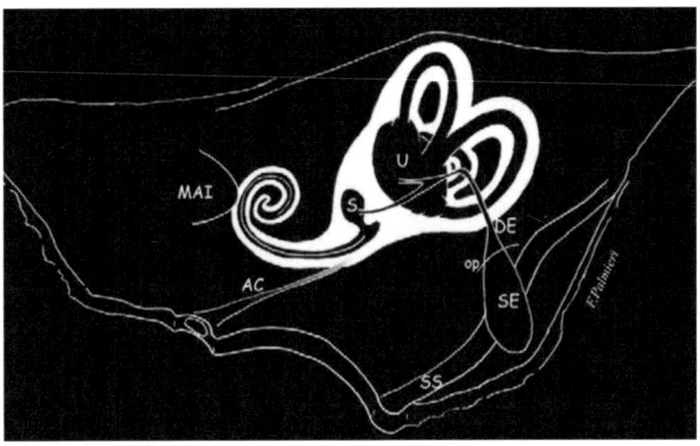

Figure 2. Schematic presentation of the labyrinth and aqueducts. AC: cochlear aqueduct; DE: endolymphatic duct; SE: endolymphatic sac; U: utricle; S: saccule; SS: sigmoid sinus; MAI: internal acoustic meatus. The white area represents the perilymphatic space; within it is the endolymphatic space in black. The endolymphatic duct is contained in the vestibular aqueduct; the perilymphatic or periotic duct is contained in the vestibular aqueduct; the endolymphatic sac protrudes from the vestibular aqueduct aperture protected by a bony operculum (op) and spreads out into the epidural space (with permission from Ref. [76]. Copyright © 2004, Springer-Verlag. All rights reserved).

3.2. Stria vascularis

The regulation of inner ear fluid homeostasis, with its parameters volume, concentration, osmolarity and pressure, is the basis for adequate response to stimulation [13]. The ion and water transport in the inner ear help maintain the proper potassium concentration required for hair cell function. Potassium is the major charge carrier for sensory transduction. It is ideal for this role, since it is by far the most abundant ion in the cytosol and responsible for the large endocochlear potential of 80 mV which is the driving force for mechanoelectrical transduction. Contrastingly, the endovestibular potential in the semicircular canals is ±1 mV [14].

The stria vascularis, located at the lateral wall of the cochlear duct, is the main structure responsible for endolymph secretion of the cochlea. It is connected to the spiral prominence, to Reissner's membrane and to the spiral ligament, which binds to the otic capsule. The stria vascularis represents one of the few epithelial types that contain capillaries. The stria vascularis has a higher oxygen consumption than brain tissue, and the strial capillaries are larger in diameter, with a higher haematocrit and a slower flow than the capillaries of any other tissue type [15]. The strial marginal cells show structural characteristics for fluid transport. They possess extensively infolded basolateral membranes with mitochondria providing the energy for active transport mechanisms, and microvilli located at the apical and basal sides increasing surface area. The stria vascularis consists of three cell layers: marginal cells, intermediate cells and basal cells. The intermediate cells, with their extensive, active transport mechanisms, are responsible for generating the endolymphatic potential. Consequently, the marginal cells possess a positive intracellular potential similar to that of the scala media [16].

A distinct pattern of tight and gap junctions, barrier and transport proteins maintains endolymph composition and generates endolymphatic potential, facilitating sensory transduction and reflecting fine regulation and a wide range of responses to stimulation. The transport proteins are regulated by purinergic, adrenergic and muscarinic receptors, steroids, vasopressin and atrial natriuretic peptide (ANP). There is evidence that the stress hormones noradrenaline and adrenaline, corticosteroids and mineralocorticosteroids possess a key role in inner ear homeostasis and sensory transduction. Besides, there exists a strongly expressed and largely non-overlapping distribution pattern for the different aquaporin (AQP) water channel subtypes in the inner ear, suggesting the existence of regional, subtype-specific water transport pathways [17–19]. The regulation of water transport in the inner ear probably requires concerted actions of multiple types of AQPs [20].

According to the tonotopy of the cochlea, potassium concentration and circulation are generally stronger at the cochlear base, and these gradients are maintained by extensive potassium recirculation cycles (**Figure 3**). In the auditory system, potassium circulation begins with the entrance of potassium into the sensory cells via the apical transduction channel. After entering the inner and outer hair cells, potassium recirculates mainly by a medial and a lateral pathway, and further smaller pathways through Reissner's membrane and the outer sulcus cells [21–23]. The medial pathway from the inner hair cells and the inner radial nerves involves inner sulcus cells, limbal fibrocytes and interdental cells. The lateral pathway from the outer hair cells consists of potassium delivery into the perilymph, absorption by the spiral ligament cells and entrance into the stria vascularis via strial intermediate cells [24, 25].

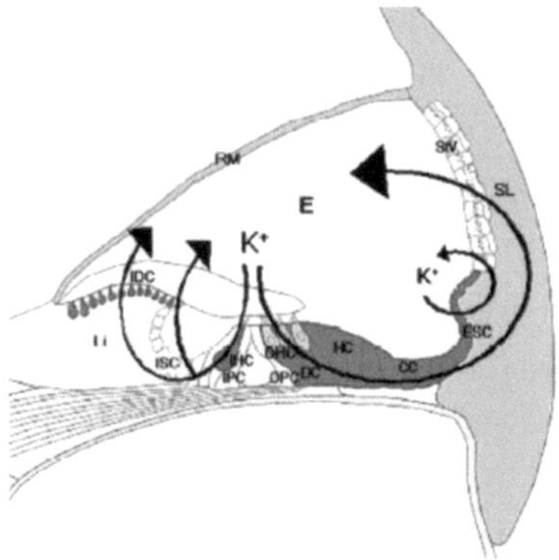

Figure 3. Schematic representation of a cochlear turn with the most significant recycling pathways of K^+ ions. Furthermore, it depicts the organ of Corti composed of sensory inner (IHC) and outer (OHC) hair cells and supporting cells. Inner pillar cells (IPC), outer pillar cells (OPC), Deiters cells (DC), Hensen cells (HC), Claudius cells (CC), external or outer sulcus cells (ESC), internal or inner sulcus cells (ISC), spiral limbus (Li), interdental cells (IDC), Reissner's membrane (RM) and stria vascularis (StV) adjacent to the fibrous spiral ligament (SL) (with permission from Professor G. van Camp, University of Antwerp, Belgium modified by Ref. [77]. Copyright © 2004, Springer-Verlag. All rights reserved).

3.3. Supporting cells

The organ of Corti encloses the outer hair cells and the inner hair cells, which are stabilized by inner sulcus and inner and outer pillar cells. The outer hair cells are placed on top of one Deiters cell each. Besides, the organ of Corti encloses two small endolymph spaces, the Nuel space and the outer tunnel, and one perilymph space, the inner tunnel. The inner sulcus cells and the interdental cells terminate the organ of Corti into the spiral limbus and the tectorial membrane. The outer sulcus cells connect to the stria vascularis and spiral ligament (**Figure 3**).

The secretory stria vascularis, the vestibular dark cells and endolymphatic sac and the non-secretory vestibular transitional cells, the Reissner's membrane, the sulcus cells, the spiral limbus cells, the Deiters cells and the lateral or outer supporting cells (Hensen and Claudius cells) are responsible for fine regulation of inner ear fluids including the maintenance of ion and osmolarity gradients and potassium recirculation. The lateral or outer supporting cells are located between the outer hair cells and outer sulcus cells. The necessity for precise fine regulation of the endolymph is underlined by the fact that basally to the Hensen cells, Boettcher cells and medioapically to the Hensen cells cover or tectal cells were distinguished [26].

4. Inner and outer hair cells – the mechanoelectrical transducers

4.1. Stereocilia

The stereocilia of the inner ear hair cells are microvilli-derived and unique cell structures that represent the gate for stimulus detection and correlate anatomically with distinct cochlear functions, including mechanoelectrical transduction, cochlear amplification, adaptation, frequency selectivity and tuning [27]. The stereocilia have a typical staircase arrangement connected with lateral and tip links stabilizing the mature hair-bundle structure. The number of stereocilia on each hair cell decreases in a linear fashion with distance from the base of the cochlea. However, stereociliary length increases as a hyperbolic function of distance along the cochlear duct [28]. Contrastingly, in the vestibular organs one kinocilium is bound to the tallest of 50–80 stereocilia, arranged in a distinct geometrical alignment [29]. Differences in ciliary gradation also exist between the three rows of stereocilia on outer hair cells and the two rows on inner hair cells, with the tallest row positioned laterally [30]. The longest stereocilia layer left imprints on the undersurface of the tectorial membrane at the region known as Hardesty's or Kimura's membrane [31]. The stereocilia of the inner hair cells do not have the same firm attachment to the tectorial membrane as the stereocilia of the outer hair cells suggesting different modes of mechanical coupling between the tectorial membrane and the inner and outer hair cell stereocilia [30].

The term stereocilia does not reflect their origin, as these microvilli-derived structures should be clearly distinguished from microtubule-based, true cilia. Stereocilia are constructed of cross-linked actin filaments in a parallel, paracrystalline array, giving stereocilia their stiffness, are rich in fimbrin and their stereociliary rootlets contain actin and tropomyosin [32]. The actin filaments insert with an electron-dense rootlet into a fibrous-anchoring structure, the cuticular plate. The cuticular plate is a network of actin filaments, which also contain myosin, α-actinin, fimbrin, tropomyosin, fodrin and calcium-binding proteins [33, 34].

When sound is induced, fluids move through the cochlear duct and vibrate the basilar membrane with the sensory hair cells against the tectorial membrane, which leads to deflection of the stereocilia and activation of the mechanoelectrical transduction channels gated by the tip links. They are extracellular, cell surface associated, fine filaments, gating the mechano-transducer channel by deflecting the hair cell bundle towards the taller row, depolarizing the hair cells and enabling potassium influx. A deflection in the opposite direction leads to hyperpolarization [35].

The stereocilia, together with the structures of the hair cell body, probably contribute actively and/or passively to cochlear amplification. They also influence the amplification properties of the outer hair cell body enabled by bending leading to a membrane potential change in outer hair cells and causing length changes [36]. These length changes feed force back to the basilar membrane on a cycle-by-cycle basis and so tune its otherwise shallow vibrations to the characteristic frequency [37]. At low frequencies, the stereociliary sensitivity is proportional to the cube of the heights of their hair bundles, whereas at high frequencies the sensitivity is proportional to the inverse of their heights [38]. Frequency and stiffness are proportional to each other [39] correlating with the height of the stereocilia [40]. The cochlear amplifier gain is the difference between the peaks in the sensitivity functions for low- and high-intensity tones [41].

4.2. Inner hair cells

The tip links of the stereocilia of the inner hair cells are the location for the mechanoelectrical transduction of the cochlea, long searched for. There exist about 3500 inner hair cells that are grouped in one row, in contrast to about 12000 outer hair cells that are grouped in three rows. 90–95 % of all innervation supplies the inner hair cells and each inner hair cell has contact with about fifteen to twenty neurons, of which about 90 % are afferent neurons [42, 43].

Inner hair cells show a characteristic 'flask' shape, displaying a constriction in the neck region. Relative to the surface of the organ of Corti, the cell body is angled towards the centre of the cochlear spiral (the modiolus) and away from the supporting pillar cell. The apical half of the cell contains the nucleus, and the infranuclear region shows an extensive and seemingly continuous network of intracellular endoplasmic reticulum membranes, associated with mitochondria and cytoplasmic vesicles. The afferent nerve endings form characteristical ribbon synapses around the entire baso-lateral region below the level of the nucleus [42]. Ribbon synapses are specialized for the precision and speed required to process auditory information and show tonotopical variation in function and form along the cochlear duct [44].

The inner hair cells are embedded for stabilization between inner sulcus cells and inner pillar cells, which shape the stiffness and elastic reactance of the travelling wave-processing structures [45]. Already, the basilar membrane and the inner and outer hair cells with their receptor potentials show tuning characteristics similar to the characteristical tuning of the cochlear afferent neurons [46].

4.3. Outer hair cells

The inner ear is not just a mechanoreceptor, but is capable to an active processing by the outer hair cells. The active component can be up to more than 100 times larger than the classical basilar membrane vibration. The outer hair cells enhance and focus the amplitude of the travelling wave by its contractions at sound pressure levels up to 60 dB (cochlear amplification) [47]. But the outer hair cells with their W-pattern-aligned stereocilia are not just a cochlear amplifier; they are three-dimensionally regulators for bone conduction and the natural exposition to bone vibrations.

To process the sound waves three-dimensionally, the outer hair cells are positioned on Deiters cells. Corresponding to the necessity for continous fast and active response to stimulation, they are surrounded by two endolymph spaces, the outer tunnel and the Nuel space.

The outer hair cells with their micromechanical properties enhance frequency selectivity and the tone intensity range. Stimulus protection, distance adjustment and sharpness enhancement in the eye are executed by the micromechanical light accommodation of the lens and the pupils and the biochemical and electrophysiological light accommodation by variation of the amount of photopigment and the open probability of transduction channels by the photoreceptors.

Hyperpolarization mediated by specific $GABA_A$ receptors (gamma aminobutyric acid A) causes expansion of prestin molecules, which elongates the outer hair cell [48]. Stimulation of ACh receptors (acetylcholine) leads to opposite outer hair cell changes [49]. Those outer hair cell changes can be measured as otoacoustic emissions (OAEs, spontaneous and evoked).

Contrastingly to the innervation of inner hair cells, the afferent nerve-receptor cell ratio is with about 1:10 negative [43, 50].

5. Afferent and efferent innervation

5.1. Afferent innervation

90–95 % of innervation to the hair cells is afferent, and 90-95 % are bipolar afferent type I neurons, which are organized in the spiral ganglion and form single ribbon synapses under inner hair cells. These specific synapses are found in retinal photoreceptors and bipolar neurons. Outer hair cells are innervated by type II afferent neurons, which are ribbonless and only excited with maximal synaptic stimulation, suggesting to be part of the sensory drive for the medial olivocochlear reflex protecting from acoustic overstimulation [51]. But the majority of outer hair cell innervation is efferent and about 90% of all efferent innervation terminates on outer hair cells [43, 52].

The first neurons of all parts of the vestibulocochlear nerve are truely bipolar, formed to the spiral ganglion in the bony modiolus, and leave the vestibule through the lamina cribrosa, which is a thin bony plate that is penetrated by the neural structures and blood vessels originating in most cases from the anterior inferior cerebellar artery. The lamina cribrosa is medially covered by dura mater and arachnoidea and forms a barrier between the inner ear and the subarachnoid space.

The excitatory afferent transmission of the auditory system is regulated by various types of glutamate receptors, ionotropic glutamate receptors of the N-methyl-D-aspartic acid (NMDA) and α-amino-3-hydroxy-5-methyl-4-isoxazolepropionic acid (AMPA) type as well as group I and II metabotropic glutamate receptors, and inhibitorily efferent modulated by GABA and dopamine [53].

Complex neural processing between afferent and efferent fibres is found in the spiral ganglion and the ventral cochlear nucleus (VCN) [54]. Not just tonotopical place coding but also periodical time coding make the signal robust, relevant for complex sounds when afferent excitation is saturated [55–57].

5.2. Efferent innervation

The efferent system of the cochlea provides stimulus protection and fine regulation, in particular noise protection, mediation of selective attention and improvement of signal-to-noise ratio, by innervating the same structures that are responsible for stimulus perception, the inner and outer hair cells. The efferent system also supports adaptation and frequency selectivity by modification of the micromechanical properties of outer hair cells. The efferent system as well as the entire human auditory system is susceptible to strengthening by training and it could be shown that efferent suppression is stronger in musicians [58].

The multipolar lateral efferent neurons originate from the lateral superior olive (LSO) and the multipolar medial efferent system from the periolivary region (medial, ventral and anterior) around the medial superior olivary (MSO) complex and the trapezoid body [59] (**Figure 4**). In human, there is no nucleus trapezoid body and the lateral efferent component is relatively small compared with other species [60–62]. By contrast, the medial superior olivary nucleus reflects a steady increase in primates corresponding to the capability of low-frequency hearing [63].

The well-developed human medial olivary nucleus seems to be the basis for extraction of interaural time and phase differences, whereas the smaller human lateral olivary nucleus probably functions in the analysis of interaural differences in frequency and intensity. The lateral and medial nuclei together form the basis for localization of a sound stimulus and enable us to function in a three-dimensional auditory world [64, 65].

The myelinated medial fibres, which innervate outer hair cells, project ipsi- and contralateral and the unmyelinated lateral fibres, which innervate the dendrites of afferent nerve fibres, project mainly ipsilateral [66]. There exists distinct but complex geometrical and functional alignment of the efferent fibres, their connections and neurotransmitters [67].

Neurotransmission of the efferent system takes place by inhibitory and excitatory transmitters reflecting fine regulation. The numerous neurotransmitters provide for the auditory system a wide operating range to enhance or depress environmental stimuli and can be co-localized as well. The neurotransmitter of the medial olivocochlear fibres includes ACh (acetylcholine), GABA (gamma aminobutyric acid), CGRP (calcitonin gene-related peptide), ATP (adenosine triphosphate), enkephalins and NO (nitric oxide) [68, 69]. The transmitter of the lateral efferent system includes ACh, GABA, CGRP, dopamine, serotonin and opioids such as dynorphin or enkephalin [70–72].

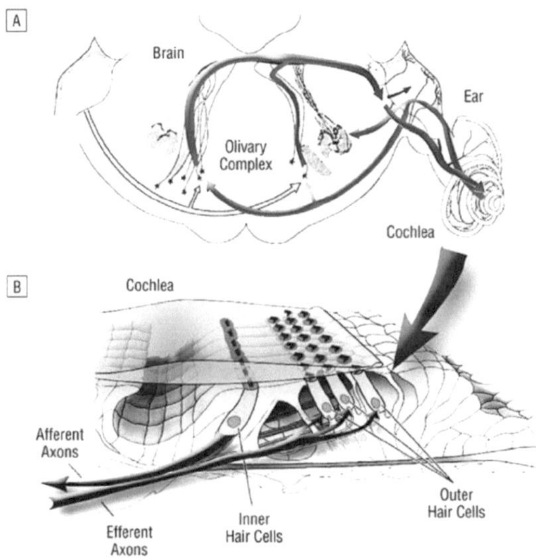

Figure 4. Course of the medial and lateral efferent systems. (**A**) The auditory brainstem section. Sound representations from the ear ascend to the olivary complex via the ventral afferent pathway and project back to the ear via dorsal crossed and uncrossed medial and lateral efferent fibres. (**B**) Cross-sectional view of the inner ear. The major ascending afferent pathway arises from inner hair cells. Descending olivocochlear projections terminate on inner and outer hair cells (with permission from Ref. [78], © 1990, Elsevier; and Ref. [79], Copyright © 2004 American Medical Association. All rights reserved).

6. Conclusion

The cochlea is a unique sense organ with regard to its qualities in continuous stimulus perception and stimulus discrimination capacity. This corresponds to the finely aligned hair cell receptors, their surrounding supporting cells and structures embedded in unique fluid spaces, and to further afferent and efferent neural processing.

	Cochlea
Perception characteristics	- continuous response to stimulation due to extensive homeostasis of the inner ear lymph spaces with a driving force of endocochlear potential of about 80 mV; - tonotopical place coding of the basilar membrane, the hair cells and the cochlear nerve (additional periodical time coding); - ossicles (lever), tympanic membrane and oval window (plane focuser) enhance the sound pressure (22–25 *x*) and together with the lymph spaces accommodate the impedance between air and receptor cells before sound stimulus perception of the mechanoreceptoric hair cells; - stimulus localization is made possible by the outer ear and bone conduction by interaural time/phase and intensity differences of both ears with up to 3° and 1 dB, respectively; - outer hair cells are the counterparts of a unique active sense organ that are not just cochlear amplifier, but three-dimensionally regulators for bone conduction and the natural exposition to bone vibrations; - predominantly fast adaptation;
Perception range	- 18 Hz to 20 kHz (acoustical fovea is 200–4000 Hz); - at 1000-Hz sound pressure levels (SPL) between 2×10^{-5} Pa = 0 dB (hearing level/HL) and 2×10^{2} Pa = 140 dB (pain threshold);
Discrimination capacity	**- frequency, colour timbre** with characteristical tuning and most sensitive areas for high-frequency sound at the cochlear base and for low-frequency sound at the cochlear apex; **loudness** by intensity (number of discharges of the hair cells and afferent nerves), **rhythm** by discharge duration of the hair cells;
Further qualities	- noise protection, mediation of selective attention and improvement of signal-to-noise ratio by efferent innervation;
	Vestibular organ
Perception characteristics	- secondary sense organ as adequate stimulation has to be centrally processed with optical or proprioceptic inputs (exception gravitation as kind of linear acceleration); - continuous response to stimulation due to extensive homeostasis of the inner ear lymph spaces with an endovestibular potential of ±1 mV; - stimulation of the vestibular organs of one site leads to contralateral inhibition with central processing; - cupula organ and endolymph have the same specific gravity; - predominantly slow adaptation in human (cupula organ needs 10–30 s to get back in resting position);
Perception range	- cut-off frequency of the semicircular canals circa 0.03 Hz for the yaw rotation [73]; yaw rotation detection threshold about 1.45 ± 0.81 °/s (3.49 ± 1.95 °/s^2) and absolute nasooccipital translation detection threshold about 2.93 ± 2.10 cm/s (7.07 ± 5.05 cm/s^2) [74];
Discrimination capacity	- perception of **linear acceleration** by macula organs in the saccule and utricule; perception of **angular acceleration** by cupula organs in the semicircular canals; **spatial resolution** by position of the semicircular canals, the saccule and utricle and the position and alignment of their hair cells, stereocilia and kinocilium;
Further qualities	- unique response to inadequate caloric stimulation, which is used for investigations;
	Optical system
Perception characteristics	- cornea, lens and vitreous body refract and accommodate the light waves before stimulus perception of the receptor cells;

	- single sense organ where receptor potential is hyperpolarization; - dark adaptation of the fovea centralis in 5–10 min, extrafoveal 45–100 min; - adaptation to darkness by the iris with its muscles sphincter and dilator pupillae, increased photopigment and spatial and time summation in the afferent nerves; in darkness the photoreceptors increase light sensitivity by increased opening of Na^+ channels;
Perception range	- 400–700 nm (highest absorption maximum for blue, 440 nm; green, 540 nm; red, 570 nm); detection threshold 1–2 nm; - flickering until 65–80 pictures/s; in darkness 20–25 pictures/s;
Discrimination capacity	- **sharpest vision** at a small area of the macula lutea, the fovea centralis, which contains only cone cells that are longer than in the periphery; sharpest vision decrease to the periphery of the retina; - **colour vision** by cone cells which decrease to the periphery of the retina and have either one of three different photopigments; neuronal processing of opposite colours already starts in the retina (colour vision and opponent colour vision theory); - **black and white vision (night vision)** by rod cells that are more light sensitive than cone cells; - **light accommodation** by different light sensitivity of the cone and rod cells and excitation of on-center (light-on) and off-center (light-off) neurons; - **contrast enhancement** by lateral inhibition (horizontal processing) of neuronal horizontal cells in the retina, but already the first step of central processing of **form and motion**;
Further qualities	- convergence reflex of the eye bulbi due to the bilateral pupil reflex and the external eye muscles; - light accommodation by the lens and the pupils for protection, sharpness, distance adjustment (comparable to the function of outer hair cells and the stapedius reflex);
	Olfactory system
Perception characteristics	- chemical receptors are slower in their time characteristics than mechano- and photoreceptors; - chemical stimulus pre-processing by dilution in the mucoepithelial film; - smell is perceived by form and size of the molecules that bind to the cell membrane (key-lock principle); - adaptation leads to no stimulus perception at all;
Perception range	- absolute threshold of about 10^7 molecules/ml; - only soluble molecules (e.g. dental metal alloy cannot be perceived) and specific molecules (key-lock principle) can be perceived; consequently absolute and relative perception thresholds are dependent on humidity and temperature;
Discrimination capacity	- perception of a few thousand smell qualities; for testing 20 standard qualities;
Further qualities	- no perceived smells can have a behavioural impact (pheromones); - trigeminal nerve for thermal and pain perception and a, hot, burning, astringent, tingling or cooling sense perception; - continuous neurogenesis of the primary sensory neurons in mammals;
	Gustatory system
Perception characteristics	- chemical receptors are slower in their time characteristics than mechano- and photoreceptors; - chemical stimulus pre-processing by dilution in seromucous saliva; - taste is perceived by form and size of the molecules that bind to the cell membrane (key-lock principle); - adaptation leads to no stimulus perception at all;
Perception range	- absolute threshold of about 10^{16} molecules/ml; - only soluble molecules (e.g. dental alloy cannot be perceived) and specific molecules (key-lock principle) can be perceived; consequently absolute and relative perception thresholds are dependent on humidity and temperature;
Discrimination capacity	- **bitter, sour, salt, sweet** with areas of highest sensitivity on the tongue; many various biochemical molecules can simulate one of these four qualities;

http://dx.doi.org/10.5772/66316

Further qualities	- trigeminal nerve for thermal and pain perception and a, hot, burning, astringent, tingling or cooling sense perception;
	Dermal receptors
Perception characteristics	- mechanoreceptors: pressure receptors are basically intensity receptors (proportional receptors), touch receptors are basically speed receptors (differential receptors) and vibration receptors are basically acceleration receptors (differential receptors), temperature receptors are proportional-differential receptors (PD receptors); - adaptation for touch leads to no stimulus perception at all; - adaptation is faster for vibration than touch and is slowest or not at all for pressure receptors; temperature receptors with few and pain receptors with no adaptation at all; - perception transmission fastest in Pacinian corpuscles (richly myelinated afferent axons) and slowest in temperature and pain receptors (poorly myelinated or unmyelinated afferent axons);
Perception range	- 40–1000 Hz for vibration (Pacinian corpuscles);
Discrimination capacity	- perception of **pain is a non-specific sensation** and can be triggered by pressure, temperature, chemicals; - **temperature/warm receptors** (40–47°C) can be triggered non-specifically by, for example, pepper; - **temperature/cold receptors** (17–36°C) can be triggered non-specifically by, for example, menthol; - **tactile sensation/pressure** by Merkel cells and Ruffini corpuscles; - **tactile sensation/touch** by Meissner tactile corpuscles and free nerve endings at hair follicles; - **tactile sensation/vibration** by Pacinian corpuscles; - **spatial resolution** by density of receptors and afferent nerves, smallest sensoric areas in tongue, lips, fingers and hands with highest number of receptor cells and amount of afferent innervation;
Further qualities	- gustatory papillae regenerate after destruction and reinnervation;

Table 1. Comparison of the perception qualities of the human sense organs.

	Cochlea
Receptor cells	- about 3500 inner and 12000 outer hair cells; - inner hair cells are the mechanoreceptors; active elongation of outer hair cells enhances the sound stimulus at sound pressure levels up to 60 dB (cochlear amplification); - inner hair cell stereocilia show linear alignment and outer hair cell stereocilia show a W-pattern; tip links of the stereocilia are the location of mechanoelectrical transduction;
Supporting structures	- supporting cells for stabilization of the inner hair cells (inner sulcus and inner and outer pillar cells) and outer hair cells (Deiters cells), which shapes the stiffness and elastic reactance of the travelling wave-processing structures; - the supporting cells of the cochlea participate in endolymph production, its fine regulation of ion and osmolarity gradients and potassium recirculation; - the stria vascularis is the main structure responsible for endolymph secretion of the cochlea; - the vestibular and cochlear aqueduct provide functionality to the cochlea and the vestibular organs by pressure equilibrium, participate in inner ear fluid regulation, make longitudinal flow feasible; pressure equilibrium may be primarily attributed to the cochlear aqueduct, whereas fluid circulation is dependent on the vestibular aqueduct;
Afferent innervation	- 90–95% of the neurons of the cochlear nerve are afferent and of them 90–95% supply inner hair cells, and only 5–10% outer hair cells; - inner and outer hair cells with bipolar afferent neurons; - Type I myelinated afferent neurons supply inner hair cells; type II myelinated afferent neurons constitute the sensory drive for the medial olivocochlear (MOC) efferent reflex on outer hair cells;

Efferent innervation	- 5–10 % of the neurons of the cochlear nerve are efferent, which predominantly terminate on outer hair cells; - medial efferent neurons that project ipsi- and contralateral and terminate directly under outer hair cells are myelinated; lateral efferent neurons that project mainly ipsilateral and innervate the dendrites of radial afferent fibres under inner hair cells are unmyelinated; - efferent innervation for noise protection, mediation of selective attention and improvement of signal-to-noise ratio; - it also supports adaptation and frequency selectivity by modification of the micromechanical properties of the outer hair cells;
	Vestibular organ
Receptor cells	- on the hair cells 50–80 stereocilia are aligned to one kinocilium; movement of the stereocilia to the kinocilium leads to neural depolarization; movement of the stereocilia into the opposite direction leads to neural hyperpolarization; - two types of hair cells with different innervation characteristics; the wider and taller type I vestibular cells possess more, taller and thicker stereocilia and a thicker cuticular plate compared with type II cells;
Supporting structures	- vestibular endolymph production and fine regulation of ion and osmolarity gradients by secretory dark cells, potassium recirculation by non-secretory transitional cells, calcium homeostasis by melanocytes; - the vestibular and cochlear aqueduct provide functionality to the cochlea and the vestibular organs by pressure equilibrium, participate in inner ear fluid regulation, make longitudinal flow feasible; pressure equilibrium is primarily the function of the cochlear aqueduct, whereas fluid circulation is dependent on the vestibular aqueduct;
Afferent innervation	- receptor cell-afferent nerve ratio of 3:1 in the cupula organs and 5:1 in the macula organs; - bipolar afferent neurons that may end as a button, dimorphic or as a cup; - excitatory glutamatergic afferent transmission;
Efferent innervation	- 5–10% are efferent neurons; - efferent nerve with direct contact to type II hair cells, but indirect contact upon afferent neuron dendrites to type I cells;
	Optical system
Receptor cells	- about 120 million rod cells and six million cone cells; - receptor cells are unipolar neurons (primary sensory cells); no elongation of receptor cells in mammals proven; - photoreceptors are characterized as well as inner hair cells by ribbon synapses with excitatory glutamatergic transmission;
Supporting structures	- supporting cells of the retina for stabilization due to localization of the first three neurons of afferent innervation within the retina; - melanin-containing cells of the stratum pigmentosum retinae increase sharpness by absorbing scattered light and extend with high light intensity deep into the photoreceptor layer;
Afferent innervation	- photoreceptor cells represent the first neuron; the second and third neurons are located in the retina as well; - one million afferent nerves with decreasing sensitivity to the periphery; photoreceptor cells in the central fovea connect to one single neuron; in the periphery up to 500 photoreceptors converge to one neuron; - the macula possesses a separate afferent nerve bundle;
Efferent innervation	- efferent innervation for light adaptation, light reflex and lateral inhibition;
	Olfactory system
Receptor cells	- receptor cells are bipolar neurons (primary sensory cells); - about 10^7 receptor cells; - 5–20 kinocilia per receptor cell;
Supporting structures	- supporting cells for stabilization, basal cells for regeneration; - Bowman glands for mucous secretion;
Afferent innervation	- the mitral cells (second afferent neuron) has contact with about 1000 primary afferent neurons (receptor cells);

Efferent innervation	- in the bulbus olfactorius, where the fila olfactoria terminate as primary afferent neurons is complex efferent inhibition localized as adaptation leads to no stimulus perception at all; the dendrites of the mitral cells can be specifically inhibited by two cell types, the periglomerular cells and granule cell interneurons (partial inhibition), which are innervated by efferent neurons;
	Gustatory system
Receptor cells	- taste perception by vallate, fungiform and foliate papillae; filiform papillae have no sensoric qualities; single gustatory papillae can be found at the soft palate, the hypopharynx and the epiglottis as well; - the gustatory papillae are formed of about 20 receptor cells;
Supporting structures	- supporting cells for stabilization; - salivatory glands for seromucous saliva production;
Afferent innervation	- about 50 afferent nerves per gustatory papilla; - facial nerve (chorda tympani) supplies the first two-thirds of the tongue; glossopharyngeal nerve (mainly bitter perception) supplies the last tongue third;
Efferent innervation	- taste adaptation after physiological food and saliva cleaning in about 5 s; efferent control dependent on concentration (salty food with longer aftertaste) and food aversion (unphysiological food such as pure vinegar with longer aftertaste); (own experiments)
	Dermal receptors
Receptor cells	- enclosed corpuscles and not enclosed free nerve endings (alone or at hair follicles); - Merkel cells are located in the corium; Ruffini corpuscles are located in the corium and the subcutis; Meissner tactile corpuscles are located in the dermal papillae; Pacinian corpuscles are located in the subcutis; free nerve endings alone or at hair follicles are located up to the highest corium layers; cold receptors are located higher in the corium than warm receptors;
Supporting structures	- Merkel cells are modified epithelial cells which are covered on the apical side by a touch meniscus representing the terminal swelling of a nerve fibre; - Meissner corpuscles are ovally formed structures built by lamellarly in layers arranged cells and surrounded by a capsula; one or more nerve fibres enter this structure and its terminating swellings are the receptoric parts; - Pacinian corpuscles are ovally formed lamellarly in layers arranged organs surrounded by a capsula, which is entered by a nerve fibre; the unmyelinated termination of the nerve fibre is the receptoric part;
Afferent innervation	- one to seven afferent nerves insert at the enclosed dermal receptors; - non-specific pain sensation and the receptoric free nerve endings with highest number of discovered different transmitters and neuropeptides (glutamate, aspartate, CGRP-calcitonin gene-related peptide, Substance P, Neurokinin A, Somatostatin, VIP-vasoactive intestinal peptide);
Efferent innervation	- indifference temperature between 31 and 36°C with few activated cold and warm receptors and efferent overweight; temperatures beneath 20°C and above 40°C lead to receptor activation and afferent overweight;

Table 2. Comparison of the structural characteristics of the human sense organs.

Cochlea Glossary

afferent innervation	*innervation that projects centrally from the effector/sense organ to the brain*
basilar membrane	*structure beneath the Corti organ consisting of the basilar lamina and a supporting fibral tissue layer*
cochlear aqueduct	*bony canal of the perilymphatic duct*
Corti organ	*all cells, tissue structures and their enclosed lymph spaces that participate in mechanoelectrical transduction, namely hair cells, supporting cells, basilar membrane, tectorial membrane, inner tunnel, outer tunnel and Nuel space*

cribrose lamina	*thin bony plate that forms the barrier between the vestibule of the inner ear and the internal auditory canal and is pierced by neurons of the cochlear nerve and blood vessels*
efferent innervation	*innervation that projects peripherally from the brain to the effector/sense organ*
endolymph	*lymph fluid in its composition close to the intracellular hair cell milieu that fills the medial scale and the outer tunnel and Nuel space in the Corti organ*
endolymphatic duct	*endolymph space that originates from the utriculosaccular duct and provides fluid circulation to the endolymphatic sac*
endolymphatic sac	*blind pouch of the endolymphatic duct with immune competence participating in the endolymph homeostasis*
helicotrema	*cochlear peak with confluence of tympanic scale and vestibulic scale*
inner hair cell	*receptor cell of the cochlea responsible for mechanoelectrical transduction*
inner tunnel	*perilymph space within the Corti organ between inner and outer pillar cells*
medial scale	*endolymph space containing the Corti organ*
modiolus	*bony spiral backbone of the cochlea*
Nuel space	*perilymph space within the Corti organ between outer pillar cells and outer hair cells*
olivocochlear bundle	*efferent innervation of the cochlea within a medial and lateral bundle can be distinguished*
outer hair cell	*receptor cell of the cochlea responsible for amplification and three-dimensionally focusing of basilar membrane vibration*
oval window	*membrane between the vestibule and the stapes*
outer tunnel	*endolymph space within the Corti organ between outer hair cells and lateral supporting cells*
perilymph	*lymph fluid in its composition close to cerebrospinal fluid that fills the tympanic scale and vestibulic scale and the inner tunnel in the Corti organ*
perilymphatic duct	*or periotic duct that originates from a pouchlike extension of the round window, containing a mesh of arachnoid-like tissue, providing communication with the subarachnoidal space and mainly pressure equilibrium to the inner ear*
reunion duct	*canal that connects the cochlear duct with the saccule*
Reissner's membrane	*cell barrier membrane between the medial scale and the vestibulic scale connected to the spiral ligament laterally and the spiral limbus medially canal that connects the cochlear duct with the saccule*
round window	*barrier membrane between the tympanic scale and the middle ear*
saccule	*vestibular endolymph space that contains one of the two macula organs and is origin of the saccular duct that combines with the utricular duct to the utriculosaccular duct, which itself is origin of the endolymphatic duct*
spiral ligament	*fibral tissue at the lateral wall of the medial scale connecting the vascular stria to the otic capsule*
spiral limbus	*fibral tissue at the medial wall of the medial scale connecting to the tectorial membrane by interdental cells and to the inner sulcus cells by forming the inner sulcus*
spiral ganglion	*first ganglion of the truely bipolar cochlear neurons located in the bony modiolus*

spiral prominence	*ledge of the lateral wall of the medial scale located at the connection between outer sulcus cells and vascular stria*
stereocilia	*microvilli derived finger-like processes of the hair cells connected by various links and location of the mechanoelectrical transduction channels within the tip links*
supporting cells	*cells within the medial scale that are located on the basilar membrane and responsible for hair cell stabilization and inner ear fluid homeostasis, comprising from medially to laterally inner sulcus cells, inner and outer pillar cells, Deiters cells, and the lateral supporting cells, namely Claudius cells, Hensen cells, Boettcher cells, tectal or cover cells and outer sulcus cells*
tectorial membrane	*structure of fibral tissue loosely covering the stereocilia of the hair cells*
tympanic scale	*perilymph space between the helicotrema and the round window*
utricle	*vestibular endolymph space that contains one of the two macula organs and is origin of the utricular duct that combines with the saccular duct to the utriculosaccular duct, which itself is origin of the endolymphatic duct*
vascular stria	*epithelial layer of the lateral wall of the medial scale between Reissner's membrane and spiral prominence covering the spiral ligament*
vestibular aqueduct	*bony canal of the endolymphatic duct*
vestibulic scale	*perilymph space between the vestibule and the helicotrema*
vestibule	*extension of the vestibulic scale between oval window and the saccule*

Author details

Raphael R. Ciuman

Address all correspondence to: ciuman.raphael@cityweb.de

Otorhinolaryngology, Natural Medicine Science, Pharmaceutical Medicine, Uranusbogen, Mülheim an der Ruhr, Germany

References

[1] Ciuman RR. Inner ear symptoms and disease: Pathophysiological understanding and therapeutic options. Med Sci Monit. 2013; 19:1195–1210. e-ISSN: 1643-3750

[2] Ciuman RR. Morbus Menière: Were the last 50 years of molecular biological research fruitless for Menière's Disease? World J Otorhinolaryngol. 2015; 5:90–92. e-ISSN: 2218-6247

[3] Ricci, AJ, Wu YC, Fettiplace R. The endogenous calcium buffer and the time course of transducer adaptation in auditory hair cells. J Neurosci. 1998; 18:8261–8277. ISSN: 0270-6474

[4] Ricci AJ, Crawford AC, Fettiplace R. Mechanisms of active hair bundle motion in auditory hair cells. J Neurosci. 2002; 22:44–52. ISSN: 0270-6474

[5] Geleoc GS, Lennan GW, Richardson GP, Kros CJ. A quantitative comparison of mechanoelectrical transduction in vestibular and auditory hair cells in neonatal mice. Proc Biol Sci. 1997; 261:611–621. ISSN: 0950-1193

[6] Kros CJ, Lennan GWT, Richardson GP. Transducer currents and bundle movements in outer hair cells of neonatal mice. In: Flock A, Ottoson D, Ulfendahl M, editors. Active Hearing. Oxford: Elsevier; 1995. pp. 113–125. ISBN: 978-0-080425-14-6

[7] Holt JR, Gillespie SK, Provance DW, Shah K, Shokat KM, Corey DP, Mercer JA, Gillespie PG. A chemical-genetic strategy implicates myosin-1c in adaptation by hair cells. Cell. 2002; 108:371–381. ISSN: 0092-8674

[8] Ciuman RR. Communication routes between intracranial spaces and inner ear: function, pathophysiologic importance and relations with inner ear diseases. Am J Otolaryngol. 2009; 30:193–202. ISSN: 0196-0709

[9] Mazzoni A. The venous drainage of the vestibular labyrinth in man. Ann Otolaryngol Chir Cervicofac. 1979; 96:211–214. ISSN: 003-438X

[10] Mazzoni A. Vein of the vestibular aqueduct. Ann Otol Rhinol Laryngol. 1979; 88:759–767. ISSN: 0003-4894

[11] Watanabe Y, Nakashima T, Yanagita N. The influence of acute venous congestion on the guinea pig cochlea. Eur Arch Otorhinolaryngol. 1990; 247:161–164. ISSN: 0937-4477

[12] Salt AN. Regulation of endolymphatic fluid volume. Ann NY Acad Sci. 2001; 942:306–312. ISSN: 0077-8923

[13] Ciuman RR. Stria vascularis and vestibular dark cells: Characterisation of main structures responsible for inner-ear homeostasis, and their pathophysiological relations. J Laryngol Otol. 2009; 123:151–162. ISSN: 0022-2151

[14] Marcus DC, Liu J, Wangemann P. Transepithelial voltage and resistance of vestibular dark cell epithelium from the gerbil ampulla. Hear Res. 1992; 73:101–118. ISSN: 0378-5955

[15] Hawkins JE Jr. Microcirculation in the labyrinth. Arch Otorhinolaryngol. 1976; 212:241–251. ISSN: 0302-9530

[16] Prazma, J. Electroanatomy of the lateral wall of the cochlea. Arch Otorhinolaryngol. 1975; 209:1–13. ISSN: 0302-9530

[17] Beitz E, Kumagami H, Krippeit-Drews P, Ruppersberg JP, Schultz JE. Expression pattern of aquaporin water channels in the inner ear of the rat. The molecular

basis for a water regulation system in the endolymphatic sac. Hear Res. 1999; 132:76–84. ISSN: 0378-5955

[18] Beitz E, Zenner HP, Schultz JE. Aquaporin-mediated fluid regulation in the inner ear. Cell Mol Neurobiol. 2003; 23:315–329. ISSN: 0272-4340

[19] Löwenheim H, Hirt B. Aquaporine. Discovery, function, and significance for otorhinolaryngology. HNO. 2004; 52:673–678 (German). ISSN: 0017-6192

[20] Huang D, Chen P, Chen S, Nagura M, Lim DJ, Lin X. Expression patterns of aquaporins in the inner ear: evidence for concerted actions of multiple types of aquaporins to facilitate water transport in the cochlea. Hear Res. 2002; 165:85–95. ISSN: 0378-5955

[21] Chiba T, Marcus DC. Nonselective cation and BK channels in apical membrane of outer sulcus epithelial cells. J Membr Biol. 2000; 174:167–179. ISSN: 0022-2631

[22] Marcus DC, Chiba T. K^+ and Na^+ absorption by outer sulcus epithelial cells. Hear Res. 1999; 134:48–56. ISSN: 0378-5955

[23] Zidanic M, Brownell WE. Fine structure of the intracochlear potential field. 1. The silent current. Biophys J. 1990; 57:1253–1268. ISSN: 0006-3495

[24] Wangemann P. K^+ cycling and its regulation in the cochlea and the vestibular labyrinth. Audiol Neurootol. 2002; 7:199–205. ISSN: 1420-3030

[25] Wangemann P. K^+ cycling and the endocochlear potential. Hear Res. 2002; 165:1–9. ISSN: 0378-5955

[26] Spicer SS, Smythe N, Schulte BA. Ultrastructure indicative of ion transport in tectal, Deiters, and tunnel cells: Differences between gerbil and chinchilla basal and apical cochlea. Anat Rec Part A. 2003; 271A:342–359. ISSN: 1552-4884

[27] Ciuman RR. Auditory and vestibular hair cell stereocilia: Relationship between functionality and inner ear disease. J Laryngol Otol. 2011; 125:991–1003. ISSN: 0022-2151

[28] Wright A. Dimensions of the cochlear stereocilia in man and the guinea pig. Hear Res. 1984; 13:89–98. ISSN: 0378-5955

[29] Morita I, Komatsuzaki A, Tatsuoka H. The morphological differences of stereocilia and cuticular plates between type I and type II hair cells of human vestibular sensory epithelia. ORL J Otorhinolaryngol Relat Spec. 1997; 59:193–197. ISSN: 0301-1569

[30] Lim DJ. Cochlear anatomy related to cochlear micromechanics. A review. J Acoust Soc Am. 1980; 67:1686–1695. ISSN: 0001-4966

[31] Gu ZP, Goodwen J. Observation on Corti's organ of entire cochlea in the guinea pig by scanning electron microscopy. Chin Med J. 1989; 102:251–256. ISSN: 0366-6999

[32] Slepecky N, Chamberlain SC. Immunoelectron microscopic and immunofluorescent localization of cytoskeletal and muscle-like contractile proteins in inner ear sensory hair cells. Hear Res. 1985; 20:245–260. ISSN: 0378-5955

[33] DeRosier DJ, Tilney LG. The structure of the cuticular plate, an in vivo actin gel. J Cell Biol. 1989; 109:2853–2867. ISSN: 0021-9525

[34] Pack AK, Slepecky NB. Cytoskeletal and calcium-binding proteins in the mammalian organ of Corti: cell type-specific proteins displaying longitudinal and radial gradients. Hear Res. 1995; 91:119–135. ISSN:0378-5955

[35] Watson GM, Mire P. A comparison of hair bundle mechanoreceptors in sea anemones and vertebrate systems. Curr Top Dev Biol. 1999; 43:51–84. ISSN: 0070-2153

[36] Brownell, WE, Bader CR, Bertrand D, deRibaupierre Y. Evoked mechanical responses of isolated outer hair cells. Science 1985; 227:641–654. ISSN: 1095-9203

[37] Bekesy G. Experiments in hearing. New York, NY: Mc-Graw Hill; 1960

[38] Shatz LF. The effect of hair bundle shape on hair bundle hydrodynamics of inner hair cells at low and high frequencies. Hear Res. 2000; 141:39–50. ISSN: 0378-5955

[39] Ehret G. Stiffness gradient along the basilar membrane as a basis for spatial frequency analysis within the cochlea. J Acoust Soc Am. 1978; 64:1723–1726. ISSN: 0001-4966

[40] Flock A, Strelioff D. Graded and nonlinear mechanical properties of sensory hairs in the mammalian hearing organ. Nature. 1984; 10:597–599. ISSN: 0028-0836

[41] Robles L, Ruggero MA. Mechanics of the mammalian cochlea. Phys Rev. 2001; 81:1305–1352. ISSN: 1522-1210

[42] Bullen A, West T, Moores C, Ashmore J, Fleck RA, MacLellan-Gibson K, Forge A. Association of intracellular and synaptic organization in cochlear inner hair cells revealed by 3D electron microscopy. J Cell Sci. 2015; 128:2529–2540. ISSN: 0370-2952

[43] Dannhof BJ, Bruns V. The innervation of the organ of Corti in the rat. Hear Res. 1993; 66:8–22. ISSN: 0378-5955

[44] Johnson SL, Forge A, Knipper M, Münkner S, Marcotti W. Tonotopic variation in the calcium dependence of neurotransmitter release and vesicle pool replenishment at mammalian auditory ribbon synapses. J Neurosci. 2008; 28:7670–7678. ISSN: 0270-6474

[45] Liu Y, Gracewski SM, Nam JH. Consequences of location-dependent organ of Corti micro-mechanics. PLoS One. 2015; 10:e0133284. e-ISSN: 1932-6203

[46] Cody AR, Russell JI. The responses of hair cells in the basal turn of the guinea pig cochlea to tones. J Physiol. 1987; 383:551–569. ISSN: 0022-3751

[47] Johnstone BM, Patuzzi R, Yates GK. Basilar membrane measurements and the travelling wave. Hear Res. 1986; 22:147–154. ISSN: 0378-5955

[48] Plinkert PK, Gitter AH, Zenner HP. GABA-receptors in cochlear outer hair cells. Eur Arch Otorhinolaryngol. 1992; 249:62–65. ISSN: 0937-4477

[49] Plinkert PK, Heilbronn E, Zenner HP. A nicotinic acetylcholine receptor-like α-bungarotoxin binding site on outer hair cells. Hear Res 1991; 53:123–130. ISSN: 0378-5955

[50] Fuchs PA, Glowatzki E. Synaptic studies inform the functional diversity of cochlear afferents. Hear Res. 2015; 330:18–25. ISSN: 0378-5955

[51] Froud KE, Wong AC, Cederholm JM, Klugmann M, Sandow SL, Julien JP, Ryan AF, Housley GD. Type II spiral ganglion afferent neurons drive medial olivocochlear reflex suppression of the cochlear amplifier. Nat Commun. 2015; 6:e7115. eISSN: 2041-1723

[52] Brown, MC. Morphology of labeled efferent fibers in the guinea pig cochlea. J Comp Neurol 1987; 260: 605–618. ISSN: 0021-9967

[53] Oestreicher E, Wolfgang A, Felix D. Neurotransmission of the cochlear inner hair cell synapse-implications for inner ear therapy. Adv Otorhinolaryngol. 2002; 59:131–139. ISSN: 0065-3071

[54] Ryan AF, Keithley EM, Wang ZX, Schwartz IR. Collaterals from lateral and medial olivocochlear efferent neurons innervate different regions of the cochlear nucleus and adjacent brainstem. J Comp Neurol. 1990; 300:572–582. ISSN: 0021-9967

[55] Evans EF. Place and time coding of frequency in the peripheral auditory system: Some physiological pros and cons. Audiology. 1978; 17:369–420. ISSN: 0020-6091

[56] Klinke R. Processing of acoustic stimuli in the inner ear—A review of recent research results. HNO. 1987; 35:139–148 (German). ISSN: 0017-6192

[57] Sachs MB. Neural coding of complex sounds: Speech. Ann Rev Physiol. 1986; 46:261–273. ISSN: 0066-4278

[58] Brashears SM, Morlet TG, Berlin CI, Hood LJ. Olivocochlear efferent suppression in classical musicians. J Am Acad Audiol. 2003; 14:314–324. ISSN: *1050-0545*

[59] Merchan-Perez A, Gil-Loyzaga P, Lopez-Sanchez J, Eybalin M, Valderrama FJ. Ontogeny of gamma-aminobutyric acid in efferent fibers to the rat cochlea. Brain Res Dev Brain Res. 1993; 76:33–41. ISSN: 0165-3806

[60] Zvorykin VP. Morphological substrate of ultrasonic and locational capacities in the dolphin. Fed Proc. 1964; 23:T647–T653. ISSN: 0430-2494

[61] Zook JM, Casseday JH. Cytoarchitecture of the auditory system in lower brainstem of the moustache bat, *Pteronotus parnellii*. J Comp Neurol. 1982; 207:1–13. ISSN: 0021-9967

[62] Warr WB. Parallel ascending pathways from the cochlear nucleus: Neuroanatomical evidence of functional specialization. Contrib Sens Physiol. 1982; 7:1–38. ISSN: 0069-9705

[63] Moore JK, Moore RY. A comparative study of the superior olivary complex in the primate brain. Folia Primat. 1971; 16:35–51. ISSN: 0015-5713

[64] Moore JK. Organization of the human superior olivary complex. Microscopy Research Technique. 2000; 51:403–412. ISSN: 1059-910X

[65] Tollin DJ. The lateral superior olive: A functional role in sound source localization. Neuroscientist. 2003; 9:127–143. ISSN: 0173-8584

[66] Wilson Jl, Henson MM, Henson OW Jr. Course and distribution of efferent fibers in the cochlea of the mouse. Hear Res. 1991; 55:98–108. ISSN: 0378-5955

[67] Ciuman RR. The efferent system or olivocochlear function bundle—fine regulator and protector of hearing perception. Int J Biomed Sci. 2010; 6:276–288. ISSN: 1550-9702

[68] Puel JL. Chemical synaptic transmission in the cochlea. Prog Neurobiol. 1995; 47:449–476. ISSN: 0278-5846

[69] Schrott-Fischer A, Kammen-Jolly K, Scholtz A, Rask-Andersen, Glueckert R, Eybalin M. Efferent neurotransmission in the human cochlea and vestibule. Acta Otolaryngol. 2007; 127:13–19. ISSN: 0001-6489

[70] Altschuler RA, Hoffman SW, Reeks KA, Fex J. Localization of dynorphin B-like and alpha-neoendorphin-like immunoreactivities in the guinea pig organ of Corti. Hear Res. 1985; 17:249–258. ISSN: 0378-5955

[71] Altschuler RA, Reeks KA, Fex J, Hoffmann DW. Lateral olivocochlear neurons contain both enkephalin and dynorphin immunoreactivities: Immunocytochemical co-localization studies. J Histochem Cytochem. 1988; 36:797–801. ISSN: 0022-1554

[72] Safiedinne S, Eybalin M. Triple immunofluorescence evidence for the coexistence of acetylcholine, enkephalins and calcitonin gene-related peptide within efferent (olivo-cochlear) neurons of rats and guinea-pigs. Eur J Neurosci. 1992; 4:981–992. ISSN: 0953-816X

[73] Lim K, Merfeld DM. Signal detection theory and vestibular perception: II. Fitting perceptual thresholds as a function of frequency. Exp Brain Res. 2012; 222:303–320. ISSN: 0014-4819

[74] MacNeilage PR, Turner AH, Angelaki DE. Canal-otolith interactions and detection thresholds of linear and angular components during curved-path self-motion. J Neurophysiol. 2010; 104:765–773. ISSN: 0022-3077

[75] Dror AA, Avraham KB. Hearing loss: Mechanisms revealed by genetics and cell biology. Annu Rev Genet 2009; 43:411–37

[76] Palmieri A, Ettore GC. Cochlear and vestibular aqueducts. Radiol Med 2004; 107:541–55.

[77] Peters TA, Monnens LAH, Cremers CWRJ, Curfs JHAJ. Genetic disorders of transporters/channels in the inner ear and their relation to the kidney. Pediatr Nephrol 2004; 19:1194–1201.

[78] Liberman MC. Effects of chronic cochlear de-differentiation on auditory-nerve response. Hear Res 1990; 49:209–224

[79] May BJ, Budelis J, Niparko JK. Behavioral studies of the olivocochlear efferent system. Arch Otolaryngol Head Neck Surg 2004; 130:660–664.

Complementary Literature to Table 1. and Table 2.

Anatomy

Kahle W, Leonhardt H, Platzer W. Color atlas of human anatomy. Vol. 3. Nervous system and sensory organs. 6th German ed. Taschenatlas der Anatomie. Band 3. Nervensystem und Sinnesorgane. Stuttgart, New York: Thieme; 1991. ISBN: 3-423-03019-4

Histology

Junqueira LC. Carneiro J. Basic Histology. 3rd German ed. Schiebler TH, Schneider F. Histologie. Berlin, Heidelberg, New York: Springer-Verlag; 1991. ISBN: 3-540-53733-3

Neuroanatomy

Trepel M. Neuroanatomy. 2nd ed. München, Stuttgart, Jena, Lübeck, Ulm: Urban und Fischer; 1999. (German). ISBN: 3-437-41296-5

Otorhinolaryngology

Maurer J. Neurootology. Stuttgart, New York: Thieme; 1999. (German). ISBN: 3-13-114681-8 Wendler J, Seidner W, Kittel G, Eysholdt U. Phoniatry and Pedaudiology. 3rd ed. Stuttgart, New York: Thieme; 1996. (German). ISBN: 3-13-102293-0 Scholtz AW, Schrott-Fischer A. Neurotransmission in the vestibular end organs. In: Stoll W, editor. Vestibular Diseases. 3rd Hennig-Symposium, Innsbruck, 2000. Stuttgart, New York: Thieme; 2000. (German). ISBN: 3-13-105821-8 Zenner HP. Hearing. Thieme Stuttgart, New York: Thieme; 1994. (German). ISBN: 3-13-139001-8

Physiology

Hick C, Hick A. Physiology. 2nd ed. Gustav Fischer, Stuttgart, Jena, Lübeck, Ulm: Gustav Fischer; 1997. (German). ISBN: 3-437-51280-3 Klinke R. (1993). Static sense, Hearing, Speaking. In: Schmidt RF, Thews G, editors. Human Physiology. 25th ed. Berlin, Heidelberg, New York: Springer-Verlag; 1993. (German). ISBN: 3-540-57104-3

Section 7

Ototoxicity

Chapter 13

Ototoxicity: Old and New Foes

Agnieszka J. Szczepek

Additional information is available at the end of the chapter

http://dx.doi.org/10.5772/66933

Abstract

Drug-induced ototoxicity has been known for centuries. Already in the seventeenth century, hearing loss was described to be a side effect of quinine. The post- World War II pharmaceutical industry boomed with the production of aminoglycoside antibiotics followed by diuretics and cytostatic drugs. Wide-spread and long-term usage of these medications brought the knowledge about their unwanted ototoxic effects. In the last decades, several new drugs appeared on the shelves of pharmacies and the hearing loss or tinnitus have been among the side effects of many of them. However, the awareness of community about new ototoxic medications is still not sufficient. New ototoxic drugs may belong to the class of phosphodiesterase-5 (PDE5) inhibitors, used to improve microcirculation and to treat erectile dysfunction. Moreover, interferons used for the therapy of hepatitis B and C, common painkiller paracetamol and hydrocodone, synthetic opioid methadone and the inhibitors of reverse transcriptase were demonstrated to induce adverse effects on hearing. Lastly, hearing loss linked to immunosuppressive drugs was documented in patients undergoing organ transplantation. Making the patients aware of adverse drug reactions and offering them audiological monitoring and intervention should be considered by respective therapists.

Keywords: ototoxic drugs, viral infections, reverse transcriptase inhibitors, interferons, PDE5 inhibitors, immunosuppressants, hearing loss, adverse reactions

1. Introduction

The sense of hearing is fundamental to the communication and proper reaction to dangerous situations. Moreover, recent studies indicated that the hearing loss increases significantly the risk of dementia [1]. Unfortunately, people's ability to hear deteriorates with time, as the human auditory epithelium is post-mitotic and unable to regenerate. In other words, the few thousand of auditory hair cells with which we are born have to last our entire life. There are several causes of hearing loss such as noise, aging, infections, tumors, neuronal degeneration or cardiovascular diseases. Another important cause of hearing loss is ototoxicity.

> Ototoxicity is defined as toxicity of chemicals (also drugs) particularly affecting cochlea or hearing nerve.

In this chapter, we will concentrate on medications that are known to induce hearing loss as an adverse effect. These medications are also known as ototoxic medications.

Clinical signs of ototoxicity may include at least one of the following symptoms:

- tinnitus
- hearing loss (unilateral or bilateral)
- vertigo.

First signs of ototoxicity usually develop during or shortly after receiving particular medication. Majority of ototoxic drugs induces irreparable damage translating into permanent hearing loss; however, **aspirin and derivatives** belong to drugs that cause most of the times **reversible hearing loss** [2]. In fact, aspirin-induced ototoxicity in form of tinnitus was used for decades by rheumatologists to adjust the maximal therapeutic dose of salicylates in the patients. This practice was abandoned because of poor correlation between salicylate blood levels and ototoxicity symptoms [3] and because of development of new drugs used for the treatment of rheumatic diseases. Nevertheless, even today there are patients occasionally admitted to the emergency room because of the salicylate-induced ototoxicity [4]. The ototoxicity of salicylate has been attributed to its capacity to bind and inhibit the action of cochlear protein **prestin**, expressed by the outer hair cells [5, 6]. In addition, salicylate can induce **death of spiral ganglion neurons** as well as cause **dysregulation in the central auditory pathway** [7].

Other groups of well-known ototoxic drugs that frequently cause **hearing loss** include:

- platinum-based cytostatic drugs
- aminoglycoside antibiotics
- loop diuretics

Platinum-based cytostatics (**cisplatin**, **carboplatin** and **oxaliplatin**) are used as single agents and in combination with other drugs for the treatment of various types of cancer (e.g., testicular carcinoma, lung carcinoma, ovarian carcinoma, head and neck carcinomas, melanomas, lymphomas and neuroblastomas) [8]. The platinum-based drugs bind DNA and induce irreversible changes that prohibit tumor cell division. However, common adverse effects of platinum-based drugs include nephrotoxicity and ototoxicity. This toxicity is being attributed to an excessive production of reactive oxygen species that leads to death of auditory hair cells [9–11]. Clinically, patients develop **permanent bilateral hearing loss that originates in high frequencies** [12]. In addition, patients may have **difficulties with speech understanding in noise** [13].

Aminoglycosides are a group of antibiotics used to treat gram-negative bacterial and mycobacterial infections. Clinically used aminoglycosides include amikacin and kanamycin (primarily cochleotoxic) as well as gentamicin, streptomycin and tobramycin (primarily vestibulotoxic) [14]. Similar to the ototoxic mechanism of platinum-based drugs, aminoglycosides induce excessive formation of free oxygen species followed by apoptosis of sensory hair cells [10, 15]. The aminoglycoside-induced hearing loss **is bilateral and permanent and starts in the high frequencies**. Precisely because of its ototoxic properties, gentamicin is frequently used for the treatment of Ménière's disease in the form of intratympanic injections to deplete the vestibular hair cells and thus, to prevent frequent vertigo attacks.

Of note: About 30% of the world population is infected with *Mycobacterium tuberculosis* [16]. The treatment of tuberculosis (especially that caused by **multiple-drug resistant *Mycobacterium tuberculosis***) includes intravenous administration of so-called ond-line antibiotics–amikacin, kanamycin and streptomycin–leaving at least 20% of the patients with serious permanent hearing impairment [17].

Loop diuretics are a group of drugs that inhibit renal reabsorption of sodium, chloride and potassium. They are often used to treat kidney insufficiency or heart failure. Loop diuretics include furosemide, bumetanide, ethacrynic acid and torsemide. Their ototoxic mechanism involves inhibition of potassium resorption occurring in the stria vascularis and consequent **decrease in the endocochlear potential** [18]. The hearing loss induced by loop diuretics is **bilateral and usually reversible;** however, since loop diuretics are known to synergize with platinum-based drugs or with aminoglycosides in their ototoxic action, in patients receiving drugs from both groups, loop diuretics may worsen the degree of permanent hearing loss [19–21].

There is a growing number of case reports and larger studies indicating that the family of ototoxic drugs is growing and embraces newly developed medications. Although the ototoxic properties of several pharmacological drugs were recently compiled in an excellent review written by Cianfrone et al. [22], the clinical information changes and requires update.

In this chapter, we review selected group of frequently used, contemporary pharmacological drugs (phosphodiesterase-5 blockers and antiviral drugs (see **Table 1**), painkillers and immunosuppressants) in aspect of audiologically important adverse reactions including hearing loss and tinnitus.

The class of medication	Type of report	Presence of tinnitus	Type of hearing loss	Measuring method	Reversibility of hearing loss	References
PDE5 inhibitors	Case report (1 subject)	Not stated	Profound bilateral sensorineural hearing loss	Pure tone audiometry; impedance audiometry; stapedial reflex absent on both sides	No	[23]
	Prospective study (21 subjects)	Not stated	Unilateral sensorineural hearing loss 1 h after injection of drug	Pure tone audiometry	Yes	[24]
	Analysis of 47 case reports (pharmacovigilance)	Not stated	Unilateral or bilateral sensorineural hearing loss	Not stated	In some cases, yes; in others long-term impairment	[26]
	Case report (2 subjects)	Yes	Unilateral sensorineural hearing loss	Pure tone audiometry, ABR	In one case, yes	[27]
Interferons	Prospective study (before/after) 49 subjects	Yes	Sensorineural hearing loss	Pure tone audiometry, tympanometry (normal)	Yes	[30]
	Case report (3 subjects)	Yes	Unilateral sensorineural hearing loss	Pure tone audiometry	Yes (2 cases), no (1 case)	[31]
	Prospective study (before/after) 73 subjects	Yes	Sensorineural hearing loss	Pure tone audiometry	Yes	[31]
PEG interferons	Prospective study (before/after) 21 subjects	Not stated	None found	Pure tone audiometry, DPOAE	Not applicable	[35]
	Case report (1 subject)	Not stated	Unilateral hearing loss	Not stated	Yes	[36]
	Case report (1 subject)	Yes	Unilateral hearing loss	Not stated	No	[37]
	Case report (6 subjects)	Yes (4 of 6)	Five subjects developed unilateral and one bilateral sensorineural hearing loss	Pure tone audiometry	No improvement in three cases, some improvement in two cases, no data in one case	[38]

Although in the industrialized countries, the hepatitis C and B therapy with pegylated or non-pegylated interferons and ribavirin is being replaced by other pharmacological regimes, one should not ignore the fact that not all countries and hospitals have adopted the new routine and that the interferons are still in use, possibly contributing to drug-related hearing loss.

Table 1. Summary of clinical reports describing hearing loss in PDE5- and interferon-treated patients.

http://dx.doi.org/10.5772/66933

2. Phosphodiesterase-5 (PDE5) inhibitors

PDE5 inhibitors block the phosphodiesterase-5 in the smooth muscle cells lining the blood vessels in the cardiovascular system. Phosphodiesterase-5 degrades cyclic GMP, regulating smooth muscle tone. The first PDE5 inhibitor–sildenafil–was introduced in the market in 1998 under the name Viagra. PDE5 inhibitors are used for the treatment of erectile dysfunctions and for pulmonary artery hypertension.

In the year 2007, an alarming report was published by Mukherjee and Shivakumar, in which a case of bilateral profound sensorineural hearing loss was described in 44-year-old man who took 50 mg/day of sildenafil for 2 weeks [23]. Based on that report, **FDA issued a warning about possible sudden hearing loss among users of PDE5 inhibitors**.

Over the past 10 years, evidence suggesting negative influence of PDE5 inhibitors on hearing has accumulated. In a clinical study, Okuyucu et al. [24] reported significant but reversible unilateral hearing loss in four of 18 patients taking PDE5 inhibitors. The hearing loss affected the right ear at 10,000 Hz ($p = 0.008$).

Much larger epidemiological study published 1 year later by McGwin [25] evaluated the relationship between hearing loss and the use of PDE5 inhibitors in a population-based sample. This USA-based study was designed using self-reported hearing impairment and PDE5i use and included over eleven thousand men who were 40 years or older. Results of this study indicated that men with hearing loss are more than twice as likely to use PDE5 inhibitors, when compared with those not reporting hearing loss. However, no causal relationship could be established in that study.

In 2011, Khan et al. [26] published a report based on data provided by pharmacovigilance agencies Europe, the Americas, East Asia and Australasia, and on published reports. The authors identified among PDE5 inhibitor users 47 cases of sensorineural hearing loss, most of them unilateral. Almost 70% of the subjects (mean age 56.6 years, men-to-women ratio 7:1) reported hearing loss within 24 h after ingestion of PDE5 inhibitors.

In 2012, unilateral sudden sensorineural hearing loss affecting two male PDE5 inhibitor users (age 37 and 43) was described by Barreto and Bahmad [27]. Unfortunately, neither the time after the hearing loss has occurred nor the dosage of PDE5 inhibitors was stated. In addition to the hearing loss, both patients were affected by vertigo and tinnitus. After combination therapy consisting of steroids administered orally and intratympanically, one of the patients recovered partially, whereas the other one was left with permanent profound sensorineural hearing loss.

The causal relationship between the PDE5 inhibitors and (sudden) sensorineural hearing loss remains to be confirmed using experimental models. Au and colleagues using the animal model (C57BL/6J mice) and sildenafil (Viagra) were unable to find the differences in hearing thresholds between the drug- and placebo-treated animals [28]. However, other functional studies in mice with the use of osmotic pumps for drug release demonstrated that the inner ear of animals exposed to sildenafil reacted with hydrops [29].

The epidemiological and case report data indicate that PDE5 inhibitors may have general negative impact on hearing. Moreover, PDE5 inhibitors may induce sudden sensorineural hearing loss that in some cases can be successfully treated with corticosteroids; in some other cases, the patients recover without any treatment; and lastly, it can also leave patients with permanent hearing impairment.

3. Antiviral medications

3.1. Interferons

Interferons (IFN) are a group of naturally occurring proteins that are released by several cell types in response to infection or tumors. There are three classes of interferons: type I, type II and type III. Type I interferons include IFN-alpha and IFN-beta. Synthetic and recombinant interferons, alpha and beta, have been used for therapy of viral infections with hepatitis C or B virus. In addition, IFN-beta can be used to treat multiple sclerosis.

One of the first reports associating interferon treatment with hearing loss was published in 1994 [30]. In that report, a group of 49 patients (32 men and 17 women, mean age 48.6, age range 23–67) receiving various brands of interferons for chronic hepatitis B or C were assessed with pure tone audiometry before the onset of treatment and then in consecutive 1-week interval. In case of IFN-alpha, the drug was administered i.m. each day for 2 weeks and then three times a week for 14–22 weeks. In case of IFN-beta, the drug was administered i.v. daily for 6 weeks. The study demonstrated that 45% (22 patients) developed auditory dysfunction: 14 patients (29%) reported having tinnitus and 18 patients (35%) were diagnosed with sudden sensorineural hearing loss. More than half (56%) of the patients treated with interferon-beta (total of 27 subjects) developed auditory disability with unilateral or bilateral hearing loss affecting various frequencies diagnosed in 11 patients (41%). In the group treated with IFN-alpha (total of 22 subjects), seven developed unilateral hearing loss affecting 8000 Hz. Progressive hearing loss leads in two cases to withdrawal from therapy. There was no association between the clinical parameters such as proteinuria, leucopenia, liver functions and the hearing loss. Interestingly, all patients recovered within 2 weeks after finishing the interferon treatment.

Published 1 year later, prospective audiological study of 73 patients treated with IFN-alpha or IFN-beta for hepatitis confirmed the above observations, including the hearing loss exclusively affecting 8000 Hz in patients receiving IFN-alpha [31]. There was, however, one difference: in the larger sample studied, the hearing abilities of one patient have not recovered after discontinuation of therapy. Later, studies confirmed majority of these observations [32] and most importantly the general reversibility of ototoxic effects of IFN-alpha [33].

Interesting mechanistic insights of IFN-alpha-induced ototoxicity were delivered from studies using mouse model [34]. There was an elevated ABR threshold in mice treated with IFN-alpha as compared to untreated control group. Moreover, histological findings of cochleae dissected from experimental animals indicated abnormalities in the number (lower) and appearance (cytoplasmic vacuolization) of the spiral limbus fibroblasts in the IFN-alpha-treated mice.

http://dx.doi.org/10.5772/66933

These findings point to direct negative effect of IFN-alpha on cochlear biology, which may result in the hearing loss.

3.2. Pegylated interferons and ribavirin

Pegylated interferons are chemically "improved" interferons bound to polyethylene glycol (PEG). Pegylation assures longer half-time of interferons in the body. There are three groups of pegylated interferons available in the market–pegylated interferon-alpha-2a (PEG-IFNa2a), pegylated interferon-alpha-2b (PEG-IFNa2b) and pegylated interferon-beta-1a.

Ribavirin is a guanosine analog (nucleoside inhibitor) that stops viral RNA synthesis. It is used to treat various viral hemorrhagic fevers, and it is the only known drug against rabies. Although new therapeutic approaches are being introduced on the healthcare market for the treatment of hepatitis C (e.g., protease inhibitor telaprevir or boceprevir), ribavirin in combination with PEG-IFN-alpha is still a part of the current standard of care (SOC) therapy in some countries and it is also included in the new therapeutic regime.

Therapeutic use of PEG-IFN and ribavirin in hepatitis C infections induces similar otological effects as the therapy with non-pegylated interferons only. However, there is one major difference: the hearing abilities do not recover in the majority of cases. Although some reports describe no hearing disabilities [35] or sudden unilateral sensorineural hearing loss resolving spontaneously within 2 weeks after the end of treatment [36], some other demonstrate that patients may develop irreversible unilateral hearing loss [37] or irreversible unilateral pantonal hearing loss (measured by pure tone audiometry) and tinnitus [38].

3.3. Inhibitors of viral reverse transcriptase

According to the United Nations AIDS organization, approximately 36.7 million people worldwide are infected with the HIV virus. The patients with HIV are treated with drugs that inhibit the virus proliferation. Since HIV virus uses very unique enzyme to copy its genome, this enzyme–reverse transcriptase–is a pharmacological target of anti-HIV therapy. The unique thing about the HIV therapy is that it should never be stopped, even if the viral load is undetectable.

The discovery and the beginning of clinical application of reverse transcriptase inhibitors date back to the eighties last century. The first reports about their negative effect on hearing appeared some 10 years later and ever since conflicting conclusions are being drawn from several studies. In some studies, authors found the hearing loss among 30% of HIV patients taking the reverse transcription inhibitors [39–41], whereas in other studies, no association between audiological impairment and antiviral medication was found [42, 43]. Various inclusion criteria, diverse outcome measure methods, sample size and many other factors could contribute to these dissimilar results.

In the controlled environment of experimental laboratory, the results look much more uniform and point at universal ototoxicity of all types of reverse transcriptase inhibitors that are on the market, as measured by the viability of auditory epithelial cell line exposed to various concentrations of 14 types of pharmacological reverse transcription inhibitors as single agents and in combination, as used in the clinics [44].

4. Paracetamol (acetaminophen) and hydrocodone

Paracetamol, also known as acetaminophen (in the USA and Canada) or APAP, is the most commonly used pain killer in North America and Europe. It inhibits selectively cyclooxygenase-2 (COX-2) and may also exert other pain-relieving functions. Recent studies on self-reported professionally diagnosed hearing loss and use of analgesics indicated that regular use of paracetamol significantly increases the risk of hearing loss in men [45] and women [46]. The large size of samples with which the studies were performed (26,917 men and 62,261 women) makes both studies particularly credible.

The main conclusion from this study was that the long-term use of paracetamol (acetaminophen) increases the risk of developing hearing loss in men and women.

The mechanism of paracetamol-induced hearing loss was experimentally addressed in vitro [47]. The authors demonstrated that in the mouse auditory epithelium cell line, paracetamol and its metabolite NAPQI (*N*-acetyl-p-benzoquinoneimine) induce ototoxicity by causing oxidative stress as well as endoplasmic reticulum (ER) stress. These basic research results possibly explain the ototoxicity seen in people who regularly consume paracetamol. The question about usage of paracetamol and its frequency should be included in the surveys/questionnaires of patients with otologic and audiologic considerations.

Hydrocodone is a semi-synthetic opioid used for pain therapy and in common anti-cough medications. Hydrocodone is often prescribed in combination with paracetamol. In a report describing 12 patients with a history of hydrocodone overuse and progressive irreversible sensorineural hearing loss, the authors implicated nonresponsiveness of this type of hearing loss to corticosteroid therapy [48]. The authors reported that seven of eight patients who underwent consecutive cochlear implantation benefited from this type of auditory rehabilitation. Similar recent case report described a patient with unilateral hearing loss attributed to abuse of hydrocodone and paracetamol [49]. Also this patient was treated with cochlear implant.

The information delivered from the in vitro model with auditory epithelial cell line suggested that the combination of hydrocodone and paracetamol results in ototoxicity not due to hydrocodone but rather due to paracetamol [50]. The authors suggested that the contribution of hydrocodone to clinically seen ototoxicity may lay in hydrocodone assisting the addiction to the drug combination.

5. Methadone

Methadone is an opioid drug for treating pain. In addition, it is used for therapy of people addicted to opioids.

In the year 2014, about 7 million US citizens were abusing prescription drugs (source: National Center for Health Statistics). One of these drugs is methadone. Six recent case reports exposed an unknown before side effect of methadone abuse–the hearing loss [51–55]. The patients described in reports were young (age range 20–37) and were admitted to the hospitals because

http://dx.doi.org/10.5772/66933

of methadone overuse. In all reported cases, the patients were deaf upon awakening (one perceived tinnitus), and in four of six cases, hearing loss was only temporary condition. The remaining two patients were unfortunately left with severe sensorineural hearing loss for the remaining observation time (2 and 9 months).

6. Immunosuppressant calcineurin inhibitors (cyclosporine A and tacrolimus)

Since the beginning of transplantology in the sixties, several people with incurable diseases of liver, kidney and other organs received the donor tissues as therapeutic procedure. This type of therapy is combined with an inevitable immune reaction against the *non-self* tissue. To prevent these reactions, immunosuppressants are used. Among them, cyclosporine A and tacrolimus (FK506) are commonly used to prevent graft rejection reaction. Both drugs decrease in various ways the activation of lymphocytes T and thus inhibit the graft rejection process. The immunosuppressants must be taken continuously.

Rifai et al. [56] performed a large study involving 521 liver transplant patients. The study was based on self-reported hearing loss and showed that of 521 individuals, 141 (27%) developed hearing loss following transplantation, particularly in those patients who were receiving tacrolimus as principal immunosuppression. This study was followed by recent trial, where instead of self-reported hearing loss, audiometric measurements were performed [57]. Of 70 liver transplant patients included in that study, 32 reported hearing loss and tinnitus following the transplantation. The types of hearing loss included sudden hearing loss and progressive hearing loss, which developed more than 3 years after transplantation. Audiometry confirmed the patients' reports and identified 12 patients with mild, 28 with moderate and 25 with severe hearing loss following the transplantation. The association between tacrolimus and hearing loss was seen again in this study.

Another group of transplant patients is the renal transplant group. Kidney transplantation is a surgical procedure performed since the mid-fifties last century; however, postsurgical survival was very low, because of the graft rejection [58]. The introduction of cyclosporine A in the eighties significantly improved the post-transplant survival rate but brought another type of problems, namely adverse reactions such as hearing loss. Renal patients are known to often have hearing impairments [59], and it was shown that the renal transplantation restores the hearing abilities, when measured 1 year after surgery. However, some renal transplant patients who are on a long-term immunosuppressant therapy such as cyclosporine A or tacrolimus develop hearing disabilities including sudden sensorineural hearing loss [60–62] or a progressive hearing loss [63].

Particularly, worrying tendency is seen among the pediatric renal transplant patients. A prospective study of 27 children (mean age 14) with normal hearing prior to kidney transplantation determined after a mean follow-up of 30 months that 17 children developed sensorineural hearing loss [60]. Two of 17 children were diagnosed with sudden hearing loss and the rest of the group with a progressive bilateral hearing loss.

It is likely that the ototoxic effect of immunosuppressants depends on the length of time of intake. Groups studying noise-induced hearing loss have successfully used cyclosporine A and tacrolimus to protect the auditory epithelium in mice from the noise-induced injury [64]. However, the dosage was single and not–like in the case of transplant patients–years long.

The treatment of hearing impairment occurring in organ transplant recipients includes hearing aids and cochlear implantation [65]. However, one should not ignore the fact that these patients are immunocompromised, and therefore, the risk of wound infection after CI should be taken under consideration during postsurgical management.

7. Mitochondrial toxicity: common denominator of ototoxic drugs

The auditory system requires a lot of energy produced in mitochondria [66–69]. Mitochondrial pathologies induced by genetic mutations are often associated with hearing loss [70–72]. Similarly, substances known to damage mitochondria such as aminoglycosides or cisplatin are known as ototoxic and contribute significantly to the hearing loss and tinnitus [73].

The substances listed in the present chapter can all damage the mitochondria. The damaging mechanism varies, and for instance, IFN-alpha impairs the transcription of mitochondrial DNA, whereas nucleoside analogues impair the replication of mitochondrial DNA [74]. In agreement with this, severe mitochondrial toxicity manifested by hyperlactatemia and pancreatitis was described in some cases involving patients with HIV/hepatitis C virus treated with pegylated interferon and ribavirin [75]. Paracetamol was also shown to have negative effect on mitochondria by inducing overproduction of reactive oxygen species (ROS) and inducing endoplasmic reticulum stress [47, 76]. Methadone was shown to impair synthesis of mitochondrial ATP leading to bioenergetics crisis of the affected organism [77]. The reverse transcriptase inhibitors used to slow down the replication of HIV virus were likewise demonstrated to induce mitochondrial toxicity [78, 79]. Lastly, cyclosporine A was shown to inhibit adenine nucleotide net transport into the mitochondria [80], whereas tacrolimus was associated with decreasing the levels of oxidative phosphorylation in mitochondria [81].

Since the negative effect of various drugs on mitochondria likely results in a damage of hearing, it is plausible that the mitochondria-supporting substances (such as coenzyme Q10, vitamin B12 with folic acid, sirtuin and many others) given as auxiliary therapy could protect the sense of hearing in patients with hepatitis, HIV, transplant patients or painkiller or PDE5 inhibitor users. In fact, targeting mitochondria is becoming increasingly popular [82], and there were some successful attempts in treatment of hearing conditions using mitochondrial supplements [83–89].

8. Conclusions

The appearance of new drugs to treat ever more conditions is an inevitable and welcomed progress of medical and pharmaceutical sciences. However, assuring the drug safety in terms of hearing disability is difficult, and it often requires very long and regular intake periods, which are outside of regular phase I, II or III clinical trials. As for the duration of phase IV (the postmarketing surveillance trials), which is usually set for 2 years, perhaps it could be extended specifically for the monitoring of audiological conditions.

The ototoxicity of prescription or over-the-counter drugs is a global problem. Collaboration between audiologists or otologists and other healthcare providers is necessary to protect the patient's auditory health. Auditory consultations ought to be a routine during the treatment of patients with viral hepatitis C or B receiving interferons and ribavirin or HIV-positive individuals taking anti-reverse transcriptase drug cocktail. Moreover, patients undergoing solid organ transplantation should be audiologically monitored. The option of audiological care for children treated for any of the above infectious diseases or undergoing transplantation should be presented to their parents. Lastly, frequent users of painkillers and recreational drugs should be informed about the risks of the medications they are reaching for every day.

During the unavoidable drug therapies, preventive means such as mitochondrial protection and supplementation during the drug treatment and audiological monitoring as well as fitting the patients with hearing aids or cochlear implants, could help to keep the hearing healthy or at least to restore it to some degree.

The good condition of hearing is as important as that of heart, lung or other organs. Informing the community about ototoxicity and keeping up to date with the case reports and other scientific communications may help to save the sense of hearing.

Glossary of terms

Cyclosporine A	Fungal metabolite that suppresses immune reaction. It inhibits the activation of lymphocytes T by binding to cyclophilin and inhibiting calcineurin
Endocochlear potential	Voltage of +80mV in the scala media, generated by the stria vascularis, essential for the auditory transduction
Interferon (IFN)-alpha	Small signaling protein produced and released mainly by white blood cells in response to viral infection
Interferon (IFN)-beta	Small signaling protein produced and released mainly by fibroblasts in response to viral infection
Intratympanic injections	Injections through the eardrum into the middle ear cavity
Mycobacterium tuberculosis	Infectious microorganism causing tuberculosis
Nucleoside	Glycosylamine (e.g., cytidine, uridine, adenosine, guanosine or thymidine), primary DNA or RNA molecule. Also known as nucleotide without phosphate group

Phosphodiesterase-5 (PDE5)	Enzyme that catalyzes the hydrolysis of cyclic GMP and regulates tonus of smooth muscle cells
PDE5i	Phosphodiesterase-5 inhibitors
Polyethylene glycol (PEG)	Polymer of ethylene oxide. PEG can be bound to proteins, therefore slowing their decay time in the body
Protease inhibitor	Inhibitor of enzymes that degrade proteins. Viral proteases are essential for viruses to complete their life cycle
Reverse transcriptase (RT)	Enzyme that synthesizes DNA using as a template RNA, a process called reverse transcription. This process is specific for viral replication and is used for instance by HIV virus
Tacrolimus (FK-506)	Bacterial derivative isolated from Streptomyces tsukubaensis. Tacrolimus inhibits activation of lymphocytes T via inhibiting calcineurin. Similar but not identical in action to cyclosporine A

Author details

Agnieszka J. Szczepek

Address all correspondence to: agnes.szczepek@charite.de

ORL Research Laboratory, Department of ORL, Head and Neck Surgery, Charité University Hospital, Berlin, Germany

References

[1] Gurgel, R.K., et al., *Relationship of hearing loss and dementia: a prospective, population-based study*. Otol Neurotol, 2014. **35**(5): p. 775–81.

[2] Jung, T.T., et al., *Ototoxicity of salicylate, nonsteroidal antiinflammatory drugs, and quinine*. Otolaryngol Clin North Am, 1993. **26**(5): p. 791–810.

[3] Halla, J.T. and J.G. Hardin, *Salicylate ototoxicity in patients with rheumatoid arthritis: a controlled study*. Ann Rheum Dis, 1988. **47**(2): p. 134–7.

[4] Kim, S.M., et al., *A case of bilateral sudden hearing loss and tinnitus after salicylate intoxication*. Korean J Audiol, 2013. **17**(1): p. 23–6.

[5] Zhang, P.C., A.M. Keleshian, and F. Sachs, *Voltage-induced membrane movement*. Nature, 2001. **413**(6854): p. 428–32.

[6] Zheng, J., et al., *Prestin is the motor protein of cochlear outer hair cells*. Nature, 2000. **405**(6783): p. 149–55.

[7] Sheppard, A., et al., *Review of salicylate-induced hearing loss, neurotoxicity, tinnitus and neuropathophysiology*. Acta Otorhinolaryngol Ital, 2014. **34**(2): p. 79–93.

[8] Apps, M.G., E.H. Choi, and N.J. Wheate, *The state-of-play and future of platinum drugs*. Endocr Relat Cancer, 2015. **22**(4): p. R219–33.

[9] Goncalves, M.S., et al., *Mechanisms of cisplatin ototoxicity: theoretical review*. J Laryngol Otol, 2013. **127**(6): p. 536–41.

[10] Rybak, L.P. and V. Ramkumar, *Ototoxicity*. Kidney Int, 2007. **72**(8): p. 931–5.

[11] Karasawa, T. and P.S. Steyger, *An integrated view of cisplatin-induced nephrotoxicity and ototoxicity*. Toxicol Lett, 2015. **237**(3): p. 219–27.

[12] Arora, R., et al., *Cisplatin-based chemotherapy: Add high-frequency audiometry in the regimen*. Indian J Cancer, 2009. **46**(4): p. 311–7.

[13] Einarsson, E.J., et al., *Severe difficulties with word recognition in noise after platinum chemotherapy in childhood, and improvements with open-fitting hearing-aids*. Int J Audiol, 2011. **50**(10): p. 642–51.

[14] Leis, J.A., J.A. Rutka, and W.L. Gold, *Aminoglycoside-induced ototoxicity*. CMAJ, 2015. **187**(1): p. E52.

[15] Sha, S.H. and J. Schacht, *Stimulation of free radical formation by aminoglycoside antibiotics*. Hear Res, 1999. **128**(1–2): p. 112–8.

[16] Kaufmann, S.H., *New issues in tuberculosis*. Ann Rheum Dis, 2004. **63 Suppl 2**: p. ii50–ii56.

[17] Garcia-Prats, A.J., H.S. Schaaf, and A.C. Hesseling, *The safety and tolerability of the second-line injectable antituberculosis drugs in children*. Expert Opin Drug Saf, 2016. **15**(11): p. 1491–1500.

[18] Rybak, L.P., *Ototoxicity of loop diuretics*. Otolaryngol Clin North Am, 1993. **26**(5): p. 829–44.

[19] Schmitz, H.M., S.B. Johnson, and P.A. Santi, *Kanamycin-furosemide ototoxicity in the mouse cochlea: a 3-dimensional analysis*. Otolaryngol Head Neck Surg, 2014. **150**(4): p. 666–72.

[20] Hirose, K., et al., *Systemic lipopolysaccharide induces cochlear inflammation and exacerbates the synergistic ototoxicity of kanamycin and furosemide*. J Assoc Res Otolaryngol, 2014. **15**(4): p. 555–70.

[21] Bates, D.E., S.J. Beaumont, and B.W. Baylis, *Ototoxicity induced by gentamicin and furosemide*. Ann Pharmacother, 2002. **36**(3): p. 446–51.

[22] Cianfrone, G., et al., *Pharmacological drugs inducing ototoxicity, vestibular symptoms and tinnitus: a reasoned and updated guide*. Eur Rev Med Pharmacol Sci, 2011. **15**(6): p. 601–36.

[23] Mukherjee, B. and T. Shivakumar, *A case of sensorineural deafness following ingestion of sildenafil*. J Laryngol Otol, 2007. **121**(4): p. 395–7.

[24] Okuyucu, S., et al., *Effect of phosphodiesterase-5 inhibitor on hearing*. J Laryngol Otol, 2009. **123**(7): p. 718–22.

[25] McGwin, G., Jr., *Phosphodiesterase type 5 inhibitor use and hearing impairment*. Arch Otolaryngol Head Neck Surg, 2010. **136**(5): p. 488–92.

[26] Khan, A.S., et al., *Viagra deafness--sensorineural hearing loss and phosphodiesterase-5 inhibitors*. Laryngoscope, 2011. **121**(5): p. 1049–54.

[27] Barreto, M.A. and F. Bahmad Jr, *Phosphodiesterase type 5 inhibitors and sudden sensorineural hearing loss*. Braz J Otorhinolaryngol, 2013. **79**(6): p. 727–33.

[28] Au, A., et al., *Ups and downs of Viagra: revisiting ototoxicity in the mouse model*. PLoS One, 2013. **8**(11): p. e79226.

[29] Degerman, E., et al., *Inhibition of phosphodiesterase 3, 4, and 5 induces endolymphatic hydrops in mouse inner ear, as evaluated with repeated 9.4T MRI*. Acta Otolaryngol, 2016: p. 1–8.

[30] Kanda, Y., et al., *Sudden hearing loss associated with interferon*. Lancet, 1994. **343**(8906): p. 1134–5.

[31] Kanda, Y., et al., *Interferon-induced sudden hearing loss*. Audiology, 1995. **34**(2): p. 98–102.

[32] Sharifian, M.R., et al., *INF-alpha and ototoxicity*. Biomed Res Int, 2013. **2013**: p. 295327.

[33] Gorur, K., et al., *The effect of recombinant interferon alpha treatment on hearing thresholds in patients with chronic viral hepatitis B*. Auris Nasus Larynx, 2003. **30**(1): p. 41–4.

[34] Akyol, M.U., et al., *Investigation of the ototoxic effects of interferon alpha2A on the mouse cochlea*. Otolaryngol Head Neck Surg, 2001. **124**(1): p. 107–10.

[35] Hagr, A., et al., *Effect of interferon treatment on hearing of patients with chronic hepatitis C*. Saudi J Gastroenterol, 2011. **17**(2): p. 114–8.

[36] Elloumi, H., et al., *Sudden hearing loss associated with peginterferon and ribavirin combination therapy during hepatitis C treatment*. World J Gastroenterol, 2007. **13**(40): p. 5411–2.

[37] Wong, V.K., et al., *Acute sensorineural hearing loss associated with peginterferon and ribavirin combination therapy during hepatitis C treatment: outcome after resumption of therapy*. World J Gastroenterol, 2005. **11**(34): p. 5392–3.

[38] Formann, E., et al., *Sudden hearing loss in patients with chronic hepatitis C treated with pegylated interferon/ribavirin*. Am J Gastroenterol, 2004. **99**(5): p. 873–7.

[39] Marra, C.M., et al., *Hearing loss and antiretroviral therapy in patients infected with HIV–1*. Arch Neurol, 1997. **54**(4): p. 407–10.

[40] Simdon, J., et al., *Ototoxicity associated with use of nucleoside analog reverse transcriptase inhibitors: a report of 3 possible cases and review of the literature*. Clin Infect Dis, 2001. **32**(11): p. 1623–7.

[41] Matas, C.G., et al., *Audiological manifestations in HIV-positive adults*. Clinics (Sao Paulo), 2014. **69**(7): p. 469–75.

[42] Luque, A.E., et al., *Hearing function in patients living with HIV/AIDS*. Ear Hear, 2014. **35**(6): p. e282–90.

[43] Schouten, J.T., et al., *A prospective study of hearing changes after beginning zidovudine or didanosine in HIV–1 treatment-naive people*. BMC Infect Dis, 2006. **6**: p. 28.

[44] Thein, P., et al., *In vitro assessment of antiretroviral drugs demonstrates potential for ototoxicity*. Hear Res, 2014. **310**: p. 27–35.

[45] Curhan, S.G., et al., *Analgesic use and the risk of hearing loss in men*. Am J Med, 2010. **123**(3): p. 231–7.

[46] Curhan, S.G., et al., *Analgesic use and the risk of hearing loss in women*. Am J Epidemiol, 2012. **176**(6): p. 544–54.

[47] Kalinec, G.M., et al., *Acetaminophen and NAPQI are toxic to auditory cells via oxidative and endoplasmic reticulum stress-dependent pathways*. Hear Res, 2014. **313**: p. 26–37.

[48] Friedman, R.A., et al., *Profound hearing loss associated with hydrocodone/acetaminophen abuse*. Am J Otol, 2000. **21**(2): p. 188–91.

[49] Novac, A., et al., *Implications of sensorineural hearing loss with hydrocodone/acetaminophen abuse*. Prim Care Companion CNS Disord, 2015. **17**(5): p. 357–359

[50] Yorgason, J.G., et al., *Acetaminophen ototoxicity after acetaminophen/hydrocodone abuse: evidence from two parallel in vitro mouse models*. Otolaryngol Head Neck Surg, 2010. **142**(6): p. 814–9, 819 e1–2.

[51] van Gaalen, F.A., E.A. Compier, and A.J. Fogteloo, *Sudden hearing loss after a methadone overdose*. Eur Arch Otorhinolaryngol, 2009. **266**(5): p. 773–4.

[52] Christenson, B.J. and A.R. Marjala, *Two cases of sudden sensorineural hearing loss after methadone overdose*. Ann Pharmacother, 2010. **44**(1): p. 207–10.

[53] Shaw, K.A., K.M. Babu, and J.B. Hack, *Methadone, another cause of opioid-associated hearing loss: a case report*. J Emerg Med, 2011. **41**(6): p. 635–9.

[54] Vorasubin, N., A.P. Calzada, and A. Ishiyama, *Methadone-induced bilateral severe sensorineural hearing loss*. Am J Otolaryngol, 2013. **34**(6): p. 735–8.

[55] Saifan, C., et al., *Methadone induced sensorineural hearing loss*. Case Rep Med, 2013. **2013**: p. 242730.

[56] Rifai, K., et al., *A new side effect of immunosuppression: high incidence of hearing impairment after liver transplantation*. Liver Transpl, 2006. **12**(3): p. 411–5.

[57] Rifai, K., et al., *High rate of unperceived hearing loss in patients after liver transplantation*. Clin Transplant, 2012. **26**(4): p. 577–80.

[58] Muntean, A. and M. Lucan, *Immunosuppression in kidney transplantation*. Clujul Med, 2013. **86**(3): p. 177–80.

[59] Bains, K.S., et al., *Cochlear function in chronic kidney disease and renal transplantation: a longitudinal study*. Transplant Proc, 2007. **39**(5): p. 1465–8.

[60] Gulleroglu, K., et al., *Hearing Status in Pediatric Renal Transplant Recipients*. Exp Clin Transplant, 2015. **13**(4): p. 324–8.

[61] Gulleroglu, K., et al., *Sudden hearing loss associated with tacrolimus after pediatric renal transplant*. Exp Clin Transplant, 2013. **11**(6): p. 562–4.

[62] Arinsoy, T., et al., *Sudden hearing loss in a cyclosporin-treated renal transplantation patient*. Nephron, 1993. **63**(1): p. 116–7.

[63] Marioni, G., et al., *Progressive bilateral sensorineural hearing loss probably induced by chronic cyclosporin A treatment after renal transplantation for focal glomerulosclerosis*. Acta Otolaryngol, 2004. **124**(5): p. 603–7.

[64] Uemaetomari, I., et al., *Protective effect of calcineurin inhibitors on acoustic injury of the cochlea*. Hear Res, 2005. **209**(1–2): p. 86–90.

[65] Patterson, D.M., et al., *Cochlear implantation in organ transplantation*. Laryngoscope, 2008. **118**(1): p. 116–9.

[66] Lalwani, A.K., et al., *Localization in stereocilia, plasma membrane, and mitochondria suggests diverse roles for NMHC-IIa within cochlear hair cells*. Brain Res, 2008. **1197**: p. 13–22.

[67] Mann, Z.F., M.R. Duchen, and J.E. Gale, *Mitochondria modulate the spatio-temporal properties of intra- and intercellular Ca2+ signals in cochlear supporting cells*. Cell Calcium, 2009. **46**(2): p. 136–46.

[68] Tao, Z.Z., T. Yamashita, and J.T. Chou, *Succinate dehydrogenase and mitochondria in the hair cells in the organ of Corti of mature and old shaker-1 mice*. J Laryngol Otol, 1987. **101**(7): p. 643–51.

[69] Spicer, S.S., et al., *Mitochondria-activated cisternae generate the cell specific vesicles in auditory hair cells*. Hear Res, 2007. **233**(1–2): p. 40–5.

[70] Subathra, M., et al., *Genetic epidemiology of mitochondrial pathogenic variants causing nonsyndromic hearing loss in a large cohort of South Indian hearing impaired individuals*. Ann Hum Genet, 2016. **80**(5): p. 257–73.

[71] Finsterer, J. and J. Fellinger, *Nuclear and mitochondrial genes mutated in nonsyndromic impaired hearing*. Int J Pediatr Otorhinolaryngol, 2005. **69**(5): p. 621–47.

[72] Ishikawa, K., et al., *Nonsyndromic hearing loss caused by a mitochondrial T7511C mutation*. Laryngoscope, 2002. **112**(8 Pt 1): p. 1494–9.

[73] Zou, J., et al., *Mitochondria toxin-induced acute cochlear cell death indicates cellular activity-correlated energy consumption*. Eur Arch Otorhinolaryngol, 2013. **270**(9): p. 2403–15.

[74] Fromenty, B. and D. Pessayre, *Impaired mitochondrial function in microvesicular steatosis. Effects of drugs, ethanol, hormones and cytokines*. J Hepatol, 1997. **26 Suppl 2**: p. 43–53.

[75] Bani-Sadr, F., et al., *Risk factors for symptomatic mitochondrial toxicity in HIV/hepatitis C virus-coinfected patients during interferon plus ribavirin-based therapy*. J Acquir Immune Defic Syndr, 2005. **40**(1): p. 47–52.

[76] Jaeschke, H., M.R. McGill, and A. Ramachandran, *Oxidant stress, mitochondria, and cell death mechanisms in drug-induced liver injury: lessons learned from acetaminophen hepatotoxicity*. Drug Metab Rev, 2012. **44**(1): p. 88–106.

[77] Perez-Alvarez, S., et al., *Methadone induces necrotic-like cell death in SH-SY5Y cells by an impairment of mitochondrial ATP synthesis*. Biochim Biophys Acta, 2010. **1802**(11): p. 1036–47.

[78] Feeney, E.R. and P.W. *Mallon, Impact of mitochondrial toxicity of HIV–1 antiretroviral drugs on lipodystrophy and metabolic dysregulation*. Curr Pharm Des, 2010. **16**(30): p. 3339–51.

[79] Apostolova, N., A. Blas-Garcia, and J.V. Esplugues, *Mitochondrial toxicity in HAART: an overview of in vitro evidence*. Curr Pharm Des, 2011. **17**(20): p. 2130–44.

[80] Henke, W., E. Nickel, and K. Jung, *Cyclosporine A inhibits ATP net uptake of rat kidney mitochondria*. Biochem Pharmacol, 1992. **43**(5): p. 1021–4.

[81] Simon, N., et al., *Tacrolimus and sirolimus decrease oxidative phosphorylation of isolated rat kidney mitochondria*. Br J Pharmacol, 2003. **138**(2): p. 369–76.

[82] Camara, A.K., E.J. Lesnefsky, and D.F. Stowe, *Potential therapeutic benefits of strategies directed to mitochondria*. Antioxid Redox Signal, 2010. **13**(3): p. 279–347.

[83] Cascella, V., et al., *A new oral otoprotective agent. Part 1: Electrophysiology data from protection against noise-induced hearing loss*. Med Sci Monit, 2012. **18**(1): p. BR1–8.

[84] Ahn, J.H., et al., *Coenzyme Q10 in combination with steroid therapy for treatment of sudden sensorineural hearing loss: a controlled prospective study*. Clin Otolaryngol, 2010. **35**(6): p. 486–9.

[85] Khan, M., et al., *A pilot clinical trial of the effects of coenzyme Q10 on chronic tinnitus aurium*. Otolaryngol Head Neck Surg, 2007. **136**(1): p. 72–7.

[86] Lasisi, A.O., F.A. Fehintola, and O.B. Yusuf, *Age-related hearing loss, vitamin B12, and folate in the elderly*. Otolaryngol Head Neck Surg, 2010. **143**(6): p. 826–30.

[87] Shemesh, Z., et al., *Vitamin B12 deficiency in patients with chronic-tinnitus and noise-induced hearing loss*. Am J Otolaryngol, 1993. **14**(2): p. 94–9.

[88] Brown, K.D., et al., *Activation of SIRT3 by the NAD(+) precursor nicotinamide riboside protects from noise-induced hearing loss*. Cell Metab, 2014. **20**(6): p. 1059–68.

[89] Mukherjea, D., et al., *Early investigational drugs for hearing loss*. Expert Opin Investig Drugs, 2015. **24**(2): p. 201–17.